GUIDELINES ON FOOD FORTIFICATION WITH MICRONUTRIENTS

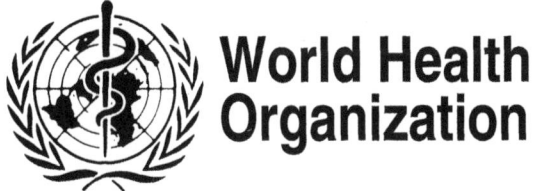

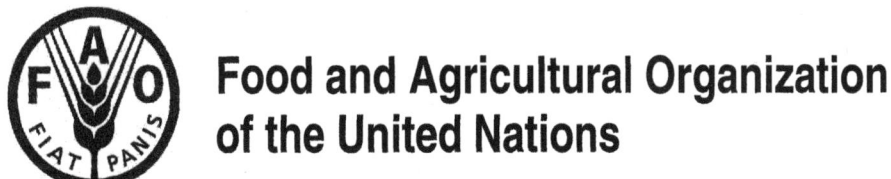

Guidelines on food fortification with micronutrients

Edited by

Lindsay Allen
*University of California,
Davis, CA, United States of America*

Bruno de Benoist
*World Health Organization,
Geneva, Switzerland*

Omar Dary
*A2Z Outreach – The USAID Micronutrient
Leadership and Support and Child Blindness Activity,
Washington, DC, United States of America*

Richard Hurrell
*Swiss Federal Institute of Technology,
Zurich, Switzerland*

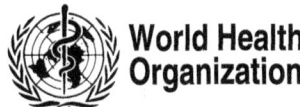
World Health Organization

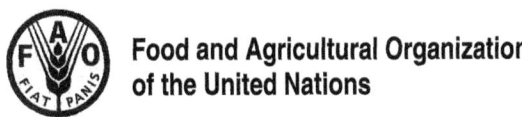
Food and Agricultural Organization of the United Nations

WHO Library Cataloguing-in-Publication Data

Guidelines on food fortification with micronutrients/edited by Lindsay Allen ... [et al.].

1. Food, Fortified. 2. Micronutrients. 3. Nutritional requirements.
4. Deficiency diseases – prevention and control. 5. Guidelines. I. Allen, Lindsay H. II. World Health Organization.

ISBN 13: 978-92-4-159401-1 (NLM classification: QU 145)

This publication is supported by funding from GAIN, the Global Alliance for Improved Nutrition. While GAIN supports the work of this publication, it cannot warrant or represent that the information contained in these Guidelines is complete and correct and GAIN shall not be liable whatsoever for any damage incurred as a result of its use.

© World Health Organization and Food and Agriculture Organization of the United Nations 2006

All rights reserved. Publications of the World Health Organization can be obtained from WHO Press, World Health Organization, 20 Avenue Appia, 1211 Geneva 27, Switzerland (tel: +41 22 791 3264; fax: +41 22 791 4857; email: bookorders@who.int). Requests for permission to reproduce or translate WHO publications – whether for sale or for noncommercial distribution – should be addressed to WHO Press, at the above address (fax: +41 22 791 4806; email: permissions@who.int), or to Chief, Publishing and Multimedia Service, Information Division, Food and Agriculture Organization of the United Nations, Viale delle di Caracalla, 00100 Rome, Italy or by email to copyright@fao.org.

The designations employed and the presentation of the material in this publication do not imply the expression of any opinion whatsoever on the part of the World Health Organization and the Food and Agriculture Organization of the United Nations concerning the legal status of any country, territory, city or area or of its authorities, or concerning the delimitation of its frontiers or boundaries. Dotted lines on maps represent approximate border lines for which there may not yet be full agreement.

The mention of specific companies or of certain manufacturers' products does not imply that they are endorsed or recommended by the World Health Organization and the Food and Agriculture Organization of the United Nations in preference to others of a similar nature that are not mentioned. Errors and omissions excepted, the names of proprietary products are distinguished by initial capital letters.

All reasonable precautions have been taken by the World Health Organization and the Food and Agriculture Organization of the United Nations to verify the information contained in this publication. However, the published material is being distributed without warranty of any kind, either express or implied. The responsibility for the interpretation and use of the material lies with the reader. In no event shall the World Health Organization and the Food and Agriculture Organization of the United Nations be liable for damages arising from its use.

Contents

List of tables	x
List of figures	xiii
Foreword	xiv
Preface	xviii
List of authors	xxi
Acknowledgements	xxiii
Abbreviations	xxiv
Glossary	xxvi

Part I. The role of food fortification in the control of micronutrient malnutrition — 1

Chapter 1 Micronutrient malnutrition: a public health problem — 3
    1.1 Global prevalence of micronutrient malnutrition — 3
    1.2 Strategies for the control of micronutrient malnutrition — 11
        1.2.1 Increasing the diversity of foods consumed — 12
        1.2.2 Food fortification — 13
        1.2.3 Supplementation — 13
        1.2.4 Public health measures — 14
    1.3 Food fortification in practice — 14
        1.3.1 Efficacy trials — 15
        1.3.2 Effectiveness evaluations — 17
    1.4 Advantages and limitations of food fortification as a strategy to combat MNM — 20

Chapter 2 Food fortification: basic principles — 24
    2.1 Terminology — 24
        2.1.1 Food fortification — 24
        2.1.2 Related codex terminology — 25
    2.2 Types of fortification — 26
        2.2.1 Mass fortification — 27
        2.2.2 Targeted fortification — 27
        2.2.3 Market-driven fortification — 28
        2.2.4 Other types of fortification — 29
    2.3 Legal considerations: mandatory versus voluntary fortification — 31
        2.3.1 Mandatory fortification — 31
        2.3.2 Voluntary fortification — 33
        2.3.3 Special voluntary fortification — 35

2.3.4 Criteria governing the selection of mandatory or voluntary fortification ... 35

Part II. Evaluating the public health significance of micronutrient malnutrition ... 39

Introduction ... 41

Chapter 3 Iron, vitamin A and iodine ... 43
    3.1 Iron deficiency and anaemia ... 43
        3.1.1 Prevalence of deficiency ... 43
        3.1.2 Risk factors for deficiency ... 44
        3.1.3 Health consequences of deficiency and benefits of intervention ... 48
    3.2 Vitamin A ... 48
        3.2.1 Prevalence of deficiency ... 49
        3.2.2 Risk factors for deficiency ... 49
        3.2.3 Health consequences of deficiency and benefits of intervention ... 51
    3.3 Iodine ... 52
        3.3.1 Prevalence of deficiency ... 52
        3.3.2 Risk factors for deficiency ... 54
        3.3.3 Health consequences of deficiency and benefits of intervention ... 54

Chapter 4 Zinc, folate, vitamin B_{12} and other B vitamins, vitamin C, vitamin D, calcium, selenium and fluoride ... 57
    4.1 Zinc ... 57
        4.1.1 Prevalence of deficiency ... 57
        4.1.2 Risk factors for deficiency ... 59
        4.1.3 Health consequences of deficiency and benefits of intervention ... 61
    4.2 Folate ... 61
        4.2.1 Prevalence of deficiency ... 61
        4.2.2 Risk factors for deficiency ... 63
        4.2.3 Health consequences of deficiency and benefits of intervention ... 63
    4.3 Vitamin B_{12} ... 64
        4.3.1 Prevalence of deficiency ... 65
        4.3.2 Risk factors for deficiency ... 66
        4.3.3 Health consequences of deficiency and benefits of intervention ... 67
    4.4 Other B vitamins (thiamine, riboflavin, niacin and vitamin B_6) ... 67
        4.4.1 Thiamine ... 68
        4.4.2 Riboflavin ... 71
        4.4.3 Niacin ... 73
        4.4.4 Vitamin B_6 ... 76
    4.5 Vitamin C ... 78
        4.5.1 Prevalence of deficiency ... 78
        4.5.2 Risk factors for deficiency ... 80

		4.5.3	Health consequences of deficiency and benefits of intervention	81

	4.6	Vitamin D		81
		4.6.1	Prevalence of deficiency	82
		4.6.2	Risk factors for deficiency	83
		4.6.3	Health consequences of deficiency and benefits of intervention	84
	4.7	Calcium		84
		4.7.1	Prevalence of deficiency	84
		4.7.2	Risk factors for deficiency	85
		4.7.3	Health consequences of deficiency and benefits of intervention	86
	4.8	Selenium		86
		4.8.1	Prevalence of deficiency	86
		4.8.2	Risk factors for deficiency	88
		4.8.3	Health consequences of deficiency and benefits of intervention	88
	4.9	Fluoride		89
		4.9.1	Prevalence of dental caries	89
		4.9.2	Risk factors for low intakes	90
		4.9.3	Health consequences of low intakes and benefits of intervention	90
	4.10	Multiple micronutrient deficiencies		91
		4.10.1	Prevalence and risk factors	91
		4.10.2	Health consequences and benefits of intervention	91

Part III. Fortificants: physical characteristics, selection and use with specific food vehicles — 93

Introduction				95
Chapter 5	Iron, vitamin A and iodine			97
	5.1	Iron		97
		5.1.1	Choice of iron fortificant	97
		5.1.2	Methods used to increase the amount of iron absorbed from fortificants	100
		5.1.3	Novel iron fortificants	102
		5.1.4	Sensory changes	104
		5.1.5	Experience with iron fortification of specific foods	104
		5.1.6	Safety issues	110
	5.2	Vitamin A and β-carotene		111
		5.2.1	Choice of vitamin A fortificant	111
		5.2.2	Experience with vitamin A fortification of specific foods	112
		5.2.3	Safety issues	117
	5.3	Iodine		118
		5.3.1	Choice of iodine fortificant	118
		5.3.2	Experience with iodine fortification of specific foods	119
		5.3.3	Safety issues	122

Chapter 6	Zinc, folate and other B vitamins, vitamin C, vitamin D, calcium, selenium and fluoride		124
	6.1	Zinc	124
		6.1.1 Choice of zinc fortificant	124
		6.1.2 The bioavailability of zinc	124
		6.1.3 Methods used to increase zinc absorption from fortificants	125
		6.1.4 Experience with zinc fortification of specific foods	125
	6.2	Folate and other B vitamins	126
		6.2.1 Choice of vitamin B fortificants	126
		6.2.2 Experience with vitamin B fortification of specific foods	128
		6.2.3 Safety issues	128
	6.3	Vitamin C (ascorbic acid)	130
		6.3.1 Choice of vitamin C fortificant	130
		6.3.2 Experience with vitamin C fortification of specific foods	130
	6.4	Vitamin D	130
		6.4.1 Choice of vitamin D fortificant	130
		6.4.2 Experience with vitamin D fortification of specific foods	130
	6.5	Calcium	131
		6.5.1 Choice of calcium fortificant	131
		6.5.2 Experience with calcium fortification	131
	6.6	Selenium	133
		6.6.1 Choice of selenium fortificant	133
		6.6.2 Experience with selenium fortification of specific foods	133
	6.7	Fluoride	134
		6.7.1 Choice of fortificant	134
		6.7.2 Experience with fluoridation	134

Part IV. Implementing effective and sustainable food fortification programmes — 135

Introduction			137
Chapter 7	Defining and setting programme		139
	7.1	Information needs	139
		7.1.1 Biochemical and clinical evidence of specific micronutrient deficiencies	139
		7.1.2 Dietary patterns	141
		7.1.3 Usual dietary intakes	142
	7.2	Defining nutritional goals: basic concepts	142
		7.2.1 The EAR cut-point method	143
		7.2.2 Dietary reference values: Estimated Average Requirements, Recommended Nutrient Intakes and upper limits	144

7.3	Using the EAR cut-point method to set goals and to evaluate the impact and safety of fortification		147
	7.3.1	Deciding on an acceptable prevalence of low intakes	149
	7.3.2	Calculating the magnitude of micronutrient additions	151
	7.3.3	Adaptations to the EAR cut-point methodology for specific nutrients	156
	7.3.4	Bioavailability considerations	161
7.4	Other factors to consider when deciding fortification levels		162
	7.4.1	Safety limits	163
	7.4.2	Technological limits	163
	7.4.3	Cost limits	164
7.5	Applying the EAR cut-point methodology to mass, targeted and market-driven fortification interventions		164
	7.5.1	Mass fortification	166
	7.5.2	Targeted fortification	169
	7.5.3	Market-driven fortification	171

Chapter 8 Monitoring and evaluation — **178**

8.1	Basic concepts and definitions		178
8.2	Regulatory monitoring		180
	8.2.1	Internal monitoring (quality control/quality assurance)	186
	8.2.2	External monitoring (inspection and technical auditing)	188
	8.2.3	Commercial monitoring	190
8.3	Household monitoring		191
	8.3.1	Aims and objectives	191
	8.3.2	Methodological considerations	192
8.4	Impact evaluation		196
	8.4.1	Impact evaluation design	196
	8.4.2	Methodological considerations	200
8.5	What is the minimum every fortification programme should have in terms of a monitoring and evaluation system?		204

Chapter 9 Estimating the cost-effectiveness and cost–benefit of fortification — **207**

9.1	Basic concepts and definitions		207
	9.1.1	Cost-effectiveness	207
	9.1.2	Cost–benefit analysis	210
9.2	Information needs		210
	9.2.1	Estimating unit costs	210
	9.2.2	Cost-effectiveness analyses	213
	9.2.3	Cost–benefit analysis	215
9.3	Estimating the cost-effectiveness and cost–benefit of vitamin A, iodine and iron interventions: worked examples		216

		9.3.1	Vitamin A supplementation: a cost-effectiveness calculation	217
		9.3.2	Iodine: a cost–benefit analysis	219
		9.3.3	Iron fortification: a cost–benefit analysis	220
		9.3.4	Iron supplementation: a cost-effectiveness calculation	222
Chapter 10	Communication, social marketing, & advocacy in support of food fortification programmes			224
	10.1	Communication strategies: the options		225
		10.1.1	Education	226
		10.1.2	Laws, policy and advocacy: communicating with policy-makers	227
		10.1.3	Social marketing	229
	10.2	Communication to support social marketing programmes		230
		10.2.1	Building collaborative partnerships	232
		10.2.2	Developing messages for government leaders	234
		10.2.3	Developing messages for industry leaders	235
		10.2.4	Developing consumer marketing strategies and consumer education	237
	10.3	Sustaining the programme		238
Chapter 11	National food law			240
	11.1	The International context		240
	11.2	National food law and fortification		241
		11.2.1	Forms of food law: legislation, regulation and complementary measures	241
		11.2.2	Regulating food fortification: general considerations	243
	11.3	Mandatory fortification		243
		11.3.1	Composition	244
		11.3.2	Labelling and advertising	247
		11.3.3	Trade considerations	249
	11.4	Voluntary fortification		250
		11.4.1	Composition	251
		11.4.2	Labelling and advertising	256
		11.4.3	Trade considerations	257
References				259
Further reading				280

Annexes		**283**
Annex A	Indicators for assessing progress towards the sustainable elimination of iodine deficiency disorders	285
Annex B	The international resource laboratory for iodine network	287
Annex C	Conversion factors for calculating Estimated Average Requirements (EARs) from FAO/WHO Recommended Nutrient Intakes (RNIs)	291
Annex D	A procedure for estimating feasible fortification levels for a mass fortification programme	294

Annex E	A quality control and monitoring system for fortified vegetable oils: an example from Morocco	313
Annex F	The Codex Alimentarius and the World Trade Organization Agreements	318
Index		331

List of tables

Table 1.1	Prevalence of the three major micronutrient deficiencies, by WHO region	4
Table 1.2	Micronutrient deficiencies: prevalence, risk factors and health consequences	6
Table 2.1	Targeted food fortification programmes	28
Table 2.2	Foods suited to fortification at the household level	30
Table 3.1	Indicators for assessing iron status at the population level	45
Table 3.2	Criteria for assessing the public health severity of anemia	47
Table 3.3	Classification of usual diets according to their iron bioavailability	47
Table 3.4	Indicators for assessing vitamin A status at the population level	50
Table 3.5	Criteria for assessing the public health severity of vitamin A deficiency	51
Table 3.6	Indicators for assessing iodine status at the population level	53
Table 3.7	Criteria for assessing the public health severity of iodine deficiency	54
Table 3.8	The spectrum of iodine deficiency disorders	55
Table 4.1	Indicators for assessing zinc status at the population level	58
Table 4.2	Classification of usual diets according to the potential bioavailability of their zinc content	60
Table 4.3	Indicators for assessing folate (vitamin B_9) status at the population level	62
Table 4.4	Indicators for assessing vitamin B_{12} (cobalamin) status at the population level	65
Table 4.5	Indicators for assessing thiamine (vitamin B_1) status at the population level	69
Table 4.6	Proposed criteria for assessing the public health severity of thiamine deficiency	70
Table 4.7	Indicators for assessing riboflavin (vitamin B_2) status at the population level	72
Table 4.8	Indicators for assessing niacin (nicotinic acid) status at the population level	75
Table 4.9	Proposed criteria for assessing public health severity of niacin deficiency	76
Table 4.10	Indicators for assessing vitamin B_6 (pyridoxine) status at the population level	77
Table 4.11	Indicators for assessing vitamin C status at the population level	79
Table 4.12	Proposed criteria for assessing the public health severity of vitamin C deficiency	80

… LIST OF TABLES

Table 4.13	Indicators for assessing vitamin D status at the population level	82
Table 4.14	Indicators for assessing calcium status at the population level	85
Table 4.15	Indicators for assessing selenium status at the population level	87
Table 4.16	Indicators for assessing fluoride status at the population level	90
Table 5.1	Key characteristics of iron compounds used for food fortification purposes: solubility, bioavailability and cost	98
Table 5.2	Suggested iron fortificants for specific food vehicles	105
Table 5.3	Commercially available forms of vitamin A, their characteristics and their main applications	112
Table 5.4	Vitamin A fortificants and their suitability for specific food vehicles	113
Table 5.5	Examples of vitamin A fortification programmes	114
Table 5.6	Iodine fortificants: chemical composition and iodine content	118
Table 5.7	Progress towards universal salt iodization in WHO regions, status as of 1999	120
Table 6.1	Vitamin B fortificants: physical characteristics and stability	127
Table 6.2	Calcium fortificants: physical characteristics	132
Table 7.1	FAO/WHO Recommended Nutrient Intakes (RNIs) for selected population subgroups	145
Table 7.2	Estimated Average Requirements (calculated values) based on FAO/WHO Recommended Nutrient Intakes	148
Table 7.3	Tolerable Upper Intake Levels (ULs)	149
Table 7.4	Predicting the effect on intake distributions of adult women of fortifying wheat flour with different levels of vitamin A	154
Table 7.5	Probability of inadequate iron intakes in selected population subgroups at different ranges of usual intake (mg/day)	158
Table 7.6	Prevalence of inadequate iron intakes for menstruating women consuming a diet from which the average bioavailability of iron is 5%: an example calculation	159
Table 7.7	Examples of micronutrients for which the bioavailability of the form used for fortification differs substantially from their bioavailability in the usual diet	162
Table 7.8	Factors that may limit the amount of fortificants that can be added to a single food vehicle	163
Table 7.9	Estimated cost of selected fortificants	165
Table 7.10	Examples of levels of micronutrients currently added to staples and condiments worldwide (mg/kg)	167
Table 7.11	Codex Nutrient Reference Values (NRVs) for selected micronutrients	172
Table 7.12	Energy densities of common food presentations	174
Table 7.13	Calculated maximum micronutrient content for a 40 kcal-sized serving, assuming no other sources of nutrient in the diet	176
Table 7.14	Factors for converting maximum micronutrient amounts for 40 kcal-sized servings to maximum amounts for different food presentations and serving sizes	176
Table 8.1	Purpose and function of the various components of monitoring and evaluation systems for fortification programmes	181
Table 8.2	Suggested criteria for measuring success at various monitoring stages for food fortification programmes	182

Table 8.3	Suggested regulatory monitoring activities for a food fortification programme	183
Table 8.4	Suggested household monitoring activities for a food fortification programme	193
Table 8.5	Evaluating the impact of fortification programmes on nutritional status: a range of appraoches	198
Table 8.6	Impact evaluation of a food fortification programme: suggested outcome indicators	201
Table 9.1	Hypothetical annual costs of wheat flour fortification with iron and zinc	212
Table 9.2	Estimated unit costs of selected micronutrient interventions	213
Table 9.3	Country-specific data required for cost-effectiveness and cost–benefit calculations, country P	216
Table 9.4	Key assumptions in estimating cost-effectiveness and cost–benefit of selected micronutrient fortification	217
Table 10.1	Nutrition promotion methods defined	225
Table 11.1	Relationship between legal minimum and maximum levels for iron, with regard to its relative bioavailability from selected fortificants	247
Table A.1	Indicators for monitoring progress towards the sustainable elimination of iodine deficiency as a public health problem	285
Table C.1	Conversion factors for calculating Estimated Average Requirements (EARs) from FAO/WHO Recommended Nutrient Intakes (RNIs)	292
Table D.1	Consumption profile of selected industrially-produced staples	301
Table D.2	Recommended composition of dietary supplements to complement fortified foods	302
Table D.3	Safety limits for vitamin A	303
Table D.4	Cost analysis of fortification with vitamin A at the estimated safety limits for sugar, oil and wheat flour	304
Table D.5	Additional intake of vitamin A at various levels of consumption of fortified foods	304
Table D.6	Production parameters for vitamin A fortification	305
Table D.7	Regulatory parameters for vitamin A fortification	305
Table D.8	Safety, technological and cost limits for wheat flour fortification	307
Table D.9	Nutritional implications of wheat flour fortification	308
Table D.10	Production and regulatory parameters for wheat flour fortification	309
Table D.11	Final formulation for the fortification of refined wheat flour and estimated associated costs for a hypothetical country	310
Table D.12	Estimating the overall cost of the proposed fortification programme and the annual investment required	311

List of figures

Figure 1.1	Effect of iron fortification of fish sauce on the iron status of non-pregnant anaemic female Vietnamese factory workers	16
Figure 1.2	Effect of dual-fortified salt (iron and iodine) on iron status of Moroccan schoolchildren	18
Figure 1.3	Effect of flour fortification with folic acid on folate status of Canadian elderly women	19
Figure 2.1	The interrelationships between the levels of coverage and compliance and the different types of food fortification	27
Figure 7.1	An example of a usual intake distribution in which the median intake is at the RNI or RDA (the formerly-used approach)	144
Figure 7.2	An example of a usual intake distribution in which only 2.5% of the group have intakes below the RNI (RDA)	150
Figure 7.3	An example of a usual intake distribution in which 2.5% of the group have intakes below the EAR (the recommended approach)	150
Figure 8.1	A monitoring and evaluation system for fortification programmes	179
Figure 8.2	Suggested frequency and intensity of sampling for monitoring compliance with standards	187
Figure 9.1	Cost-effectiveness of micronutrient supplementation and fortification	209
Figure 9.2	Cost-effectiveness of selected interventions affecting children	209
Figure 10.1	Relationship between individual decision-making and the perceived costs and benefits of any new behavior, idea or product	226

Foreword

Interest in micronutrient malnutrition has increased greatly over the last few years. One of the main reasons for the increased interest is the realization that micronutrient malnutrition contributes substantially to the global burden of disease. In 2000, the *World Health Report*[1] identified iodine, iron, vitamin A and zinc deficiencies as being among the world's most serious health risk factors. In addition to the more obvious clinical manifestations, micronutrient malnutrition is responsible for a wide range of non-specific physiological impairments, leading to reduced resistance to infections, metabolic disorders, and delayed or impaired physical and psychomotor development. The public health implications of micronutrient malnutrition are potentially huge, and are especially significant when it comes to designing strategies for the prevention and control of diseases such as HIV/AIDS, malaria and tuberculosis, and diet-related chronic diseases.

Another reason for the increased attention to the problem of micronutrient malnutrition is that, contrary to previous thinking, it is not uniquely the concern of poor countries. While micronutrient deficiencies are certainly more frequent and severe among disadvantaged populations, they do represent a public health problem in some industrialized countries. This is particularly true of iodine deficiency in Europe, where it was generally assumed to have been eradicated, and of iron deficiency, which is currently the most prevalent micronutrient deficiency in the world. In addition, the increased consumption in industrialized countries (and increasingly in those in social and economic transition) of highly-processed energy-dense but micronutrient-poor foods, is likely to adversely affect micronutrient intake and status.

Measures to correct micronutrient deficiencies – at least the major ones – are, however, well known, and moreover relatively cheap and easy to implement. The control of iodine deficiency disorders through salt iodization, for example, has been a major accomplishment in public health nutrition over the last 30 years.

---

[1] World *health report, 2000*. Geneva, World Heath Organization, 2000.

The best way of preventing micronutrient malnutrition is to ensure consumption of a balanced diet that is adequate in every nutrient. Unfortunately, this is far from being achievable everywhere since it requires universal access to adequate food and appropriate dietary habits. From this standpoint, food fortification has the dual advantage of being able to deliver nutrients to large segments of the population without requiring radical changes in food consumption patterns. In fact, fortification has been used for more than 80 years in industrialized countries as a means of restoring micronutrients lost by food processing, in particular, some of the B vitamins, and has been a major contributory factor in the eradication of diseases associated with deficiencies in these vitamins. Because of the increased awareness of the widespread prevalence and harmful effects of micronutrient malnutrition, and in consideration of changes in food systems (notably an increased reliance on centrally processed foods), and successful fortification experiences in other regions, increasing numbers of developing countries are now committed to, or are considering, fortification programmes.

With so much accumulated experience, the conditions under which food fortification can be recommended as a strategic option for controlling micronutrient malnutrition are now better understood. Its limitations are also well known: food fortification alone cannot correct micronutrient deficiencies when large numbers of the targeted population, either because of poverty or locality, have little or no access to the fortified food, when the level of micronutrient deficiency is too severe, or when the concurrent presence of infections increases the metabolic demand for micronutrients. Various safety, technological and cost considerations can also place constraints on food fortification interventions. Thus, proper food fortification programme planning not only requires assessment of its potential impact on the nutritional status of the population but also of its feasibility in a given context.

The success of a fortification programme can be measured through its public health impact and its sustainability. The latter implies an intersectoral approach where, in addition to competent national public health authorities, research, trade, law, education, nongovernmental organizations and the commercial sector are all involved in the planning and implementation of the programme. It has taken time to appreciate the role of the private sector, in particular industry, and the importance of civil society in this process. These are now fully acknowledged and this recognition should strengthen the capability of interventions to combat micronutrient malnutrition.

The main purpose of these Guidelines is to assist countries in the design and implementation of appropriate food fortification programmes. Drawing on several recent high quality publications on the subject and on programme experience, information on food fortification has been critically analysed and then translated into scientifically sound guidelines for application in the field. More specifically, the Guidelines provide information relating to the benefits, limitations, design, implementation, monitoring, evaluation, cost–benefit and regulation of food fortification, particularly in developing countries. They are intended to be a resource for governments and agencies that are currently implementing, or considering food fortification, and a source of information for scientists, technologists and the food industry. The Guidelines are written from a nutrition and public health perspective, to provide practical guidance on how food fortification should be implemented, monitored and evaluated within the general context of the need to control micronutrient deficiencies in a population. They are primarily intended for nutrition-related public health programme managers, but should also be useful to all those working to control micronutrient malnutrition, including industry.

The document is organized into four complementary sections. Part I introduces the concept of food fortification as a potential strategy for the control of micronutrient malnutrition. Part II summarizes the prevalence, causes and consequences of micronutrient deficiencies, and the public health benefits of micronutrient malnutrition control. It lays the groundwork for public health personnel to assess the magnitude of the problem, and the potential benefits of fortification, in their particular situation. Part III provides technical information on the various chemical forms of micronutrients that can be used to fortify foods, and reviews experience of their use in specific food vehicles. Part IV describes the key steps involved in designing, implementing and sustaining fortification programmes, starting with the determination of the amount of nutrients to be added to foods, followed by the implementation of monitoring and evaluating systems, including quality control/quality assurance procedures, before moving on to the estimation of cost-effectiveness and cost–benefit ratios. The importance of, and strategies for, regulation and international harmonization, communication, advocacy, consumer marketing and public education are also explained in some detail.

The production of the Guidelines has been the result of a long process that started in 2002. Under the aegis of the World Health Organization (WHO), an expert group was established and charged with the task of developing a set of guidelines on food fortification practice. A draft version of the guidelines was reviewed in 2003 by a multidisciplinary panel of experts who collectively represented the range of knowledge and experience required for developing such guidelines. The panel members included experts in public health, nutrition sciences and food technology, from both the public and the private sectors. Afterwards, the draft of the guidelines was circulated among field nutritionists and public health practitioners and also tested in a number of countries. All of the comments received through this process were considered for this finalized version of the guidelines.

We are all committed to the elimination of micronutrient malnutrition. We hope that these Guidelines will help countries to meet this goal and therefore enable their population to achieve its full social and economic potential.

Lindsay Allen
Bruno de Benoist
Omar Dary
Richard Hurrell

Preface

More than 2 billion people in the world today suffer from micronutrient deficiencies caused largely by a dietary deficiency of vitamins and minerals. The public health importance of these deficiencies lies upon their magnitude and their health consequences, especially in pregnant women and young children, as they affect fetal and child growth, cognitive development and resistance to infection. Although people in all population groups in all regions of the world may be affected, the most widespread and severe problems are usually found amongst resource poor, food insecure and vulnerable households in developing countries. Poverty, lack of access to a variety of foods, lack of knowledge of appropriate dietary practices and high incidence of infectious diseases are key factors. Micronutrient malnutrition is thus a major impediment to socio-economic development contributing to a vicious circle of underdevelopment and to the detriment of already underprivileged groups. It has long-ranging effects on health, learning ability and productivity and has high social and public costs leading to reduced work capacity due to high rates of illness and disability.

Overcoming micronutrient malnutrition is therefore a precondition for ensuring rapid and appropriate national development. This was the consensus reached at the FAO/WHO International Conference on Nutrition (ICN) in December 1992, where 159 countries endorsed the World Declaration on Nutrition, pledging "to make all efforts to eliminate . . . iodine and vitamin A deficiencies" and "to reduce substantially . . . other important micronutrient deficiencies, including iron." Since then, FAO and WHO have continued to work to achieve this goal and in doing so have adopted four main strategies improving dietary intakes through increased production, preservation and marketing of micronutrient-rich foods combined with nutrition education; food fortification; supplementation; and global public health and other disease control measures. Each of these strategies have a place in eliminating micronutrient malnutrition. For maximum impact, the right balance or mix of these mutually reinforcing strategies need to be put in place to ensure access to consumption and utilization of an adequate variety and quantity of safe, good-quality foods for all people of the world. Underpinning these strategies is the realisation that when there is a dietary deficiency in any one nutrient, there are likely to be other nutrient deficiencies as well. Consequently in the long-term, measures for the prevention and control of micronutrient deficiencies should be based on diet diversification and consumer education about how to choose foods that provide a balanced diet, including the necessary vitamins and minerals.

These guidelines are meant to assist countries in the design and implementation of appropriate food fortification programmes as part of a comprehensive food-based strategy for combating micronutrient deficiencies. Fortification of food can make an important contribution to the reduction of micronutrient malnutrition when and where existing food supplies and limited access fail to provide adequate levels of certain nutrients in the diet. To ensure that the target population will benefit from a food fortification programme, an appropriate food vehicle must be selected that is widely consumed throughout the year by a large portion of the population at risk of a particular deficiency. In order to reach different segments of the population who may have different dietary habits, selecting more than one food vehicle may be necessary. Fortification of a staple food affects everyone, including the poor, pregnant women, young children and populations that can never be completely covered by social services. In addition, fortification reaches secondary at-risk groups, such as the elderly and those who have an unbalanced diet. Food fortification is usually socially acceptable, requires no change in food habits, does not alter the characteristics of the food, can be introduced quickly, can produce nutritional benefits for the target population quickly, is safe, and can be a cost-effective way of reaching large target populations that are at risk of micronutrient deficiency.

However, there are limitations on the benefits of fortification and difficulties in its implementation and effectiveness. There may, for example, be concerns raised about the possibility of overdose or a reluctance to fortify on human rights grounds where consumer choice may be an issue. There may be reluctance on the part of the food industry to fortify out of fear of insufficient market demand for fortified foods or concern about consumer perceptions that the food product has been altered. Food fortification also raises production costs through such expenses as initial equipment purchases, equipment maintenance, increased production staff needs and quality control and assurance facilities. Economically marginalised households may not have access to such foods and other vulnerable population groups, particularly children under five years of age, may not be able to consume large enough quantities of the fortified food to satisfy an adequate level of their daily requirements. All these issues need to be carefully assessed and these are discussed in detail.

This publication is a useful guide to assist decision makers in ensuring that the nutritionally vulnerable and at-risk populations benefit from food fortification programmes and FAO and WHO would like to express our thanks to all who have been involved in this process. We reaffirm our support to achieve the Millennium Development Goals set by governments for overall nutrition improvement and will collaborate with international and national agencies so as to accelerate the planning and implementation of comprehensive and sustainable food fortification programmes as one element of national nutrition improvement policies, plans and programmes.

Kraisid Tontisirin,
Director,
Nutrition and Consumer Protection Division,
Food and Agriculture Organization

Denise C. Coitinho,
Director,
Department of Nutrition for Health and Development,
World Health Organization

List of authors

Lindsay Allen
Center Director
USDA, Agricultural Research Service
Western Human Nutrition Research Center
University of California
Davis, California 95616, United States of America

Bruno de Benoist
Coordinator, Micronutrient Unit
Department of Nutrition for Health and Development
World Health Organization
CH 1201, Geneva 27, Switzerland

Omar Dary
Food fortification specialist
A2Z Outreach/The USAID Micronutrient Leadership and Support and Child Blindness Activity
Academy for Educational Development (AED)
Washington D.C. 20009-5721, United States of America

Richard Hurrell
Head, Human Nutrition Laboratory
Food science and Nutrition, Human Nutrition,
ETH (Swiss Federal Institute of Technology)
CH 8092 Zurich, Switzerland

Sue Horton
Professor and Chair Division of Social Sciences
Department of Economics
Munk Center for International Studies
University of Toronto (UTSC)
Toronto, Ontario M5S 3K7, Canada

Janine Lewis
Principal Nutritionist, Nutrition and Labelling programme
Food Standards Australia New Zealand
PO Box 7186
Canberra BC ACT 2610, Australia

Claudia Parvanta
Chair and Professor
Department of Social Sciences
University of the Sciences in Philadelphia
Philadelphia, Pennsylvania, United States of America

Mohammed Rahmani
Département des sciences alimentaires et nutritionnelles
Institut agronomique et vétérinaire Hassan II
BP 6202-Instituts
10101 Rabat, Morocco

Marie Ruel
Division Director
Food Consumption and Nutrition Division
International Food Policy Research Institute
Washington D.C. 20006, United States of America

Brian Thompson
Senior Officer
Nutrition and Consumer Protection Division
Food and Agriculture Organization
Via delle Terme di Caracalla
00100 Rome, Italy

Acknowledgements

Special acknowledgement is given to the following experts for their invaluable contribution to the text and the refinement of the manuscript: Jack Bagriansky, Rune Blomhoff, François Delange, Sean Lynch, Basil Mathioudakis, Suzanne Murphy.

These guidelines were also improved by the experts who participated in the Technical Consultation to review and comment on the manuscript convened by WHO in Geneva in April 2003. Their valuable advice greatly improved the clarity of the text. Those who participated were Maria Andersson, Douglas Balentine, Denise Bienz, André Briend, Rolf Carriere, Ian Darnton-Hill, Jose Chavez, Jose Cordero, Hector Cori, Ines Egli, Dana Faulkner, Olivier Fontaine, Wilma Freire, Cutberto Garza, Rosalind Gibson, Joyce Greene, Graeme Clugston, Michael Hambidge, Pieter Jooste, Venkatesh Mannar, Reynaldo Martorell, Penelope Nestel, Ibrahim Parvanta, Poul Petersen, Peter Ranum, Beatrice Rogers, Richard Smith, Aristide Sagbohan, Bahi Takkouche, Tessa Tan Torres, Robert Tilden, Barbara Underwood, Tina Van Den Briel, Anna Verster, Emorn Wasantwisut and Trudy Wijnhoven. We acknowledge with gratitude Irwin Rosenberg for chairing the meeting in such a way that the ensuing debate added much to the content of the guidelines.

We would like to give a special thanks to Sue Hobbs, Erin McLean, Grace Rob and Afrah Shakori who dedicated so much of their time and patience to make the production of the guidelines possible and to Victoria Menezes Miller for her artistic design of the cover illustration.

We would like also to express our deep appreciation to the Government of Luxembourg for the generous financial support it has provided for the development of these guidelines on food fortification. This contribution has enabled the step-by-step process that was required to establish appropriate normative criteria for guiding WHO and FAO Member States in the implementation of their food fortification programmes. This process included the organization of several expert meetings to develop the guidelines and a technical consultation to review and consolidate the guidelines.

Lastly, we wish to thank the Global Alliance for Improved Nutrition for its support to the publication of the guidelines.

Abbreviations

AI	Adequate Intake
CDC	Centers for Disease Control
CHD	Coronary heart disease
DALY	Disability-adjusted life year
DFE	Dietary folate equivalents
DRI	Dietary Recommended Intake
DRV	Dietary Reference Value
EAR	Estimated Average Requirement
EDTA	Ethylenediaminetetraacetic acid
FAO	Food and Agriculture Organization of the United Nations
FFL	Feasible Fortification Level
FNB	Food and Nutrition Board
GAIN	Global Alliance for Improved Nutrition
GDP	Gross domestic product
GMP	Good manufacturing practice
HACCP	Hazard analysis critical control point
ICCIDD	International Council for Control of Iodine Deficiency Disorders
IDD	Iodine deficiency disorders
IIH	Iodine-induced hyperthroidism
ILO	International Labour Organization
INACG	International Nutritional Anemia Consultative Group
IOM	Institute of Medicine
IRLI	International Resource Laboratory for Iodine
IVACG	International Vitamin A Consultative Group
IZiNCG	International Zinc Nutrition Consultative Group
LmL	Legal Minimum Level
LQAS	Lot quality assurance sampling
mFL	Minimum Fortification Level
MI	Micronutrient Initiative
MMR	Maternal mortality rate
MNM	Micronutrient malnutrition
MTL	Maximum Tolerable Level
MW	Molecular weight

NGO	Nongovernmental organization
NRV	Nutrient Reference Value
PAHO	Pan American Health Organization
PAR	Population attributable risk
PEM	Protein–energy malnutrition
QA	Quality assurance
QC	Quality control
RBV	Relative bioavailability
RDA	Recommended Dietary Allowance
RE	Retinol equivalents
RNI	Recommended Nutrient Intake
RR	Relative risk
SUSTAIN	Sharing United States Technology to Aid in the Improvement of Nutrition
TBT	(Agreement on) Technical Barriers to Trade
UNICEF	United Nations Children's Fund
UL	Tolerable Upper Intake Level
USI	Universal salt iodization
VAD	Vitamin A deficiency
WFP	World Food Programme
WHO	World Health Organization

Glossary

The **Average Intake (AI)** is a recommended intake value based on observed or experimentally determined approximations or estimates of nutrient intake by a group or groups of apparently healthy people that are assumed to be adequate.

Cost limit refers to the maximum acceptable increment in price of a food due to fortification.

A **Dietary Recommended Intake (DRI)** is a quantitative estimate of a nutrient intake that is used as a reference value for planning and assessing diets for apparently healthy people. Examples include AIs, EARs, RDAs and ULs.

Effectiveness refers to the impact of an intervention in practice. Compared to efficacy, the effectiveness of a fortification programme will be limited by factors such as non- or low consumption of the fortified food.

Efficacy refers to the capacity of an intervention such as fortification to achieve the desired impact under ideal circumstances. This usually refers to experimental, well-supervised intervention trials.

Enrichment is synonymous with fortification and refers to the addition of micronutrients to a food irrespective of whether the nutrients were originally in the food before processing or not.

Essential micronutrient refers to any micronutrient, which is needed for growth and development and the maintenance of healthy life, that is normally consumed as a constituent of food and cannot be synthesized in adequate amounts by the body.

The **Estimated Average Requirement (EAR)** is the average (median) daily nutrient intake level estimated to meet the needs of half the healthy individuals in a particular age and gender group. The EAR is used to derive the Recommended Dietary Allowance.

Evaluation refers to the assessment of the effectiveness and impact of the programme on the targeted population. The aim of an evaluation is to provide evidence that the programme is achieving its nutritional goals.

Feasible Fortification Level (FFL) is that which is determined, subject to cost and technological constraints, as the level that will provide the greatest number of at-risk individual with an adequate intake without causing an unacceptable risk of excess intakes in the whole population.

Food commodities are staple foods, condiments and milk.

Fortification is the practice of deliberately increasing the content of an essential micronutrient, i.e. vitamins and minerals (including trace elements) in a food, so as to improve the nutritional quality of the food supply and provide a public health benefit with minimal risk to health.

Legal Minimum level (LmL) is the minimum amount of micronutrient that a fortified food must contain according to national regulations and standards. This value is estimated by adding the intrinsic content of a micronutrient in the food to the selected level of fortification.

Market-driven fortification refers to the situation where the food manufacturer takes the initiative to add one or more micronutrients to processed foods, usually within regulatory limits, in order to increase sales and profitability.

Mass fortification refers to the addition of micronutrients to foods commonly consumed by the general public, such as cereals, condiments and milk.

Maximum Tolerable Level (MTL) is the maximum micronutrient content that a fortified food can present as it is established in food law, in order to minimize the risk of excess intake. It should coincide or be lower than the safety limit.

Minimum Fortification Level (mFL) is the level calculated by reducing the Feasible Fortification Level by three standards deviations (or coefficients of variation) of the fortification process, in order that the average coincides or is lower than the calculated Feasible Fortification Level.

Monitoring refers to the continuous collection and review of information on programme implementation activities for the purposes of identifying problems (such as non-compliance) and taking corrective actions so that the programme fulfils its stated objectives.

Nutritional equivalence is achieved when an essential nutrient is added to a product that is designed to resemble a common food in appearance, texture, flavour and odour in amounts such that the substitute product has a similar nutritive value, in terms of the amount and bioavailability of the added essential nutrient.

Nutrient Reference Values (NRVs) are dietary reference values defined by the Codex Alimentarius Commission with the aim of harmonizing the labelling of processed foods. It is a value applicable to all members of the family aged

3 years and over. These values are constantly reviewed based on advances in scientific knowledge.

Nutrient requirement refers to the lowest continuing intake level of a nutrient that will maintain a defined level of nutriture in an individual for a given criterion of nutritional adequacy.

Processed foods are those in which food raw materials have been treated industrially so as to preserve them. Some may be formulated by mixing several different ingredients.

A **premix** is a mixture of a micronutrient(s) and another ingredient, often the same food that is to be fortified, that is added to the food vehicle to improve the distribution of the micronutrient mix within the food matrix and to reduce the separation (segregation) between the food and micronutrient particles.

Quality assurance (QA) refers to the implementation of planned and systematic activities necessary to ensure that products or services meet quality standards. The performance of quality assurance can be expressed numerically as the results of quality control exercises.

Quality control (QC) refers to the techniques and assessments used to document compliance of the product with established technical standards, through the use of objective and measurable indicators.

Relative bioavailability is used to rank the absorbability of a nutrient by comparing its absorbability with that of a reference nutrient that is considered as having the most efficient absorbability.

Restoration is the addition of essential nutrients to foods to restore amounts originally present in the natural product, but unavoidably lost during processing (such as milling), storage or handling.

Recommended Dietary Allowances (RDAs) are defined by the United States Food and Nutrition Board and are conceptually the same as the Recommended Nutrient Intake (RNI), but may have a slightly different values for some micronutrients.

The **Recommended Nutrient Intake (RNI)** is the daily intake that meets the nutrient requirements of almost all apparently healthy individuals in an age- and sex-specific population group. It is set at the Estimated Average Requirement plus 2 standard deviations.

Safety limit is the greatest amount of a micronutrient that can be safely added to specific foods. It considers the UL for the nutrient and the 95th percentile of consumption of a food, and makes allowances for the fact that the nutrient is also consumed in unfortified foods, and may be lost during storage and distribution, and/or cooking.

Targeted fortification refers to the fortification of foods designed for specific population subgroups, such as complementary weaning foods for infants.

The **technological limit** is the maximum level of micronutrient addition that does not change the organoleptic or physical properties of the food.

The **Tolerable Upper Intake Level (UL)** is to the highest average daily nutrient intake level unlikely to pose risk of adverse health effects to almost all (97.5%) apparently healthy individuals in an age- and sex-specific population group.

Universal fortification is equivalent to mass fortification.

Universal salt iodization (USI) refers to the addition of iodine to all salt for both human and animal consumption.

Usual intake refers to an individual's average intake over a relatively long period of time.

PART I
The role of food fortification in the control of micronutrient malnutrition

CHAPTER 1
Micronutrient malnutrition: a public health problem

1.1 Global prevalence of micronutrient malnutrition

Micronutrient malnutrition (MNM) is widespread in the industrialized nations, but even more so in the developing regions of the world. It can affect all age groups, but young children and women of reproductive age tend to be among those most at risk of developing micronutrient deficiencies. Micronutrient malnutrition has many adverse effects on human health, not all of which are clinically evident. Even moderate levels of deficiency (which can be detected by biochemical or clinical measurements) can have serious detrimental effects on human function. Thus, in addition to the obvious and direct health effects, the existence of MNM has profound implications for economic development and productivity, particularly in terms of the potentially huge public health costs and the loss of human capital formation.

Worldwide, the three most common forms of MNM are iron, vitamin A and iodine deficiency. Together, these affect at least one third of the world's population, the majority of whom are in developing countries. Of the three, iron deficiency is the most prevalent. It is estimated that just over 2 billion people are anaemic, just under 2 billion have inadequate iodine nutrition and 254 million preschool-aged children are vitamin A deficient (**Table 1.1**).

From a public health viewpoint, MNM is a concern not just because such large numbers of people are affected, but also because MNM, being a risk factor for many diseases, can contribute to high rates of morbidity and even mortality. It has been estimated that micronutrient deficiencies account for about 7.3% of the global burden of disease, with iron and vitamin A deficiency ranking among the 15 leading causes of the global disease burden (*4*).

According to WHO mortality data, around 0.8 million deaths (1.5% of the total) can be attributed to iron deficiency each year, and a similar number to vitamin A deficiency. In terms of the loss of healthy life, expressed in disability-adjusted life years (DALYs), iron-deficiency anaemia results in 25 million DALYs lost (or 2.4% of the global total), vitamin A deficiency in 18 million DALYs lost (or 1.8% of the global total) and iodine deficiency in 2.5 million DALYs lost (or 0.2% of the global total) (*4*).

The scale and impact of deficiencies in other micronutrients is much more difficult to quantify, although it is likely that some forms of MNM, including

TABLE 1.1
Prevalence of the three major micronutrient deficiencies by WHO region

WHO region	Anaemia[a] (total population)		Insufficient iodine intake[b] (total population)		Vitamin A deficiency[c] (preschool children)	
	No. (millions)	% of total	No. (millions)	% of total	No. (millions)	% of total
Africa	244	46	260	43	53	49
Americas	141	19	75	10	16	20
South-East Asia	779	57	624	40	127	69
Europe	84	10	436	57	No data available	
Eastern Mediterranean	184	45	229	54	16	22
Western Pacific	598	38	365	24	42	27
Total	2030	37	1989	35	254	42

[a] Based on the proportion of the population with haemoglobin concentrations below established cut-off levels.
[b] Based on the proportion of the population with urinary iodine <100 µg/l.
[c] Based on the proportion of the population with clinical eye signs and/or serum retinol ≤0.70 µmol/l.

Sources: references (*1–3*).

zinc, folate and vitamin D deficiency, make a substantial contribution to the global burden of disease. However, there are few data on the prevalence of deficiencies in these micronutrients, and as their adverse effects on health are sometimes non-specific, the public health implications are less well understood.

In the poorer regions of the world, MNM is certain to exist wherever there is undernutrition due to food shortages and is likely to be common where diets lack diversity. Generally speaking, whereas wealthier population groups are able to augment dietary staples with micronutrient-rich foods (such as meat, fish, poultry, eggs, milk and dairy products) and have greater access to a variety of fruits and vegetables, poorer people tend to consume only small amounts of such foods, relying instead on more monotonous diets based on cereals, roots and tubers. The micronutrient content of cereals (especially after milling), roots and tubers is low, so these foods typically provide only a small proportion of the daily requirements for most vitamins and minerals. Fat intake among such groups is also often very low and given the role of fat in facilitating the absorption of a range of micronutrients across the gut wall, the low level of dietary fat puts such populations at further risk of MNM. Consequently, populations that consume few animal source foods may suffer from a high prevalence of several micronutrient deficiencies simultaneously.

In the wealthier countries, higher incomes, greater access to a wider variety of micronutrient-rich and fortified foods, and better health services, are all factors that contribute to the lowering of the risk and prevalence of MNM.

However, consumption of a diet that contains a high proportion of energy-dense but micronutrient-poor processed foods can put some population groups at risk of MNM. Although at present this practice is more common in industrialized countries, it is rapidly becoming more prevalent among countries undergoing social and economic transition.

Table 1.2 provides an overview of the prevalence, risk factors, and health consequences of deficiencies in each of the 15 micronutrients covered in thesee guidelines. For reasons stated above, prevalence estimates are only provided for iron vitamin A and iodine deficiencies. Further information is available from the WHO Vitamin and Mineral Nutrition Information System[1].

Up until the 1980s, efforts to alleviate undernutrition in developing countries were focused on protein–energy malnutrition (PEM). While PEM certainly remains an important concern, we have since come to appreciate the significance of micronutrient malnutrition in terms of its effect on human health and function. As a result, the past two decades have seen an increase in activities that seek to understand and control specific micronutrient deficiencies (7). Efforts to control iodine deficiency in developing countries, for example, were given new impetus in the early 1980s when it was recognized that iodine deficiency was the most common cause of preventable brain damage and mental retardation in childhood (8,9). There were also reports of increased risks of stillbirths and low-birth-weight infants in iodine deficient areas (10,11). Importantly, the technology to prevent iodine deficiency – salt iodization – already existed and, moreover, was easy to implement and affordable even by governments with limited health budgets. It therefore seemed likely that salt iodization could be a feasible option for preventing iodine deficiency on a global scale.

Similarly, having established that vitamin A status is an important determinant of child survival – in addition to preventing and treating eye disorders, supplementation of vitamin A-deficient children lowers their risk of morbidity (particularly that related to severe diarrhoea), and reduces mortality from measles and all-cause mortality (12,13) – measures to control vitamin A deficiency have been initiated in several world regions. Reports that iron supplementation of iron-deficient individuals can improve cognitive function, school performance and work capacity (14,15), and that severe anaemia increases the risk of maternal and child mortality (16), have provided a strong rationale for iron interventions. Intervention trials have also revealed that zinc supplementation improves the growth of stunted, zinc-deficient children (17), lowers rates of diarrhoea and pneumonia (the two leading causes of child death), and shortens the duration of diarrhoeal episodes (18,19).

In the wake of such accumulated evidence, the international community has increasingly come to recognize the public health importance of MNM. In 1990,

---

[1] See http://www.who.int/nutrition/en

TABLE 1.2
Micronutrient deficiencies: prevalence, risk factors and health consequences

Micronutrient[a]	Prevalence of deficiency	Risk factors	Health consequences
Iron	There are an estimated 2 billion cases of anaemia worldwide In developing countries, anaemia prevalence rates are estimated to be about 50% in pregnant women and infants under 2 years, 40% in school-aged children and 25–55% in other women and children Iron deficiency is estimated to be responsible for around 50% of all anaemia cases There are approximately 1 billion cases of iron-deficiency anaemia and a further 1 billion cases of iron deficiency without anaemia worldwide	Low intakes of meat/fish/poultry and high intakes of cereals and legumes Preterm delivery or low birth weight Pregnancy and adolescence (periods during which requirements for iron are especially high) Heavy menstrual losses Parasite infections (i.e. hookworm, schistosomiasis, ascaris) which cause heavy blood losses Malaria (causes anaemia not iron deficiency) Low intakes of vitamin C (ascorbic acid)	Reduced cognitive performance Lower work performance and endurance Impaired iodine and vitamin A metabolism Anaemia Increased risk of maternal mortality and child mortality (with more severe anaemia)
Vitamin A	An estimated 254 million preschool children are vitamin A deficient	Allergy to cow's milk Low intakes of dairy products, eggs and β-carotene from fruits and vegetables Presence of helminth infection, ascaris	Increased risk of mortality in children and pregnant women Night blindness, xerophthalmia

Nutrient	Prevalence	Risk factors	Health consequences
Iodine	An estimated 2 billion people have inadequate iodine nutrition and therefore are at risk of iodine deficiency disorders	Residence in areas with low levels of iodine in soil and water Living in high altitude regions, river plains or far from the sea Consumption of non-detoxified cassava	Birth defects Increased risk of stillbirth and infant mortality Cognitive and neurological impairment including cretinism Impaired cognitive function Hypothyroidism Goitre
Zinc	Insufficient data, but prevalence of deficiency is likely to be moderate to high in developing countries, especially those in Africa, South-East Asia and the Western Pacific	Low intakes of animal products High phytate intakes Malabsorption and infection with intestinal parasites Diarrhoea, especially persistent Genetic disorders	Non-specific if marginal deficiency Possibly poor pregnancy outcomes Impaired growth (stunting) Decreased resistance to infectious diseases Severe deficiency results in dermatitis, retarded growth, diarrhoea, mental disturbance, delayed sexual maturation and/or recurrent infections
Folate (vitamin B_9)	Insufficient data	Low intakes of fruits and vegetables, legumes and dairy products Malabsorption and intestinal parasites infections (e.g. *Giardia Lamblia*) Genetic disorder of folic acid metabolism	Megaloblastic anaemia Risk factor for: — neural tube defects and other birth defects (oro-facial clefts, heart defects) and adverse pregnancy outcomes; — elevated plasma homocysteine; — heart disease and stroke — impaired cognitive function — depression

TABLE 1.2
Micronutrient deficiencies: prevalence, risk factors and health consequences (*Continued*)

Micronutrient[a]	Prevalence of deficiency	Risk factors	Health consequences
Vitamin B_{12} (cobalamin)	Insufficient data	Low intakes of animal products Malabsorption from food due to gastric atrophy induced by *Helicobacter pylori*, or bacterial overgrowth Genetic disorder of vitamin B_{12} metabolism	Megaloblastic anaemia Severe deficiency can cause developmental delays, poor neurobehavioral performance and growth in infants and children, nerve demyelination and neurological dysfunction Risk factor for: — neural tube defects; — elevated plasma homocysteine; — impaired cognitive function
Vitamin B_1 (thiamine)	Insufficient data on marginal deficiency Severe deficiency (beriberi) is reported in parts of Japan and north-east Thailand Regularly reported in famine situations and among displaced populations	High consumption of refined rice and cereals Low intakes of animal and dairy products, and legumes Consumption of thiaminase (found in raw fish) Breastfeeding (from deficient mothers) Chronic alcoholism Genetic disorder of thiamine metabolism	Beriberi presents in two forms: — a cardiac form with risk of heart failure (predominant in neonates) — a neurological form with chronic peripheral neuropathy (loss of sensation and reflexes) Wernicke-Korsakov syndrome (usually in alcoholics) with confusion, lack of coordination and paralysis
Vitamin B_2 (riboflavin)	Insufficient data, but some evidence that it might be very common in developing countries	Low intakes of animal and dairy products Chronic alcoholism	Symptoms are non-specific and can include fatigue, eye changes and in more severe cases, dermatitis (stomatitis, cheilosis), brain dysfunction and microcytic anaemia Impaired iron absorption and utilization

Vitamin B$_3$ (niacin)	Insufficient data on marginal deficiency Severe deficiency (pellagra) still common in Africa, China and India and recently reported among displaced populations (south-eastern Africa) and in famine situations	Low intakes of animal and dairy products High consumption of refined cereals Maize-based diets (not lime treated)	Severe deficiency results in pellagra, which is characterized by: — dermatitis (symmetrical pigmented rash on skin areas exposed to sunlight); — digestive mucosa disorders (diarrhoea and vomiting); — neurological symptoms, depression and loss of memory
Vitamin B$_6$	Insufficient data, but recent reports from Egypt and Indonesia suggest deficiency is likely to be widespread in developing countries Rather uncommon in isolation, being typically associated with deficiencies in the other B vitamins	Low intakes of animal products High consumption of refined cereals Chronic alcoholism	Symptoms are non-specific and may include: — neurological disorders with convulsions; — dermatitis (stomatitis and cheilosis) Anaemia (possibly) Deficiency is a risk factor for elevated plasma homocysteine
Vitamin C (ascorbic acid)	Insufficient data on moderate deficiencies Severe deficiency (scurvy) regularly reported in famine situations (e.g. east Africa) and among displaced people dependent on food aid for long periods (e.g. east Africa, Nepal)	Low intakes of fresh vitamin C-rich fruits and vegetables Prolonged cooking	Severe deficiency results in scurvy with haemorrhagic syndrome (i.e. bleeding gums, joint and muscle pain, peripheral oedema) Anaemia
Vitamin D	Insufficient data, but likely to be common in both industrialized and developing countries Higher at more northerly and southerly latitudes where daylight hours are limited during the winter months	Low exposure to ultra-violet radiation from the sun Wearing excess clothing Having darkly pigmented skin	Severe forms result in rickets in children and osteomalacia in adults

TABLE 1.2
Micronutrient deficiencies: prevalence, risk factors and health consequences (*Continued*)

Micronutrient[a]	Prevalence of deficiency	Risk factors	Health consequences
Calcium	Insufficient data, but low intakes very common	Low intakes of dairy products	Decreased bone mineralization Increased risk of osteoporosis in adults Increased risk of rickets in children
Selenium	Insufficient data on moderate deficiency Severe deficiency reported in some regions of China, Japan, Korea, New Zealand, Scandinavia and Siberia	Residing in low selenium environments Low intakes of animal products Some evidence that symptoms are not due to selenium deficiency alone, but also to the presence of the cocksackie virus (Keshan disease) or mycotoxins (Kaschin-Beck disease)	Severe deficiency presents as: — cardiomyopathy (Keshan disease), or — osteoarthropathy in children (Kaschin-Beck disease) Increased risk of cancer and cardiovascular disease Exacerbation of thyroid dysfunction caused by iodine deficiency
Fluoride	NA	Residing in areas with low fluoride levels in water	Increased risk of dental decay

NA, not applicable.
[a] Micronutrients are listed in order of their public health significance.

Sources: adapted from references (*1–3,5,6*).

the World Health Assembly passed a landmark resolution urging action by Member States "to prevent and control iodine deficiency disorders" (20). Later that year, at the World Summit for Children, the world's leaders endorsed the "virtual elimination of iodine and vitamin A deficiency and a reduction of the prevalence of iron-deficiency anaemia in women by one third". These goals have been reiterated at a number of subsequent international fora, including the Montreal conference on Ending Hidden Hunger in 1991, the 1992 FAO/WHO International Conference on Nutrition held in Rome, the 1993 World Health Assembly held in Geneva, and the Special Session on Children of the United Nations General Assembly, which was held in New York in 2002. There has been remarkable degree of consensus and support for MNM control between governments, United Nations agencies, multilateral and bilateral agencies, academic and research institutions, nongovernmental organizations (NGOs) and donor foundations. More recently, following recognition of the essential role played by industry – in particular, the salt, food and drug industries – stronger links with the private sector have been forged. This is reflected by the implementation of several public–private coalitions aimed at addressing the main micronutrient deficiencies, which include the Global Alliance for Improved Nutrition[1] and The Global Network for Sustained Elimination of Iodine Deficiency[2].

1.2 Strategies for the control of micronutrient malnutrition

The control of vitamin and mineral deficiencies is an essential part of the overall effort to fight hunger and malnutrition. Countries need to adopt and support a comprehensive approach that addresses the causes of malnutrition and the often associated "hidden hunger" which rest intinsic to in poverty and unsustainable livelihoods. Actions that promote an increase in the supply, access, consumption and utilization of an adequate quantity, quality and variety of foods for all populations groups should be supported. The aim is for all people to be able to obtain from their diet all the energy, macro- and micronutrients they need to enjoy a healthy and productive life.

Policy and programme responses include food-based strategies such as dietary diversification and food fortification, as well as nutrition education, public health and food safety measures, and finally supplementation. These approaches should be regarded as complementary, with their relative importance depending on local conditions and the specific mix of local needs.

Of the three options that are aimed at increasing the intake of micronutrients, programmes that deliver micronutrient supplements often provide the fastest improvement in the micronutrient status of individuals or targeted population

---

[1] See http://www.gainhealth.org.
[2] See http://www.iodinenetwork.net.

groups. Food fortification tends to have a less immediate but nevertheless a much wider and more sustained impact. Although increasing dietary diversity is generally regarded as the most desirable and sustainable option, it takes the longest to implement.

1.2.1 Increasing the diversity of foods consumed

Increasing dietary diversity means increasing both the quantity and the range of micronutrient-rich foods consumed. In practice, this requires the implementation of programmes that improve the availability and consumption of, and access to, different types of micronutrient-rich foods (such as animal products, fruits and vegetables) in adequate quantities, especially among those who at risk for, or vulnerable to, MNM. In poorer communities, attention also needs to be paid to ensuring that dietary intakes of oils and fats are adequate for enhancing the absorption of the limited supplies of micronutrients.

Increasing dietary diversity is the preferred way of improving the nutrition of a population because it has the potential to improve the intake of many food constituents – not just micronutrients – simultaneously. Ongoing research suggests that micronutrient-rich foods also provide a range of antioxidants and probiotic substances that are important for protection against selected non-communicable diseases and for enhancing immune function. However, as a strategy for combating MNM, increasing dietary diversity is not without its limitations, the main one being the need for behaviour change and for education about how certain foods provide essential micronutrients and other nutritive substances. A lack of resources for producing and purchasing higher quality foods can sometimes present a barrier to achieving greater dietary diversity, especially in the case of poorer populations. The importance of animal source foods for dietary quality is increasingly being recognized, and innovative approaches to increase their production and consumption in poorer regions of the world are currently being explored (21). Efforts are also underway to help poorer communities identify, domesticate and cultivate traditional and wild micronutrient-rich foods as a simple and affordable means of satisfying micronutrient needs (22–24).

For infants, ensuring a diet of breast milk is an effective way of preventing micronutrient deficiencies. In much of the developing world, breast milk is the main source of micronutrients during the first year of life (with the exception of iron). Exclusive breastfeeding for the first 6 months of life and continuation into the second year should thus be promoted. Moreover, all lactating women should be encouraged to consume a healthful and varied diet so that adequate levels of micronutrients are secreted in their milk. After the age of 6 months, it is important that the complementary foods provided to breast-fed infants are as diverse and as rich in micronutrients as possible.

1.2.2 Food fortification

Food fortification refers to the addition of micronutrients to processed foods. In many situations, this strategy can lead to relatively rapid improvements in the micronutrient status of a population, and at a very reasonable cost, especially if advantage can be taken of existing technology and local distribution networks. Since the benefits are potentially large, food fortification can be a very cost-effective public health intervention. However, an obvious requirement is that the fortified food(s) needs to be consumed in adequate amounts by a large proportion of the target individuals in a population. It is also necessary to have access to, and to use, fortificants that are well absorbed yet do not affect the sensory properties of foods. In most cases, it is preferable to use food vehicles that are centrally processed, and to have the support of the food industry.

Fortification of food with micronutrients is a valid technology for reducing micronutrient malnutrition as part of a food-based approach when and where existing food supplies and limited access fail to provide adequate levels of the respective nutrients in the diet. In such cases, food fortification reinforces and supports ongoing nutrition improvement programmes and should be regarded as part of a broader, integrated approach to prevent MNM, thereby complementing other approaches to improve micronutrient status.

1.2.3 Supplementation

Supplementation is the term used to describe the provision of relatively large doses of micronutrients, usually in the form of pills, capsules or syrups. It has the advantage of being capable of supplying an optimal amount of a specific nutrient or nutrients, in a highly absorbable form, and is often the fastest way to control deficiency in individuals or population groups that have been identified as being deficient.

In developing countries, supplementation programmes have been widely used to provide iron and folic acid to pregnant women, and vitamin A to infants, children under 5 years of age and postpartum women. Because a single high-dose vitamin A supplement improves vitamin A stores for about 4–6 months, supplementation two or three times a year is usually adequate. However, in the case of the more water-soluble vitamins and minerals, supplements need to be consumed more frequently. Supplementation usually requires the procurement and purchase of micronutrients in a relatively expensive pre-packaged form, an effective distribution system and a high degree of consumer compliance (especially if supplements need to be consumed on a long-term basis). A lack of supplies and poor compliance are consistently reported by many supplementation programme managers as being the main barriers to success.

1.2.4 Public health measures

In addition to the specific interventions outlined above, public health measures of a more general nature are often required to help prevent and correct MNM, because MNM is often associated with poor overall nutritional status and with a high prevalence of infection. Such measures include infection control (e.g. immunization, malaria and parasite control), and improvement of water and sanitation. Other factors, such as the quality of child care and maternal education, also need to be taken into consideration when developing public health responses to MNM.

1.3 Food fortification in practice

Food fortification has a long history of use in industrialized countries for the successful control of deficiencies of vitamins A and D, several B vitamins (thiamine, riboflavin and niacin), iodine and iron. Salt iodization was introduced in the early 1920s in both Switzerland (25) and the United States of America (26) and has since expanded progressively all over the world to the extent that iodized salt is now used in most countries. From the early 1940s onwards, the fortification of cereal products with thiamine, riboflavin and niacin became common practice. Margarine was fortified with vitamin A in Denmark and milk with vitamin D in the United States. Foods for young children were fortified with iron, a practice which has substantially reduced the risk of iron-deficiency anaemia in this age group. In more recent years, folic acid fortification of wheat has become widespread in the Americas, a strategy adopted by Canada and the United States and about 20 Latin American countries.

In the less industrialized countries, fortification has become an increasingly attractive option in recent years, so much so that planned programmes have moved forward to the implementation phase more rapidly than previously thought possible. Given the success of the relatively long-running programme to fortify sugar with vitamin A in Central America, where the prevalence of vitamin A deficiency has been reduced considerably, similar initiatives are being attempted in other world regions. Currently, the first sugar fortification experience in sub-Saharan Africa is taking place in Zambia, and if successful will be emulated elsewhere. Darnton-Hill and Nalubola (27) have identified at least 27 developing countries that could benefit from programmes to fortify one or more foods.

Despite apparent past successes, to date, very few fortification programmes have formally evaluated their impact on nutritional status. However, without a specific evaluation component, once a fortification programme has been initiated, it is difficult to know whether subsequent improvements in the nutritional status of a population are due to the intervention or to other changes, such as, improvements in socioeconomic status or in public health provision, that occurred over the same period of time. Evidence that food fortification programmes do indeed improve nutritional status has therefore tended to come from either efficacy trials and/or reports of programme effectiveness. Efficacy trials, i.e. trials conducted in controlled feeding situations, are relatively numerous and have usefully documented the impact of fortified foods on nutritional status and other outcomes. Evidence of programme effectiveness, which is obtained by assessing changes in nutritional status and other outcomes once a programme has been implemented, is less widely available. Of the few effectiveness studies that have been conducted, even fewer included a non-intervention control group, an omission that weakens the evidence that can be obtained from studies of this type.

1.3.1 Efficacy trials

As indicated above, efficacy trials evaluate the impact of a test intervention under ideal circumstances. In the case of food fortification, this typically involves all test subjects consuming a known amount of the fortified food. In the majority of efficacy trials conducted to date, fortified foods have been shown to improve micronutrient status. Selected examples, involving a range of micronutrients, are briefly described below. The general principles of programme impact evaluation, including the design of efficacy trials, are discussed in greater detail in Chapter 8 of these guidelines.

1.3.1.1 Iron fortification

In Viet Nam, 6-month efficacy trials have established that fortification of fish sauce with iron can significantly improve iron status and reduce anaemia and iron deficiency (28). The subjects were non-pregnant anaemic female factory workers who consumed 10 ml per day of a sauce that was fortified with 100 mg iron (as NaFeEDTA) per 100 ml. **Figure 1.1** illustrates the effect of the intervention on iron deficiency and iron-deficiency anaemia; both were significantly reduced after 6 months in the group receiving the fortified sauce relative to the placebo control group.

In China, a series of studies have been conducted to assess the efficacy, effectiveness and feasibility of fortifying soy sauce with iron (in the form of NaFeEDTA). Daily consumption of 5 mg or 20 mg iron in the fortified sauce was reported to be very effective in the treatment of iron-deficiency anaemia in children; positive effects were seen within 3 months of the start of the intervention (J. Chen, cited in (29). In a double-blind placebo-controlled effectiveness trial of the iron-fortified sauce, involving about 10 000 children and women, a reduction in the prevalence of anaemia was observed within 6 months (see also section 1.3.2.2).

FIGURE 1.1
Effect of iron fortification of fish sauce on iron status of non-pregnant anaemic female Vietnamese factory workers

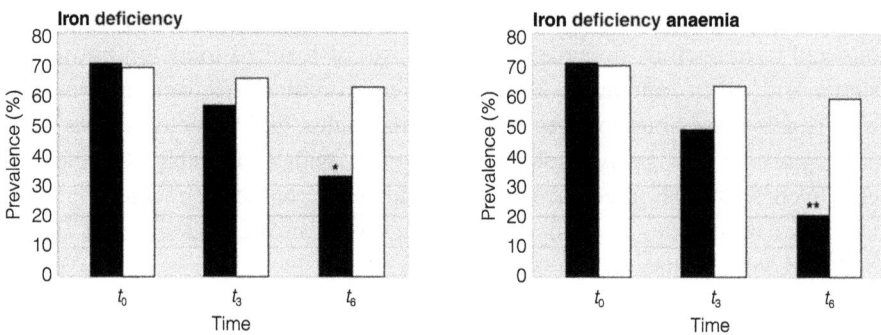

Prevalence of iron deficiency and iron deficiency anaemia at baseline, and after 3 and 6 months of intervention in the iron intervention group ■ (10 mg iron/day in NaFeEDTA-fortified fish sauce (n = 64)) and the control group □ (n = 72) in anaemic Vietnamese women.

Source: reproduced from reference (*28*), with the permission of the publishers.

In an iron-deficient Indian population in South Africa, fortification of curry powder with NaFeEDTA produced significant improvements in blood haemoglobin, ferritin levels and iron stores in women, and in ferritin levels in men (*30*). During the 2-year study, the prevalence of iron-deficiency anaemia in women fell from 22% to just 5%.

Regrettably, well-designed trials of the impact of iron fortification of flour are lacking at the present time.

1.3.1.2 Vitamin A fortification

Trials conducted in the Philippines have revealed that fortification of monosodium glutamate with vitamin A produces positive effects on child mortality, and improved growth and haemoglobin levels in children (*31*). Later studies with preschool-aged children, who consumed 27 g of vitamin A-fortified margarine per day for a period of 6 months, reported a reduction in the prevalence of low serum retinol concentrations from 26% to 10% (*32*). Wheat flour fortified with vitamin A and fed as buns to Filipino schoolchildren for 30 weeks had the effect of halving the number that had low liver stores of the vitamin (*33*).

1.3.1.3 Multiple fortification

A number of trials have evaluated the efficacy of specially-formulated foods and beverages as vehicles for multiple fortification. In South Africa, for example, fortification of biscuits with iron, β-carotene and iodine improved the status of all of these nutrients in schoolchildren (*34*). Vitamin A and iron status deteriorated during the long school holidays when the biscuits were not fed. Fortification of a flavoured beverage with 10 micronutrients increased serum retinol and reduced iron deficiency in Tanzanian schoolchildren, and also improved their growth rates (*35*). Similarly, in Botswana, regular consumption of a 12-micronutrient enriched beverage by school-aged children increased their weight gain and mid-upper arm circumference, and improved their iron, folate, riboflavin and zinc status (*36*).

1.3.2 Effectiveness evaluations

The aim of an effectiveness evaluation is to assess the impact of an intervention or programme in actual practice, as opposed to under controlled conditions. Because of factors such as the lack of consumption of the fortified food, the magnitude of the impact of an intervention is likely to be less than that in an efficacy trial (see also Chapter 8: Monitoring and evaluation).

1.3.2.1 Iodine fortification

Numerous studies, particularly from the developed world, have clearly established that salt iodization is an effective means of controlling iodine deficiency. In the United States, large-scale iodization of salt in Michigan reduced the goitre rate from about 40% to below 10% (*26*). In the early 20th century almost all Swiss schoolchildren had goitre and 0.5% of the population had cretinism. When salt iodization was introduced in 1922, the prevalence of goitre and deaf mutism in children dropped dramatically. Since then, a sustained salt iodization programme has ensured an adequate iodine status among the whole Swiss population (*25*). Despite such convincing evidence in support of salt iodization, in as recently as 2003, it was estimated that 54 countries still have inadequate iodine nutrition (i.e. median urinary iodine < 100 µg/l) (*2*).

1.3.2.2 Iron fortification

The effectiveness of iron fortification has been demonstrated in several world regions. Iron fortification of infant formulas has been associated with a fall in the prevalence of anaemia in children aged under 5 years in the United States (*37,38*). In Venezuela, wheat and maize flours have been fortified with iron (as a mixture of ferrous fumarate and elemental iron), vitamin A and various B vitamins since 1993. A comparison of the prevalence of iron deficiency and anaemia pre- and post-intervention showed a significant reduction in the prevalence of these conditions in children (*39*). Fortification of milk with iron and vitamin C (ascorbic acid) in Chile produced a rapid reduction in the prevalence of iron deficiency in infants and young children (*40,41*). The effectiveness of the fortification of soy sauce with iron is currently being evaluated in a population of 10 000 Chinese women and children with a high risk of anaemia. Preliminary results of the 2-year double-blind placebo-controlled study have shown a reduction in anaemia prevalence rates for all age groups after the first 6 months (J. Chen, cited in (*29*)).

Unfortunately, very few other iron fortification programmes have been evaluated. Information about the efficacy and effectiveness of flour fortification in particular is urgently needed (*42*).

1.3.2.3 Combined iron and iodine fortification

A randomized, double-blind effectiveness trial in Moroccan schoolchildren (n = 367) has demonstrated that the dual fortification of salt with iron and iodine can improve both iron and iodine status (*43*). Results of the 40-week trial, in which salt was fortified with iron at a level of 1 mg Fe/g salt (as ferrous sulfate microencapsulated with partially hydrogenated vegetable oil) are summarized in **Figure 1.2**. In addition to improved iron status, by the end of the trial the iron-fortified group had significantly lower thyroid volumes. Because iron is required for thyroxine synthesis, iron deficiency reduces the efficacy of iodine prophylaxis. Thus, by supplying both iodine and iron, the impact of iodine fortification is maximized.

FIGURE 1.2

Effect of dual-fortified salt (iron and iodine) on the iron status of Moroccan schoolchildren

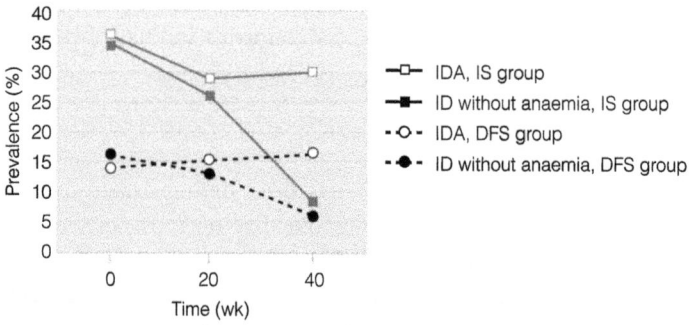

The probability of iron deficiency anaemia (IDA) and iron deficiency without anaemia (ID) was significantly less in 6–15 year-old children receiving dual-fortified salt (DFS) containing both iron and iodine (n = 183) than in those receiving iodized salt (IS) (n = 184). For both IDA and ID without anaemia, the difference between the IS and DFS groups increased significantly with time (P < 0.01).

Source: reproduced from reference (*44*).

1.3.2.4 Vitamin A fortification

Fortification of sugar with vitamin A is a strategy that has been used extensively throughout Central America. Starting in Guatemala in 1974, and extending to other countries in the region in subsequent years, the effect of this programme has been to reduce the prevalence of low serum retinol values – from 27% in 1965 to 9% in 1977 (*45,46*). There is also evidence to suggest that sugar fortification substantially increases the concentration of vitamin A in breast milk (*47*). When the programme was temporarily discontinued in parts of the region, the prevalence of low serum retinol again increased. Vitamin A fortification of sugar is, however, still ongoing in Guatemala.

1.3.2.5 Folic acid fortification

The introduction of the mandatory fortification of wheat flour with folic acid in the United States in 1998 was accompanied by a significant reduction in the prevalence of neural tube defects (*48*) and in plasma levels of homocysteine. (Elevated plasma homocysteine has been identified as a risk factor for cardiovascular disease and other health problems (*49*). Even though these outcomes may have been due to other factors, there was certainly an increase in folate intakes (*50*) and an improvement in folate status (*49*) among the population in the period immediately following the implementation of the new legislation. Similar improvements in folate status have been seen after the commencement of folic acid fortification of wheat flour in Canada (*51*) (see **Figure 1.3**).

FIGURE 1.3

Effect of flour fortification with folic acid on the folate status of elderly Canadian women

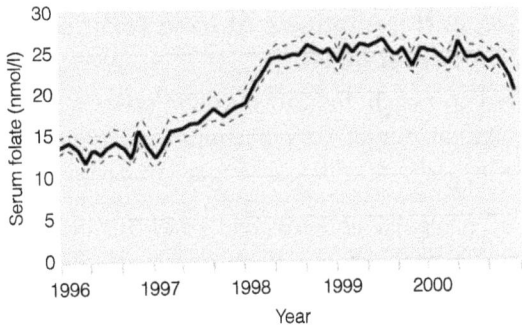

Serum folate concentrations in a cross-section of 15 664 Canadian women aged 65 years and older in relation to the introduction of flour fortification in mid-1997. Data are presented as mean values (solid line) with 95% confidence limits (dotted lines)

Source: reproduced from reference (*53*), with the permission of the publishers.

Likewise, in Chile, a national programme of flour fortification with folic acid increased serum folate and reduced serum homocysteine in a group of elderly people (52).

1.3.2.6 Fortification with other B vitamins

Beriberi, riboflavin deficiency, pellagra and anaemia were relatively widespread public health problems during the 1930s in several countries, including the United States. In an attempt to reduce the prevalence of these conditions, a decision was taken to add thiamine, riboflavin, niacin and iron to wheat flour. With the implementation of fortification programmes for these micronutrients during the early 1940s in the United States and in some European countries, these deficiencies largely disappeared (54). While it can be argued that other factors – such as improved dietary diversity – also played a role, enriched flour continues to make an important contribution to meeting recommended nutrient intakes for the B-complex vitamins and iron in these and many other countries today.

1.3.2.7 Vitamin D fortification

The virtual elimination of childhood rickets in the industrialized countries has been largely attributed to the addition of vitamin D to milk, a practice that commenced in the 1930s in Canada and the United States. However, there are some signs that rickets is re-emerging as a public health problem in these countries (55). In a recent study of African American women, a low intake of vitamin D fortified milk was found to be a significant predictor of a high prevalence of vitamin D deficiency (56). Vitamin D fortification of milk also reduces the risk of osteoporosis in the elderly, especially in higher latitude regions where levels of incident ultraviolet light are lower during the winter months (57,58).

1.4 Advantages and limitations of food fortification as a strategy to combat MNM

Being a food-based approach, food fortification offers a number of advantages over other interventions aimed at preventing and controlling MNM. These include:

- If consumed on a regular and frequent basis, fortified foods will maintain body stores of nutrients more efficiently and more effectively than will intermittent supplements. Fortified foods are also better at lowering the risk of the multiple deficiencies that can result from seasonal deficits in the food supply or a poor quality diet. This is an important advantage to growing children who need a sustained supply of micronutrients for growth and development, and to women of fertile age who need to enter periods of pregnancy and lactation with adequate nutrient stores. Fortification can be an excellent way of increasing the content of vitamins in breast milk and thus reducing the need for supplementation in postpartum women and infants.

- Fortification generally aims to supply micronutrients in amounts that approximate to those provided by a good, well-balanced diet. Consequently, fortified staple foods will contain "natural" or near natural levels of micronutrients, which may not necessarily be the case with supplements.

- Fortification of widely distributed and widely consumed foods has the potential to improve the nutritional status of a large proportion of the population, both poor and wealthy.

- Fortification requires neither changes in existing food patterns – which are notoriously difficult to achieve, especially in the short-term – nor individual compliance.

- In most settings, the delivery system for fortified foods is already in place, generally through the private sector. The global tendency towards urbanization means that an ever increasing proportion of the population, including that in developing countries is consuming industry-processed, rather than locally-produced, foods. This affords many countries the opportunity to develop effective strategies to combat MNM based on the fortification of centrally-processed dietary staples that once would have reached only a very small proportion of the population.

- Multiple micronutrient deficiencies often coexist in a population that has a poor diet. It follows that multiple micronutrient fortification is frequently desirable. In most cases, it is feasible to fortify foods with several micronutrients simultaneously.

- It is usually possible to add one or several micronutrients without adding substantially to the total cost of the food product at the point of manufacture.

- When properly regulated, fortification carries a minimal risk of chronic toxicity.

- Fortification is often more cost-effective than other strategies, especially if the technology already exists and if an appropriate food distribution system is in place (59,60).

Although it is generally recognized that food fortification can have an enormous positive impact on public health, there are, however, some limitations to this strategy for MNM control:

- While fortified foods contain increased amounts of selected micronutrients, they are not a substitute for a good quality diet that supplies adequate amounts of energy, protein, essential fats and other food constituents required for optimal health.

- A specific fortified foodstuff might not be consumed by all members of a target population. Conversely, everyone in the population is exposed to increased levels of micronutrients in food, irrespective of whether or not they will benefit from fortification.

- Infants and young children, who consume relatively small amounts of food, are less likely to be able to obtain their recommended intakes of all micronutrients from universally fortified staples or condiments alone; fortified complementary foods may be appropriate for these age groups. It is also likely that in many locations fortified foods will not supply adequate amounts of some micronutrients, such as iron for pregnant women, in which case supplements will still be needed to satisfy the requirements of selected population groups.

- Fortified foods often fail to reach the poorest segments of the general population who are at the greatest risk of micronutrient deficiency. This is because such groups often have restricted access to fortified foods due to low purchasing power and an underdeveloped distribution channel. Many undernourished population groups often live on the margins of the market economy, relying on own-grown or locally produced food. Availability, access and consumption of adequate quantities and a variety of micronutrient-rich foods, such as animal foods and fruits and vegetables, is limited. Access to the food distribution system is similarly restricted and these population groups will purchase only small amounts of processed foods. Rice production, in particular, tends to be domestic or local, as does maize production. In populations who rely on these staples, it may be difficult to find an appropriate food to fortify. Fortification of sugar, sauces, seasonings and other condiments may provide a solution to this problem in some countries, if such products are consumed in sufficient amounts by target groups.

- Very low-income population groups are known to have coexisting multiple micronutrient deficiencies, as a result of inadequate intakes of the traditional diet. Although multiple micronutrient fortification is technically possible, the reality is that the poor will be unable to obtain recommended intakes of all micronutrients from fortified foods alone.

- Technological issues relating to food fortification have yet to be fully resolved, especially with regard to appropriate levels of nutrients, stability of fortificants, nutrient interactions, physical properties, as well as acceptability by consumers including cooking properties and taste (see Part III).

- The nature of the food vehicle, and/or the fortificant, may limit the amount of fortificant that can be successfully added. For example, some iron fortificants change the colour and flavour of many foods to which they are added, and can cause the destruction of fortificant vitamin A and iodine. Ways of solving some of these problems (e.g. microencapsulation of fortificants with protective coatings) have been developed, but some difficulties remain (see Part III).

- While it is generally possible to add a mixture of vitamins and minerals to relatively inert and dry foods, such as cereals, interactions can occur between fortificant nutrients that adversely affect the organoleptic qualities of the food or the stability of the nutrients. Knowledge is lacking about the quantitative impact of interactions among nutrients that are added as a mixture on the absorption of the individual nutrients. This complicates the estimation of how much of each nutrient should be added. For example, the presence of large amounts of calcium can inhibit the absorption of iron from a fortified food; the presence of vitamin C has the opposite effect and increases iron absorption.

- Although often more cost-effective than other strategies, there are nevertheless significant costs associated with the food fortification process, which might limit the implementation and effectiveness of food fortification programmes. These typically include start-up costs, the expense of conducting trials for micronutrient levels, physical qualities and taste, a realistic analysis of the purchasing power of the expected beneficiaries, the recurrent costs involved in creating and maintaining the demand for these products, as well as the cost of an effective national surveillance system to ensure that fortification is both effective and safe (see Chapter 9).

To ensure their success and sustainability, especially in resource-poor countries, food fortification programmes should be implemented in concert with poverty reduction programmes and other agricultural, health, education and social intervention programmes that promote the consumption and utilization of adequate quantities of good quality nutritious foods among the nutritionally vulnerable. Food fortification should thus be viewed as a complementary strategy for improving micronutrient status.

CHAPTER 2
Food fortification: basic principles

Food fortification is usually regarded as the deliberate addition of one or more micronutrients to particular foods, so as to increase the intake of these micronutrient(s) in order to correct or prevent a demonstrated deficiency and provide a health benefit. The extent to which a national or regional food supply is fortified varies considerably. The concentration of just one micronutrient might be increased in a single foodstuff (e.g. the iodization of salt), or, at the other end of the scale, there might be a whole range of food–micronutrient combinations. The public health impact of food fortification depends on a number of parameters, but predominantly the level of fortification, the bioavailability of the fortificants, and the amount of fortified food consumed. As a general rule, however, the more widely and regularly a fortified food is consumed, the greater the proportion of the population likely to benefit from food fortification.

2.1 Terminology

2.1.1 Food fortification

For the purpose of these guidelines, food fortification is defined as the practice of deliberately increasing the content of essential[1] micronutrients – that is to say, vitamins and minerals (including trace elements) – in a food so as to improve the nutritional quality of the food supply and to provide a public health benefit with minimal risk to health. The public health benefits of fortification may either be demonstrable, or indicated as potential or plausible by generally accepted scientific research, and include:

- Prevention or minimization of the risk of occurrence of micronutrient deficiency in a population or specific population groups.

- Contribution to the correction of a demonstrated micronutrient deficiency in a population or specific population groups.

---

[1] The word "essential" means any substance that is normally consumed as a constituent of food which is needed for growth and development and the maintenance of healthy life and which cannot be synthesized in adequate amounts by the body (61).

- A potential for an improvement in nutritional status and dietary intakes that may be, or may become, suboptimal as a result of changes in dietary habits/lifestyles.

- Plausible beneficial effects of micronutrients consistent with maintaining or improving health (e.g. there is some evidence to suggest that a diet rich in selected anitoxidants might help to prevent cancer and other diseases).

The Codex *General Principles for the Addition of Essential Nutrients to Foods* (*61*) defines "fortification", or synonymously "enrichment", as "the addition of one or more essential nutrients to a food whether or not it is normally contained in the food, for the purpose of preventing or correcting a demonstrated deficiency of one or more nutrients in the population or specific population groups". The Codex General Principles go on to state that the first-mentioned condition for the fulfilment of any fortification programme "should be a demonstrated need for increasing the intake of an essential nutrient in one or more population groups. This may be in the form of actual clinical or subclinical evidence of deficiency, estimates indicating low levels of intake of nutrients or possible deficiencies likely to develop because of changes taking place in food habits" (*61*).

The broad definition of fortification used in these guidelines extends the interpretation of public health need prescribed by the Codex *General Principles for the Addition of Essential Nutrients to Foods* (*61*) in that it also incorporates plausible public health benefits that may be derived from increased micronutrient intakes (as opposed to merely demonstrable benefits), based on new and evolving scientific knowledge. The broader definition thus encompasses the growing range of different types of food fortification initiatives that have been implemented in recent years in response to an increasingly diverse set of public health circumstances.

Clearly, the public health significance of the potential benefits of food fortification is primarily a function of the extent of the public health problem. Generally speaking, therefore, when deciding to implement a fortification programme, priority should be given to controlling those nutrient deficiencies that are most common in the population and that have the greatest adverse effect on health and function. In Part II of these guidelines, appropriate criteria that can be applied to the determination of the significance of the public health problem are described; these criteria are largely expressed in terms of the prevalence and severity of MNM. Ideally this should be determined at the country or regional level.

2.1.2 Related codex terminology

The following definitions are used in these guidelines as follows:

- *Restoration* is the addition of essential nutrients to foods to restore amounts originally present in the natural product that are unavoidably lost during processing (e.g. milling), storage or handling.

- *Nutritional equivalence* is achieved when an essential nutrient is added to a product that is designed to resemble a common food in appearance, texture, flavour and odour in amounts such that the substitute product has a similar nutritive value, in terms of the amount and bioavailability of the added essential nutrient. An example is the addition of vitamin A to margarine sold as a butter substitute, in an amount equal to butter's natural content.

- *Appropriate nutrient composition of a special purpose food* describes the addition of an essential nutrient to a food that is designed to perform a specific function (such as meal replacement or a complementary food for young children), or that is processed or formulated to satisfy particular dietary requirements, in amounts that ensure that the nutrient content of the food is adequate and appropriate for its purpose.

Whereas restoration and nutritional equivalence are strategies aimed at correcting food supply changes that could otherwise adversely affect public health, the term "fortification" tends to be reserved for essential nutrient additions that address specific public health needs. Nevertheless, all the Codex categories of nutrient additions adopt, albeit to a varying degree, the general aim of providing a public health benefit.

2.2 Types of fortification

Food fortification can take several forms. It is possible to fortify foods that are widely consumed by the general population (mass fortification[1]), to fortify foods designed for specific population subgroups, such as complementary foods for young children or rations for displaced populations (targeted fortification) and/or to allow food manufacturers to voluntarily fortify foods available in the market place (market-driven fortification[2]).

Generally speaking, mass fortification is nearly always mandatory, targeted fortification can be either mandatory or voluntary depending on the public health significance of the problem it is seeking to address, and market-driven fortification is always voluntary, but governed by regulatory limits (**Figure 2.1**). The choice between mandatory or voluntary food fortification usually depends on national circumstances. For example, in countries where a large proportion of maize flour is produced by small mills, enforcement of mandatory fortifica-

---

[1] Mass fortification is sometimes called "universal fortification".
[2] Market-driven fortification is sometimes called "industry-driven fortification", "open-market" or "free-market" fortification.

FIGURE 2.1

The interrelationships between the levels of coverage and compliance and the different types of food fortification

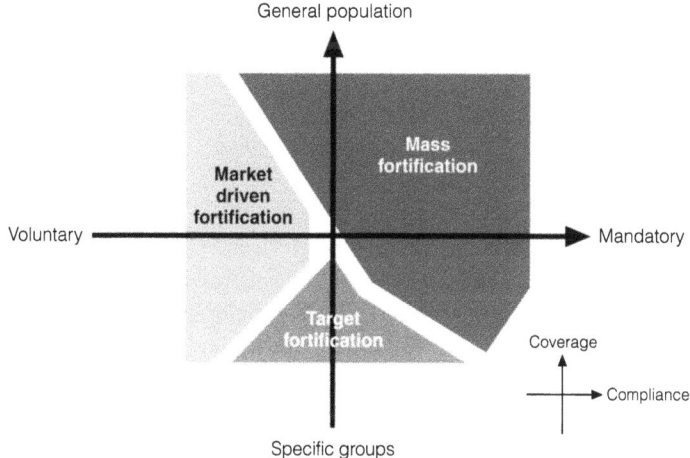

tion might be impractical. Under such circumstances, one option would be, if feasible, to allow small mills to fortify their product on a voluntary basis but following specified regulations.

2.2.1 Mass fortification

As indicated above, mass fortification is the term used to describe the addition of one or more micronutrients to foods commonly consumed by the general public, such as cereals, condiments and milk. It is usually instigated, mandated and regulated by the government sector.

Mass fortification is generally the best option when the majority of the population has an unacceptable risk, in terms of public health, of being or becoming deficient in specific micronutrients. In some situations, deficiency may be demonstrable, as evidenced by unacceptably low intakes and/or biochemical signs of deficiency. In others, the population may not actually be deficient according to usual biochemical or dietary criteria, but are likely to benefit from fortification. The mandatory addition of folic acid to wheat flour with a view to lowering the risk of birth defects, a practice which has been introduced in Canada and the United States, and also in many Latin American countries, is one example of the latter scenario.

2.2.2 Targeted fortification

In targeted food fortification programmes, foods aimed at specific subgroups of the population are fortified, thereby increasing the intake of that particular group

TABLE 2.1
Targeted food fortification programmes

Country	Food	Target population
Guatemala	Incaparina	
Indonesia	Complementary foods	Infants
Mexico	Progresa	
Peru	Ali Alimentu	Schoolchildren
South Africa	Biscuits	Schoolchildren

rather than that of the population as a whole. Examples include complementary foods for infants and young children, foods developed for school feeding programmes, special biscuits for children and pregnant women, and rations (blended foods) for emergency feeding and displaced persons (**Table 2.1**). In some cases, such foods may be required to provide a substantial proportion of daily micronutrient requirements of the target group.

The majority of blended foods for feeding refugees and displaced persons are managed by the World Food Programme (WFP) and guidelines covering their fortification (including wheat soy blends and corn soy blends) are already available (*62*). Although blended foods usually supply all or nearly all of the energy and protein intake of refugees and displaced individuals, especially in the earlier stages of dislocation, for historical reasons such foods may not always provide adequate amounts of all micronutrients. Therefore, other sources of micronutrients may need to be provided. In particular, it may be necessary to add iodized salt to foods, provide iron supplements to pregnant women or supply high-dose vitamin A supplements to young children and postpartum women. Whenever possible, fresh fruits and vegetables should be added to the diets of displaced persons relying on blended foods (see Chapter 4: section 4.5). Fortified foods for displaced persons are often targeted at children and pregnant or lactating women.

2.2.3 Market-driven fortification

The term "market-driven fortification" is applied to situations whereby a food manufacturer takes a business-oriented initiative to add specific amounts of one or more micronutrients to processed foods. Although voluntary, this type of food fortification usually takes place within government-set regulatory limits (see Chapter 11: National food law).

Market-driven fortification can play a positive role in public health by contributing to meeting nutrient requirements and thereby reducing the risk of micronutrient deficiency. In the European Union, fortified processed foods have been shown to be a substantial source of micronutrients such as iron, and vitamins A and D (*63,64*). Market-driven fortification can also improve the supply of micronutrients that are otherwise difficult to add in sufficient amounts through the mass fortification of staple foods and condiments because of safety, technological or cost constraints. Examples include certain minerals (e.g. iron, calcium) and sometimes selected vitamins (e.g. vitamin C, vitamin B_2).

Market-driven fortification is more widespread in industrialized countries, whereas in most developing countries the public health impact of market-driven food interventions is still rather limited. However, their importance is likely to be greater in the future, because of increasing urbanization and wider availability of such foods.

The predicted increase in the availability of fortified processed foods in developing countries has given rise to a number of concerns. Firstly, these fortified foods – especially those that are attractive to consumers – could divert consumers from their usual dietary pattern and result in, for example, an increased consumption of sugar, or a lower consumption of fibre. Secondly, because in most developing countries foods fortified through market-driven fortification currently receive scant regulatory attention even though such foods are intended for wide-scale consumption (see section 2.3), there is a potential risk that unnecessarily high levels of micronutrients may be delivered to children if the same serving size of the fortified food (such as breakfast cereals, beverages and nutrition bars) is intended for all members of a household. Regulation is thus necessary to ensure that the consumption of these foods will not result in an excessive intake of micronutrients. Furthermore, manufacturers of processed fortified foods should be encouraged to follow the same quality control and assurance procedures as those that are prescribed for mandatory mass-fortified products (see Chapter 8: Monitoring and evaluation).

2.2.4 Other types of fortification
2.2.4.1 Household and community fortification

Efforts are under way in a number of countries to develop and test practical ways of adding micronutrients to foods at the household level, in particular, to complementary foods for young children. In effect, this approach is a combination of supplementation and fortification, and has been referred to by some as "complementary food supplementation" (*65*).

The efficacy and effectiveness of several different types of products, including soluble or crushable tablets, micronutrient-based powder ("sprinkles") and micronutrient-rich spreads are currently being evaluated (**Table 2.2**). Crushable tablets, and especially micronutrient-based powder, are relatively expensive ways of increasing micronutrient intakes, certainly more costly than mass fortification, but may be especially useful for improving local foods fed to infants and young children, or where universal fortification is not possible (*66*). The

TABLE 2.2
Foods for fortification at the household level

Product	Comments
Micronutrient powder which can be sprinkled onto food	■ Contain several micronutrients, including iron, encapsulated to minimize adverse interactions between micronutrients and sensory changes to the food to which they are added; available in sachets
Soluble micronutrient tablets which can be dissolved in water and fed as a drink	■ Suitable for young children; ■ Tested by WHO
Crushable micronutrient tablets for adding to foods	■ For infants and young children ■ Tested by UNICEF
Fat-based spread fortified with micronutrient	■ Popular with children ■ Can be produced locally as the technology required is easy to implement

Sources: references (66,67).

micronutrient-dense fortified spreads have been found to be very popular with children (67).

Fortification of foods at the community level is also still at the experimental stage. One such approach involves the addition of a commercial micronutrient premix, available in sachets, to small batches of flour during the milling process (68). Although feasible in theory, major challenges to local-scale fortification programmes include the initial cost of the mixing equipment, the price of the premix (which would need to be imported in most cases), achieving and maintaining an adequate standard of quality control (e.g. in uniformity of mixing), and sustaining monitoring and distribution systems.

2.2.4.2 Biofortification of staple foods

The biofortification of staple foods, i.e. the breeding and genetic modification of plants so as to improve their nutrient content and/or absorption is another novel approach that is currently being considered. The potential for plant breeding to increase the micronutrient content of various cereals, legumes and tubers certainly exists; for instance, it is possible to select certain cereals (such as rice) and legumes for their high iron content, various varieties of carrots and sweet potatoes for their favourable β-carotene levels, and maizes for their low phytate content (which improves the absorption of iron and zinc) (69–71). However, much more work still needs to be done before the efficacy and effectiveness of these foods are proven, and current concerns about their safety, cost and impact on the environment are alleviated (72).

2.3 Legal considerations: mandatory versus voluntary fortification

The huge diversity in national circumstances and public health goals worldwide has resulted in the development of many different approaches to the regulation of food fortification. In most industrialized countries, food fortification parameters are established by law or through cooperative arrangements. Elsewhere, and representing the other end of the spectrum, fortified foods are produced without any form of governmental guidance or control at all. Since it is the role of government to protect public health, it is generally recommended that all forms of food fortification be appropriately regulated in order to ensure the safety of all consumers and the maximum benefit to target groups.

Within the legal context, fortification can be categorized as either mandatory or voluntary. These terms refer to the level of obligation required of food producers to comply with government intentions expressed in law.

The fundamental distinction between mandatory and voluntary regulation as it applies to food fortification is the level of certainty over time that a particular category of food will contain a pre-determined amount of a micronutrient. By providing a higher level of certainty, mandatory fortification is more likely to deliver a sustained source of fortified food for consumption by the relevant population group, and, in turn, a public health benefit.

2.3.1 Mandatory fortification

2.3.1.1 Key characteristics

Mandatory fortification occurs when governments legally oblige food producers to fortify particular foods or categories of foods with specified micronutrients. Mandatory fortification, especially when supported by a properly resourced enforcement and information dissemination system, delivers a high level of certainty that the selected food(s) will be appropriately fortified and in constant supply.

In deciding the precise form of mandatory fortification regulation, governments are responsible for ensuring that the combination of the food vehicle and the fortificants will be both *efficacious* and *effective* for the target group, yet safe for target and non-target groups alike. Food vehicles range from basic commodities, such as various types of flour, sugar and salt which are available on the retail market for use by consumers as well as ingredients of processed foods, to processed foods that are fortified at the point of manufacture. Given their widespread and regular consumption, basic commodities are more suited to mass fortification (i.e. intended to reach the whole population), whereas certain processed formulated foods are usually the better vehicle for targeted fortification initiatives (i.e. those aimed at specific population groups).

Globally, mandatory regulations are most often applied to the fortification of food with micronutrients such as iodine, iron, vitamin A, and increasingly folic acid. Of these, the iodization of salt is probably the most widely adopted form of mandatory mass fortification. In the Philippines, for example, the legal standard for iodized salt, which is appended to the Philippine Act Promoting Salt Iodization Nationwide, requires a minimum level of iodine fortification of all food-grade salt destined for human consumption (6). This form of mandatory regulation is used in many other countries. Other examples of mandatory mass fortification include the addition of vitamin A to sugar and margarine, and the fortification of flour with iron (usually together with restoration of vitamins B_1, B_2 and niacin), and, more recently, with folic acid and vitamin B_{12}.

The types of food vehicles that are subjected to mandatory fortification are usually characterized by either a physical or an intrinsic attribute, or a specific purpose. A requisite flour, for example, could be described as either white or wholemeal and/or milled from a particular grain, or destined for bread making. Alternatively, the prescribed fortification requirements may apply only to a food that is identified and labelled in a certain way. In the United States, for instance, only those flours and other grain products identified and labelled as "enriched" are required by law to contain added folic acid (and some other essential micronutrients). Similarly, Australia and New Zealand mandate the addition of iodine only to salt identified and labelled as "iodized salt". Although the potential public health impact is more variable, mass fortification can be achieved under these conditions, particularly if the labelled fortified foods constitute a major and stable share of the market for that food class as a whole.

2.3.1.2 Mandatory fortification in relation to public health

Governments tend to institute mandatory fortification in situations where a proportion of the general population – either the majority (mass fortification) or an identified population group (target fortification) – has a significant public health need, or is at risk of being, or becoming, deficient in a specific micronutrient(s), and where such needs or risks can be ameliorated or minimized by a sustained supply and regular consumption of particular fortified food(s) containing those micronutrients.

Mandatory fortification is usually prompted by evidence that a given population is deficient or inadequately nourished, such as clinical or biochemical signs of deficiency and/or unacceptably low levels of micronutrient intake. In some circumstances, a demonstrated public health benefit of an increased consumption of a given micronutrient might be considered sufficient grounds to warrant mandatory fortification even if the population is not considered to be seriously at risk according to conventional biochemical or dietary intake criteria. The mandatory addition of folic acid to flour to reduce the risk of birth defects is a case in point.

2.3.2 Voluntary fortification

2.3.2.1 Key characteristics

Fortification is described as voluntary when a food manufacturer freely chooses to fortify particular foods in response to permission given in food law, or under special circumstances, is encouraged by government to do so.

The impetus for voluntary fortification usually stems from industry and consumers seeking to obtain possible health benefits through an increase in micronutrient intakes. Occasionally, however, government provides the driving force. Given this diversity in the circumstances that drive voluntary fortification, it is not surprising that the public health impacts range from negligible to substantial. Indeed, depending on the nutritional quality of their basic diet, those individuals who regularly consume fortified foods might well gain discernable benefits.

However, it is important that governments exercise an appropriate degree of control over voluntary fortification through food laws or other cooperative arrangements, such as industry codes of practice. The degree of control should at least be commensurate with the inherent level of risk. Regulatory controls of this nature should also ensure the safety of fortified foods for all consumers, as well as provide opportunities for industry to produce fortified foods that offer consumers nutritional and/or other health benefits. The potential benefits may be demonstrable, or indicated as potential or plausible by generally accepted scientific data.

When instituting voluntary fortification arrangements, governments have a duty to ensure that consumers are not misled or deceived by fortification practices and may also wish to be satisfied that market promotion of fortified foods does not conflict with, or compromise, any national food and nutrition policies on healthy eating. This could be achieved through regulations on the range of foods eligible for voluntary fortification and on the permitted combinations of particular micronutrients and foods (see Chapter 11: National food law).

Currently many countries permit voluntary fortification, but the range of foods that may be fortified varies considerably from country to country. Some Scandinavian countries allow only a narrow range of foods to be fortified, whereas the range of products that can be fortified is much greater in the United States. Similarly, the permitted fortificants range from a select few to almost all micronutrients that are considered essential.

The level of industry uptake of fortification practice is greatly influenced by prevailing market conditions. For example, in many industrialized countries, the vast majority of processed breakfast cereals are moderately fortified with various combinations of micronutrients, sometimes differentiated according to the target market; the remaining few are either highly or extensively fortified (where permitted) and/or unfortified. Other food categories, such as fruit juices or dairy products, tend to exhibit a greater variability in fortification rates, this being influenced by market differentiation and brand identity. For some permitted categories there may be no industry interest in fortification.

2.3.2.2 Voluntary fortification in relation to public health

Voluntary fortification tends to be used when there are lower order risks to public health, i.e. when the risks to public health are not as serious or demonstrable so as to warrant mass fortification. Inadequate micronutrient intakes that arise because of changes in lifestyles that tend to follow changing social and economic circumstances are more likely to be associated with lower order public health risks than inadequate intakes that arise because of significantly modified eating habits and dietary behaviour. In addition, for certain nutrients, dietary requirements have been reappraised in light of evolving scientific knowledge about their physiological role and the beneficial effects on certain physiological processes and health conditions.

Because of uncertainty about the level of industry uptake of fortification within each food product category, and the fact that regular consumers of a given fortified food may vary over time and thus do not constitute a readily identifiable group, voluntary fortification is less likely than mandatory fortification to deliver a guaranteed favourable outcome in terms of increased intakes of micronutrients across a target population. Apart from the extent to which a given food category is fortified, the public health impact of voluntary fortification depends on the contribution of that food category to the diet of the population as whole, and also whether or not those individuals who would benefit most from fortification regularly consume and have access to that food category.

Despite these inherent difficulties, a consistent supply of appropriately regulated, voluntarily-fortified foods, produced under free-market conditions and widely and regularly consumed by a given population group, can have a beneficial impact on public health by positively contributing to micronutrient balance and thereby reducing the risk of deficiency. For example, in the European Union where fortification of margarine is voluntary, it is estimated that the addition of vitamins A and D to margarine and spreadable fats contributes about 20% of the reference nutrient intake for vitamin A and 30% of that for vitamin D (63). It has also been reported that by the 1990s fortified breakfast cereals had become the principal source of iron for young children in the United Kingdom (64).

2.3.3 Special voluntary fortification

Some voluntary fortification programmes are capable of achieving similar outcomes to mandatory fortification, thus avoiding the need for complex mandatory legal requirements. A notable example is the Swiss programme of salt iodization. Circumstances that contribute to the success of voluntary fortification in Switzerland and elsewhere include the existence of an industry that comprises only a few producers or manufacturers and a strong government interest in industry practice (e.g. one that provides subsidies and ensures sustainable fortification practices). Voluntary fortification initiatives are also more likely to succeed when supported by public education activities that increase public awareness of the importance of consuming the fortified food (see Chapter 10: Communication, social marketing and advocacy).

2.3.4 Criteria governing the selection of mandatory or voluntary fortification

For any given population group, which may be either the entire population or a specific subgroup(s), there are five key factors that together determine whether mandatory or voluntary fortification is likely to be the most appropriate option for the prevailing conditions. In brief, they are: the significance of the public health need; the size and scale of the food industry sector; the level of awareness among the population about nutritional needs; the political environment; and food consumption patterns. These five factors are described in more detail below, and in each case, an indication given of the circumstances that favour one or the other of the two main regulatory mechanisms.

1. *The significance of the public health need or risk of deficiency, as determined by the severity of the problem and its prevalence within a population group.* The significance of the public health problem is of primary importance and should be determined at the country or regional level, ideally with reference to set criteria that describe the severity of the public health problem. The public health need or risk can be assessed according to evidence of clinical or subclinical deficiency, inadequate nutrient intake, or potential health benefit (see Part II: Evaluating the public health significance of micronutrient malnutrition).

- ■ **Mandatory fortification** is more suited to cases of serious public health need or risk, and **voluntary fortification** to cases of lower order public health need or risk, or where the potential exists for some individuals to benefit from, or to exercise, consumer choice.
- ■ Under certain conditions, **voluntary fortification** can achieve similar public health impacts as mandatory fortification.

2. *The features of the food industry sector that will responsible for the production of the proposed food vehicle.* The aspects of the food industry sector that are especially relevant in this context are the number, capacity and geographical distribution of the producers, the presence of any government support or control, and the prevailing commercial environment.

> ■ In developing countries in particular, **mandatory fortification** is more likely to succeed when the industry sector in question is either relatively centralized (i.e confined to a handful of major producers) and/or well organized. If it consists of numerous small, widely dispersed producers, mandatory fortification will be more difficult to achieve, unless these small units have some form of collective arrangement in place, such as an established industry association. It is also the better option in settings where governments seeking high rates of industry participation do not have any alternative legal or administrative arrangements that could potentially be used to institute voluntary cooperative arrangements within the industry.
>
> ■ **Voluntary fortification** does not need to take account of industry arrangements but where there is a monopoly or a government-sponsored industry, the impact of voluntary arrangements can match those achieved by mandatory fortification.

3. *The relevant population's present level of knowledge about the importance of consuming fortified foods or their interest in consuming fortified foods.* The level of resources available for implementing and sustaining specific nutrition education programmes is also an important factor to consider when choosing the most suitable regulatory environment for a food fortification programme.

> ■ **Mandatory fortification** is likely to be the more effective option when consumer knowledge is poor or demand for voluntarily-fortified products is low, and there are few opportunities for community nutrition education.
>
> ■ **Voluntary fortification** generally relies on consumer interest and/or demand for fortified foods. Although consumer behaviour is influenced by many factors, it could be engendered by commercial promotion or specific nutrition education programmes.

4. *The political environment.* In terms of the political environment, the acceptable level of government intervention and the value placed on informed consumer choice are probably the most significant factors that affecting regulatory decisions.

- In environments where consumer choice is highly valued, both **voluntary and mandatory fortification** could be appropriate. In such settings, **mandatory fortification** tends to be limited to a subset of products within one or more proposed food categories, in order to maintain some degree of consumer choice.

- **Voluntary fortification** usually confers a higher level of consumer choice; however, this is not the main issue in many developing countries, where poverty remains the limiting factor to access to processed foods for the majority of the population.

5. *Food consumption patterns.* Clearly, food consumption patterns, especially in terms of the relative contributions of certain foods to the diet of the target population, will have a bearing on the choice of mandatory or voluntary fortification. Linked to this factor is the issue of the technical suitability of the candidate food as a vehicle for fortification.

- Foods considered for **mandatory fortification** should be widely and regularly consumed by the population group that the fortification is intended to benefit. In addition, the fortification itself should be technically feasible.

- The likelihood of all at-risk consumers increasing their usual micronutrient intake through **voluntary fortification** is lower than with mandatory fortification. However, the likelihood rises as the particular micronutrient is added to a wider range of voluntarily-fortified foods, assuming they are accessible to consumers.

PART II

Evaluating the public health significance of micronutrient malnutrition

Introduction

The chapters in Part II of these guidelines provide more detailed background information on the prevalence, causes and health consequences of various micronutrient deficiencies, and review the available evidence regarding the benefits of their control. They are intended to assist planners not only in their evaluation of the micronutrient deficiency situation in their own country, but also to assess the need for, and potential benefits of, food fortification with specific micronutrients.

Chapter 3 looks at iron, vitamin A and iodine deficiencies, which, owing to their widespread occurrence globally, have received the most attention to date. A large amount of information is now available regarding the prevalence, the causes and the control of deficiencies in these three micronutrients. Various studies on the efficacy and effectiveness of interventions to control deficiencies in iron, vitamin A and iodine, are briefly described here (and in the opening chapter of this document; see section 1.3), but are reviewed in greater depth elsewhere (*73*). Chapter 4 focuses on a range of other micronutrients, which, in comparison, have hitherto been somewhat neglected. Deficiencies in at least some of these "neglected" micronutrients (i.e. in zinc, vitamins B_2 and B_{12}, niacin, vitamin D and calcium) are likely to be common throughout much of the developing world and among the poorest populations in the industrialized nations. Fortification provides a means of lowering the prevalence of deficiencies in all of these micronutrients, and their inclusion in mass fortification programmes, in particular, could produce significant public health benefits. Since there is less information about these micronutrient deficiencies in the literature, a concerted effort has been made to summarize what is known about them in these guidelines.

In both chapters, micronutrients are discussed in order of their perceived public health significance, and in each case the recommended or the most commonly used biochemical status indicators are critically reviewed. For some micronutrients, however, biochemical data reflecting nutritional status will be inadequate for assessing the prevalence of deficiencies. Suggestions for dealing with this situation, for example, by using food intake data to estimate the prevalence of inadequate intakes, are provided in Part IV of these guidelines (see section 7.3.2).

Other than a low dietary intake, important causes of MNM include poor bioavailability from foods (especially for minerals), frequent infection with parasites, diarrhoea, and various malabsorption disorders. The presence of any of these risk factors can lead to an underestimation of the prevalence of deficiency in a population if this is calculated on the basis of micronutrient intakes alone.

Risk factors for micronutrient malnutrition

- Monotonous diet resulting in low micronutrient intake, and poor bioavailability, especially of minerals.
- Low intake of animal source foods.
- Low prevalence of breastfeeding.
- Low micronutrient density of complementary foods.
- Increased physiological demands for growth during pregnancy and lactation.
- Increased demand due to acute infection (especially if infection episodes are frequent), chronic infection (e.g. tuberculosis, malaria and HIV/AIDS) and disease (e.g. cancer).
- Poor general nutritional status, in particular, protein–energy malnutrition.
- Malabsorption due to diarrhoea or the presence of intestinal parasites (e.g. *Giardia lamblia*, hookworms).
- Increased excretion (e.g. due to schistosomiasis).
- Seasonal variations in food availability, food shortages.
- Social deprivation, illiteracy, low education.
- Poor economic status and poverty.

CHAPTER 3
Iron, vitamin A and iodine

3.1 Iron deficiency and anaemia

Most of the iron in the human body is present in the erythrocytes as haemoglobin, where its main function is to carry oxygen from the lungs to the tissues. Iron is also an important component of various enzyme systems, such as the cytochromes, which are involved in oxidative metabolism. It is stored in the liver as ferritin and as haemosiderin.

Iron deficiency is the most common and widespread nutritional disorder in the world, and is a public health problem in both industrialized and non-industrialized countries. Iron deficiency is the result of a long-term negative iron balance; in its more severe stages, iron deficiency causes anaemia. Anaemia is defined as a low blood haemoglobin concentration. Haemoglobin cut-off values that indicate anaemia vary with physiological status (e.g. age, sex) and have been defined for various population groups by WHO (*1*).

3.1.1 Prevalence of deficiency

The terms, "iron deficiency" and "iron-deficiency anaemia" are often used synonymously although they are in fact not the same conditions. About 40% of the world's population (i.e. more than 2 billion individuals) is thought to suffer from anaemia, i.e. low blood haemoglobin (**see Table 1.1**). The mean prevalences among specific population groups are estimated to be:

— pregnant women, infants and children aged 1–2 years, 50%;

— preschool-aged children, 25%;

— schoolchildren, 40%;

— adolescents, 30–55%;

— non-pregnant women, 35%.

These average figures obscure the fact that iron deficiency and iron-deficiency anaemia are even more prevalent in some parts of the world, especially in the Indian subcontinent and in sub-Saharan Africa, where, for example, up to 90% of women become anaemic during pregnancy.

The prevalence of anaemia caused by iron deficiency, usually referred to as iron-deficiency anaemia, is less certain because the specific indicators of iron status, such as serum ferritin, transferrin saturation, zinc protoporphyrin and serum transferrin receptors, are measured less often than blood haemoglobin (**Table 3.1**). Most indicators of iron status – with the possible exception of serum transferrin receptors – are also affected by the presence of infection and can therefore be misleading (*74*). Indeed, every indicator listed in Table 3.1 has its own set of limitations, and so iron status is best assessed by a combination of indicators (*74*).

It is generally assumed that, on average, around 50% of the cases of anaemia are due to iron deficiency, as opposed to malaria (which causes anaemia because the malaria parasite destroys erythrocytes), the presence of infection or other nutrient deficiencies. However, the proportion is probably higher in infants and preschool-aged children than in older children or women (*75*), and is likely to vary by location. Although anaemia usually occurs when iron stores are depleted, the prevalence of iron deficiency will often be substantially higher than the prevalence of iron-deficiency anaemia. However, in iron-deficient populations with endemic malaria, the prevalence of anaemia will be greater than, or similar to, the prevalence of iron deficiency (*75*). Furthermore, the use of serum ferritin as an indicator of iron status may well *overestimate* the prevalence of iron deficiency in malaria endemic areas; this is because serum ferritin levels are elevated by the presence of infections such as malaria (Table 3.1), and also the reason why, traditionally, the cut-off level that defined iron deficiency in individuals with malaria was higher (<30 µg/l) than that used for individuals free from infection (<15 µg/l).

Anaemia is considered to be a public health problem when the prevalence of low haemoglobin concentrations exceeds 5% in the population (*1*). The severity of the public health problem of anaemia is classified as mild, moderate or severe according to the prevalence of anaemia (**Table 3.2**).

3.1.2 Risk factors for deficiency

The main risk factors for iron deficiency have been summarized in **Table 1.2**. They include:

- a low intake of haem iron (which is present in meat, poultry and fish);

- an inadequate intake of vitamin C (ascorbic acid) from fruit and vegetables (the presence of vitamin C enhances the absorption of iron from the diet);

- poor absorption of iron from diets high in phytate (including legumes and cereals) or phenolic compounds (present in coffee, tea, sorghum and millet);

TABLE 3.1
Indicators for assessing iron status at the population level[a]

Indicator	Sample	Population group	Cut-off to define deficiency		Comments
			Mild	Severe	
Haemoglobin[b]	Blood	Children 6–59 months	110 g/l	Not defined	Blood haemoglobin is primarily an indicator of anaemia but can provide useful information regarding iron status, as follows:
		Children 5–11 years	115 g/l		— An increase of at least 10 g/l in blood haemoglobin after 1 or 2 months of iron supplementation is indicative of baseline iron deficiency.
		Children 12–14 years	120 g/l		
		Men over 15 years	130 g/l		
		Women over 15 years (non-pregnant)	120 g/l		— Where poor availability of dietary iron is the main cause of anaemia, children and women have disproportionately low haemoglobin values, while those of adult men are virtually unaffected. Where other factors, such as parasites, contribute significantly, adult men are more likely to also have low haemoglobin values.
		Pregnant women	110 g/l	<70 g/l	
Ferritin	Serum or plasma	Under 5 years	<12 µg/l	Not defined	Useful indicator of iron status and also for monitoring interventions for iron deficiency.
		Over 5 years	<15 µg/l	Not defined	Reflects total body iron stores and is decreased in deficient subjects.
					Elevated in the presence of infection or inflammatory process and should thus be measured, if possible, in combination with another acute phase protein (CRP or AGP), which indicate the presence of infection.
					Levels of >200 µg/l in adult males (or 150 µg/l in adult females) indicates severe risk of iron overload.

TABLE 3.1
Indicators for assessing iron status at the population level[a] *(Continued)*

Indicator	Sample	Population group	Cut-off to define deficiency		Comments
			Mild	Severe	
Transferrin receptors	Serum	Can be applied to all population groups	Cut-off values vary with method used		Useful indicator of iron status; not affected by infection and thus can be used in combination with measurement of serum ferritin to confirm deficiency in cases of infection. No universally agreed cut-offs; reference materials still need to be standardized.
Transferrin saturation	Serum	Can be applied to all population groups	<16%	Not defined	Pronounced diurnal variation and not very specific. Elevated in the presence of infection. No universally agreed cut-offs.
Erythrocyte protoporphyrin	Erythrocytes (RBC)	Under 5 years Over 5 years	Normal Normal	>70 µg/dl >80 µg/dl	Elevated when iron supply is inadequate for haem production. Elevated in the presence of infection, lead poisoning and haemolytic anaemia.

AGP, Alpha 1 acid glycoprotein; CRP, C-reactive protein; RBC, red blood cell.
[a] Every indicator of iron status has limitations so the best way to assess iron status is to use a combination of indicators.
[b] Haemoglobin values for populations living at sea level require adjustment for selected variables, including altitude and tobacco consumption.

Sources: reference (*1*,*74*).

TABLE 3.2
Criteria for assessing the public health severity of anaemia

Severity of the public health problem	Prevalence of anaemia[a] (% of the population)
None	≤4.9
Mild	5.0–19.9
Moderate	20.0–39.9
Severe	≥40

[a] Anaemia is defined on the basis of blood haemoglobin concentrations (see **Table 3.1**)

Source: reference (1).

TABLE 3.3
Classification of usual diets according to their iron bioavailability

Category	Iron bioavailability (%)	Dietary characteristics
Low	1–9	Simple, monotonous diet based on cereals, roots or tubers, with negligible amounts of meat, fish, poultry or ascorbic acid-rich foods. Diet high in foods that inhibit iron absorption such as maize, beans, whole wheat flour and sorghum.
Intermediate	10–15	Diet of cereals, roots or tubers, with some foods of animal origin (meat, fish or poultry) and/or containing some ascorbic acid (from fruits and vegetables).
High	>15	Diversified diet containing greater amounts of meat, fish, poultry and/or foods high in ascorbic acid.

Sources: adapted from references (78,79).

- periods of life when iron requirements are especially high (i.e. growth and pregnancy);
- heavy blood losses as a result of menstruation, or parasite infections such as hookworm, ascaris and schistosomiasis.

As mentioned above, acute or chronic infections, including malaria, can also lower haemoglobin concentrations (76). The presence of other micronutrient deficiencies, especially of vitamins A and B_{12}, folate and riboflavin, also increases the risk of anaemia (77).

The dietary habits of a population group strongly affect the bioavailability of both dietary iron and added fortificant iron. Estimates of the average bioavailability of iron from different types of diets are provided in **Table 3.3**. Although the efficiency of iron absorption increases substantially as iron stores become depleted, the amount absorbed from foods, especially where diets are low in meat, fish, fruit and vegetables, is not enough to prevent iron deficiency in many women and children, especially in the developing world.

3.1.3 Health consequences of deficiency and benefits of intervention

The main consequences of iron deficiency are anaemia, impaired cognitive and physical performance, and increased maternal and child mortality (see **Table 1.2**). Iron deficiency has been shown to reduce physical endurance, even in the absence of anaemia (*80*), and severe anaemia has been associated with an increased risk of both maternal and child mortality (*81,82*). As indicated previously (see section 1.1), there is now substantial evidence to suggest that iron supplementation can reverse the adverse effects of iron deficiency on work capacity and productivity, and on pregnancy outcome and child development (*14–16*). In a study in the United States, for example, iron supplementation during pregnancy reduced the number of preterm deliveries and low-birth-weight infants (*83*).

Improving iron status may have other, but as yet poorly appreciated, benefits for health, most noticeably with respect to the utilization of vitamin A and iodine. That vitamin A (retinol) is mobilized from the liver by an iron-dependent enzyme is well-established fact, but more recently, experimental studies have suggested that in cases of iron deficiency the vitamin is trapped in the liver and thus may be less accessible to other tissues and organs (*84*). Furthermore, iron supplementation of iron-deficient individuals increased plasma retinol in some studies through mechanisms that are as yet incompletely understood (*85*). Similarly, iron is required by the enzymes that synthesize thyroxine, and thus a low iron status may have implications for iodine metabolism. Studies in Côte d'Ivoire have demonstrated that recovery from goitre after iodine treatment is slower in iron-deficient individuals (*86*). In a population of children with a high prevalence of anaemia and goitre, iron supplementation improved the response to iodized oil or iodized salt (*87*) (see also section 1.3.2.3). On the basis of the above findings, it is reasonable to assume that improvements in the iron status of a population may well have benefits for vitamin A and iodine metabolism.

3.2 Vitamin A

Vitamin A is an essential nutrient that is required in small amounts by humans for the normal functioning of the visual system, the maintenance of cell function for growth, epithelial cellular integrity, immune function and reproduction. Dietary requirements for vitamin A are normally provided as a mixture of preformed vitamin A (retinol), which is present in animal source foods, and provitamin A carotenoids, which are derived from foods of vegetable origin and which have to be converted into retinol by tissues such as the intestinal mucosa and the liver in order to be utilized by cells.

Aside from the clinical ocular signs, i.e. night blindness and xerophthalmia, symptoms of vitamin A deficiency (VAD) are largely non-specific. Nevertheless, accumulated evidence suggests that VAD is an important determinant of child survival and safe motherhood (see section 3.2.3). The non-specificity of symptoms, however, means that, in the absence of biochemical measures of vitamin A status, it is difficult to attribute non-ocular symptoms to VAD and it also complicates the definition of VAD. With these considerations in mind, WHO has defined VAD as tissue concentrations of vitamin A low enough to have adverse health consequences, even if there is no evidence of clinical xerophthalmia (5). In more recent years, the term "vitamin A deficiency disorders" has been coined to reflect the diversity of adverse outcomes caused by vitamin A deficiency (88).

3.2.1 Prevalence of deficiency

As vitamin A deficiency affects visual function, indicators of vitamin A status have traditionally relied on changes in the eye, specifically night blindness and xerophthalmia (5) (**Table 3.4**). Worldwide, about 3 million preschool-aged children present ocular signs of VAD (3). Vitamin A deficiency is, however, more commonly assessed using serum or plasma retinol levels. WHO estimates that 254 million preschool-aged children throughout the world have low serum retinol levels and can therefore be considered to be clinically or subclinically vitamin A deficient (3). In the developing world, prevalence rates in this age group range from 15% up to as high as 60%, with Latin America, the Eastern Mediterranean and the Western Pacific being at the low end of this range, and Africa and South-East Asia occupying the high end (3,89) (see also Table 1.1). The prevalence of night blindness is also high among pregnant women in many poor regions of the world, with rates varying between 8% and 24% (89). Night blindness tends to be accompanied by a high prevalence of low concentrations of retinol in breast milk (<1.05 µmol/l or 30 µg/dl) (89,90).

According to WHO criteria (5), a greater than 1% prevalence of night blindness in children aged 24–71 months, or the presence of serum retinol concentrations of less than 0.70 µmol/l in 10% or more of children aged 6–71 months indicates a public health problem (**Table 3.5**). It has been suggested recently that a prevalence of night blindness of more than 5% in pregnant women should be added to the list of criteria that signify a public health problem (88).

3.2.2 Risk factors for deficiency

Usually vitamin A deficiency develops in an environment of ecological, social and economical deprivation, in which the key risk factors for vitamin A

TABLE 3.4
Indicators for assessing vitamin A status at the population level

Indicator	Sample	Population group	Cut-off to define deficiency		Comments
			Mild	Severe	
Prevalence of night blindness (%)	Clinical examination	Children 6–71 months	>1%	>5%	
		Pregnant women	>5%	Not defined	Night blindness prevalence is assessed by interview about reported occurrence during last pregnancy.
Retinol	Serum or plasma[a]	Preschool-age children	0.35–0.7 µmol/l	<0.35 µmol/l	Good indicator of vitamin A status at population level. Also depressed by infection.
Retinol	Breast milk	Lactating women	<1.05 µmol/l (<87 µg/g milk fat)	Not defined	Directly related to the vitamin A status of the mother. Provides information about the vitamin A status of both the mother and her breast-fed infant. Should be measured after the first month postpartum, i.e. once the milk composition has become stable.

[a] Ethylene diamine tetraacetic acid (EDTA) should not be used as the anticoagulant.

Sources: references (5,91).

TABLE 3.5
Criteria for assessing the public health severity of vitamin A deficiency

Indicator	Population group	Prevalence indicating a public health problem (% of the population)
Night blindness	Pregnant women	>5
Night blindness	Children 24–71 months	>1
Bitot's spots	Children 24–71 months	>0.5
Serum retinol <0.7 µmol/l (<20 µg/dl)	Children 6–71 months	≥10

Sources: references (5,88).

deficiency are a diet low in sources of vitamin A (i.e. dairy products, eggs, fruits and vegetables), poor nutritional status, and a high rate of infections, in particular, measles and diarrhoeal diseases (see **Table 1.2**).

The best sources of vitamin A are animal source foods, in particular, liver, eggs and dairy products, which contain vitamin A in the form of retinol, i.e in a form that can be readily used by the body. It is not surprising then that the risk of vitamin A deficiency is strongly inversely related to intakes of vitamin A from animal source foods. In fact, it is difficult for children to meet their requirements for vitamin A if their diet is low in animal source foods (92), especially if their diet is also low in fat. Fruits and vegetables contain vitamin A in the form of carotenoids, the most important of which is β-carotene. In a mixed diet, the conversion rate of β-carotene to retinol is approximately 12:1 (higher, i.e. less efficient than previously believed). The conversion of the other provitamin-A carotenoids to retinol is less efficient, the corresponding conversion rate being of the order of 24:1 (91,93). Various food preparation techniques, such as cooking, grinding and the addition of oil, can improve the absorption of food carotenoids (94–96). Synthetic β-carotene in oil, which is widely used in vitamin A supplements, has a conversion rate to retinol of 2:1, and the synthetic forms of β-carotene that are commonly used to fortify foods, a conversion rate of 6:1 (93).

3.2.3 Health consequences of deficiency and benefits of intervention

Vitamin A deficiency is the leading cause of preventable severe visual impairment and blindness in children, and significantly increases their risk of severe illness and death. An estimated 250000–500000 vitamin A-deficient children become blind every year, approximately half of which die within a year of becoming blind. Subclinical vitamin A deficiency is also associated with an increased risk of child mortality, especially from diarrhoea and measles. A meta-analysis demonstrated that high dose vitamin A supplementation can reduce mortality from measles by as much as 50%. Another analysis found that improvement of vitamin A status, whether by supplementation or fortification, decreased all-cause mortality in children aged between 6 months and 5 years by 23% (*12*).

In addition to causing night blindness, vitamin A deficiency is probably an important contributor to maternal mortality and other poor outcomes in pregnancy and lactation. According to the results of one study, in which vitamin A-deficient pregnant women received vitamin A or β-carotene supplements at doses equivalent to their weekly requirement for the vitamin, maternal mortality was reduced by 40% and 49%, respectively, relative to a control group (*97*). Other studies have shown night blindness to be a risk factor for maternal mortality and morbidity: in Nepal, for example, the death rate from infections was about five times higher among unsupplemented pregnant women who reported night blindness compared with those who did not (*98*). Vitamin A deficiency also increases vulnerability to other disorders, such as iron deficiency (*see section 3.1.3*). Providing an iron supplement with vitamin A to pregnant women in Indonesia increased haemoglobin concentrations by approximately 10 g/l more than did supplementation with iron alone (*99*).

3.3 Iodine

Iodine is present in the body in minute amounts, mainly in the thyroid gland. Its only confirmed role is in the synthesis of thyroid hormones. Iodine deficiency is a major public health problem for populations throughout the world, but particularly for young children and pregnant women, and in some settings represents a significant threat to national social and economic development. The most devastating outcome of iodine deficiency is mental retardation: it is currently one of the world's main causes of preventable cognitive impairment. This is the primary motivation behind the current worldwide drive to eliminate iodine deficiency disorders (IDD).

3.3.1 Prevalence of deficiency

The recommended indicators for assessing the extent of iodine deficiency within a population are median urinary iodine and total goitre prevalence (**Table 3.6**). According to generally accepted criteria, iodine deficiency is a public health problem in populations where the median urinary iodine concentration is below 100 µg/l, or in areas where goitre is endemic, that is to say, where more than 5% of children aged 6–12 years have goitre (**Table 3.7**).

As the median urinary iodine concentration reflects current iodine intake and responds relatively rapidly to the correction of iodine deficiency, it is usually the preferred indicator for monitoring the impact of interventions for IDD control. An expanded set of indicators for assessing national progress towards the goal of the sustainable elimination of IDDs is given in Annex A. This indicator set,

TABLE 3.6
Indicators for assessing iodine status at the population level

Indicator	Sample	Population group	Cut-off to define deficiency		Comments
			Mild	Severe	
Iodine	Urine	Children 6–12 years	Median <100 µg/l	Median <20 µg/l	Recommended indicator for monitoring or evaluating iodine status at the population level. As urinary iodine distribution is not normal, cut-off is defined on the basis of median values.
Total goiter prevalence	Clinical examination	Children 6–12 years	>5%	>30%	Reflects past or current thyroid dysfunction and can be measured by clinical examination or by ultrasonography. Not recommended for monitoring the impact of interventions as goitre response to iodine status correction is delayed.

Source: reference (6).

TABLE 3.7
Criteria for assessing the public health severity of iodine deficiency

Severity of public health problem	Indicator	
	Median urinary iodine (µg/l)	Total goitre prevalence (%)
Mild	50–99	5.0–19.9
Moderate	20–49	20–29.9
Severe	<20	>30

Source: reference (6).

which has been recommended by WHO, relates not just to the population's iodine status (as measured by urinary concentrations) but includes various programmatic indicators which measure the sustainability of the salt iodization programme itself.

According to recent WHO estimates, some 1989 million people have inadequate iodine nutrition (2). The WHO regions, ranked by the absolute number of people affected are, in decreasing order of magnitude, South-East Asia, Europe, the Western Pacific, Africa, the Eastern Mediterranean and the Americas (see Table 1.1). In some parts of the world, for example, in parts of eastern and western Europe, iodine deficiency, in its subclinical form, is re-emerging, having previously been eliminated. This underscores the need to sustain efforts to control iodine deficiency on a global scale.

3.3.2 Risk factors for deficiency

The main factor responsible for the development of iodine deficiency is a low dietary supply of iodine (100). This tends to occur in populations living in areas where the soil has been deprived of iodine as the result of past glaciation, and subsequently, because of the leaching effects of snow, water and heavy rainfall.

Iodine deficiency is exacerbated by a high consumption of natural goitrogens that are present in some staple foods such as cassava. The antithyroid action of goitrogens is related to the presence of thiocyanate which inhibits thyroid iodide transport and, at higher doses, competes with iodide in the synthesis of thyroid hormones (101). Goitrogenicity is determined by the balance between the dietary supply of iodine and thiocyanate: goitre develops when the urinary iodine (µg): thiocyanate (mg) ratio falls below 3.

3.3.3 Health consequences of deficiency and benefits of intervention

Iodine deficiency is associated with a large range of abnormalities, grouped under the heading of "iodine deficiency disorders", that reflect thyroid

TABLE 3.8
The spectrum of iodine deficiency disorders

Fetus	Abortions
	Stillbirths
	Congenital abnormalities
Neonate	Increased infant mortality
	Cognitive impairment and neurological disorders, including endemic cretinism and endemic mental retardation
	Hypothyroidism
	Increased susceptibility of the thyroid gland to nuclear radiation
Child, adolescent and adult	Hypothyroidism
	Goitre
	Retarded physical development in child and adolescent
	Impaired mental function
	Decreased fertility
	Iodine-induced hyperthyroidism in adults
	Increased susceptibility of the thyroid gland to nuclear radiation
	Spontaneous hyperthyroidism in the elderly
	Goitre with its complications

Source: adapted from reference (9).

dysfunction (9). Goitre and cretinism are the most visible manifestations of iodine deficiency; others include hypothyroidism, decreased fertility rate, increased perinatal death and infant mortality (**Table 3.8**).

When iodine intake is abnormally low, an adequate production of thyroid hormones may still be achieved by increased secretion of thyroid stimulating hormone (TSH). However, a prolonged stimulation of the thyroid gland by TSH will result in goitre. This condition is indicative of thyroid hyperplasia, which occurs because of the thyroid's inability to synthesize sufficient thyroid hormones.

Irreversible mental retardation is the most serious disorder induced by iodine deficiency (9,102,103). A deficit in iodine resulting in thyroid failure during the critical period of brain development, that is, from fetal life up to the third month after birth, will result in irreversible alterations in brain function (104,105). In areas of severe endemic iodine deficiency, cretinism may affect up to 5–15% of the population. Some individuals living in regions of mild or moderate iodine deficiency exhibit neurological and intellectual deficits that are similar to, but less marked, than those found in overt cretins. A meta-analysis of 19 studies conducted in regions of severe deficiency showed that iodine deficiency is responsible for a mean IQ loss of 13.5 points among affected populations (104).

Correction of iodine deficiency, when carried out at the right time, reduces or eliminates all consequences of iodine deficiency. The validity of this statement is borne out by the sharp reduction in the incidence of IDD that is consistently observed when iodine is added to the diet (*see section 1.3*), and the recurrence of IDD when an effective IDD control programme is interrupted in a previously iodine-deficient population (*106*).

CHAPTER 4

Zinc, folate, vitamin B_{12} and other B vitamins, vitamin C, vitamin D, calcium, selenium and fluoride

4.1 Zinc

Zinc is an essential component of a large number of enzymes, and plays a central role in cellular growth and differentiation in tissues that have a rapid differentiation and turnover, including those of the immune system and those in the gastrointestinal tract. The positive impact of zinc supplementation on the growth of some stunted children, and on the prevalence of selected childhood diseases such as diarrhoea, suggests that zinc deficiency is likely to be a significant public health problem, especially in developing countries. However, the extent of zinc deficiency worldwide is not well documented. All population age groups are at risk of zinc deficiency, but infants and young children are probably the most vulnerable. Pregnant and lactating women are also likely to be very susceptible to zinc deficiency, and there is an urgent need for more information on the implications of low zinc status in these particular population groups (*107,108*).

4.1.1 Prevalence of deficiency

The lack of reliable and widely accepted indicators of zinc status of adequate sensitivity means that the global prevalence of zinc deficiency is uncertain. Those indicators that are available, such as zinc concentration in plasma and hair (see **Table 4.1**), detect changes in zinc status only in cases of severe deficiency, and may fail to detect marginal deficiency.

As suggested above, there are, however, several good reasons to suspect that zinc deficiency is common, especially in infants and children. Firstly, a high prevalence of low plasma zinc, which is a reasonable indicator of relatively severe depletion, has been observed in some population groups. Secondly, several randomized control trials have demonstrated that stunted children, and/or those with low plasma zinc, respond positively to zinc supplementation, a finding that suggests that zinc deficiency was a limiting factor in their growth. Growth stunting affects about a third of children in less wealthy regions of the world and is very common in settings where diets are of poor quality. This is not too say that zinc deficiency affects up to one third of children in the developing world since zinc deficiency is only but one of several possible causes of growth stunting.

TABLE 4.1
Indicators for assessing zinc status at the population level

Indicator	Sample	Population group	Cut-off to define deficiency	Comments
Zinc	Serum or plasma	Applies to all population groups	<70 µg/dl	No universally agreed cut-offs. Plasma zinc is homeostatically regulated and therefore may not detect marginal deficiency. Values change diurnally. Plasma zinc is decreased by pregnancy, hypoalbuminemia (PEM) and infection.
Zinc	Erythrocytes (RBC)	Applies to all population groups	No universally agreed cut-offs at this time	May be used as a secondary supportive indicator.
Zinc	Hair	Applies to all population groups	No universally agreed cut-offs at this time	Needs further research before this can be used as a supportive indicator. Not widely used as an indicator in population surveys.

PEM, protein energy malnutrition; RBC, red blood cell.
Sources: references (*91,93*).

Using estimates of zinc intake and bioavailability derived from FAO's food balance data, it has been calculated that about 20% of the world's population could be at risk of zinc deficiency. The geographical regions most affected are believed to be, in descending order of severity, south Asia (in particular, Bangladesh and India), Africa and the western Pacific (*109*). It is probable that the occurrence of zinc deficiency is strongly associated with that of iron deficiency, because both iron and zinc are found in the same foods (i.e. meat, poultry and fish) and, in both cases, their absorption from foods is inhibited by the presence of phytates. The minerals differ in that zinc is not as affected by blood loss as is iron.

4.1.2 Risk factors for deficiency

The central role of zinc in cell division, protein synthesis and growth means that an adequate supply is especially important for infants, and pregnant and lactating women. Principal risk factors for zinc deficiency include diets low in zinc or high in phytates, malabsorption disorders (including the presence of intestinal parasites and diarrhoea), impaired utilization of zinc and genetic diseases (e.g. acrodermatitis enteropathica, sickle-cell anaemia) (**Table 1.2**).

The bioavailability of zinc is dependent on dietary composition, in particular, on the proportion of high-phytate foods in the diet (i.e. selected cereals and legumes). The molar ratio of phytate:zinc in meals or diets provides a useful measure of zinc bioavailability. At high ratios (i.e. above 15:1), zinc absorption from food is low, that is to say, less than 15% (*110,111*). The inclusion of animal proteins can improve the total zinc intake and the efficiency of zinc absorption from a phytate-containing diet (*112*). For instance, the addition of animal source foods to a diet based on rice and wheat approximately doubled the amount of zinc that was absorbed by young Chinese women (*113*). Using data obtained from experimental zinc absorption studies, various criteria have been developed to differentiate between diets likely to have high, moderate and low zinc bioavailability; these are summarized in **Table 4.2**.

The extent to which the presence of phytates inhibits the absorption of zinc is not precisely known at the present time. It is interesting to note that several studies have shown that zinc absorption from some legume-based diets is comparable to that from a diet based on animal products, despite the relatively high phytate content of the former (*112,114*), and that in adult women, approximately 30% of dietary zinc is absorbed across a wide range of different diets (*93*). In a controlled experiment, infants absorbed nearly 45% of the zinc from a wheat-soy complementary food, regardless of whether it contained 0.77% or 0.3% phytic acid (*115*). In Malawi, 24% of the zinc was absorbed from high-phytate maize meals consumed by children, again a relatively high proportion given the phytate content (*116*).

Competitive interactions can occur between zinc and other minerals that have similar physical and chemical properties, such as iron and copper. When present in large amounts (e.g. in the form of supplements) or in aqueous solution, these minerals reduce zinc absorption. However, at the levels present in the usual diet and in fortified foods, zinc absorption is not generally affected (*93*). On the other hand, high levels of dietary calcium (i.e. >1 g per day), which might be consumed by some individuals, can inhibit zinc absorption, especially in the presence of phytates. The degree of impairment varies depending on the type of diet and the source of the calcium (*93*). Unlike iron, zinc absorption is neither inhibited by phenolic compounds, nor enhanced by vitamin C.

TABLE 4.2

Classification of usual diets according to the potential bioavailability of their zinc content

Bioavailability[a]	Main dietary characteristics
High	Refined diets low in cereal fibre, low in phytic acid content, and with a phytate:zinc molar ratio <5; adequate protein content principally from non-vegetable sources, such as meats and fish.
	Includes semi-synthetic formula diets based on animal protein.
Moderate	Mixed diets containing animal or fish protein.
	Lacto-ovo, ovovegetarian or vegan diets not based primarily on unrefined cereal grains or high-extraction-rate flours.
	Phytate:zinc molar ratio of total diet within the range 5–15 or not in excess of 10 if more than 50% of energy intake is from unfermented unrefined cereal grains and flours, and the diet is fortified with inorganic calcium salts (>1 g Ca^{2+}/day).
	Bioavailability of zinc improves when the diet includes animal protein sources (including milk).
Low	Diets high in unrefined, unfermented and ungerminated cereal grains[b], especially when fortified with inorganic calcium salts and when intake of animal protein is negligible.
	Phytate: zinc molar ratio of total diet exceeds 15[c].
	High-phytate soy protein products constitute the primary protein source.
	Diets in which, singly or collectively, approximately 50% of the energy intake is from the following high-phytate foods: high-extraction-rate (≥90%) wheat, rice, maize, grains and flours, oatmeal, and millet; chapatti flours and *tanok*; and sorghum, cowpeas, pigeon peas, grams, kidney beans, blackeyed beans, and groundnut flours.
	High intakes of inorganic calcium salts (>1 g Ca^{2+}/day), either as supplements or as adventitious contaminants (e.g. from calcareous geophagia), potentiate the inhibitory effects; low intakes of animal protein exacerbate these effects.

[a] At intakes adequate to meet the average normative requirements for absorbed zinc the three bioavailability levels correspond to 50%, 30% and 15% absorption. With higher zinc intakes, the fractional absorption is lower.
[b] Germination of such grains or fermentation of many flours can reduce antagonistic potency; if cereal grains have been germinated then the diet should then be classified as having moderate zinc bioavailability.
[c] Vegetable diets with phytate:zinc ratios >30 are not unknown; for such diets, an assumption of 10% bioavailability of zinc or less may be justified, especially if the intake of protein is low, or the intake of inorganic calcium salts is excessive, or both.

Source: reference (*93*).

The influence of all of the above-mentioned risk factors for zinc deficiency is difficult to integrate in any coherent way. In particular, further research is needed to evaluate the bioavailability of zinc from usual diets in developing countries and to better understand the relationship between dietary patterns and zinc supply.

4.1.3 Health consequences of deficiency and benefits of intervention

Zinc deficiency is often hard to identify as its clinical manifestations are largely non-specific (**Table 1.2**). The symptoms of severe deficiency include dermatitis, retarded growth, diarrhoea, mental disturbances and recurrent infections. Moderate and mild deficiencies are even more difficult to diagnose, not only because they are characterized by a diversity of symptoms, but also on account of the fact that there are no suitable biomarkers of zinc deficiency (117).

In children, impaired growth (stunting) is one of the possible consequences of zinc deficiency. Zinc supplementation trials conducted over the last few decades in children from developing countries have clearly demonstrated the positive benefits of improved zinc status, including improved growth rates and reductions in the incidence of various infectious diseases (17,18,118). For example, a meta-analysis of randomized controlled supplementation trials reported an 18% decrease in diarrhoea incidence, a 25% reduction in diarrhoea prevalence, and a 41% fall in the incidence of pneumonia (18). Zinc supplementation also led to fewer episodes of malaria and fewer clinic visits due to complications of malaria in Papua New Guinea (118), but not in Burkina Faso (119).

The effect of maternal zinc status on pregnancy outcomes is unclear at the present time (120). Although severe zinc deficiency has been associated with poor maternal pregnancy outcomes (121), studies involving moderate deficiency have proved inconclusive (122). Maternal zinc supplementation in Peru improved fetal neurobehavioral development (123), but had no effect on size at birth or pregnancy duration (124). In India, zinc supplements helped to reduce mortality among low-birth-weight infants (125). Interestingly, the zinc content of breast milk has not been shown to correlate with maternal zinc intake and appears to be unaffected by supplementation (126,127).

4.2 Folate

Folate (vitamin B_9) plays a central role in the synthesis and methylation of nucleotides that intervene in cell multiplication and tissue growth. Its role in protein synthesis and metabolism is closely interrelated to that of vitamin B_{12}. The combination of severe folate deficiency and vitamin B_{12} deficiency can result in megaloblastic anaemia. Low intakes of folate are also associated with a higher risk of giving birth to infants with neural tube defects and possibly other birth defects, and with an increased risk of cardiovascular diseases, cancer and impaired cognitive function in adults.

4.2.1 Prevalence of deficiency

Serum folate is a good indicator of recent dietary folate intake, and the most widely used method of assessing folate status (128). Erythrocyte folate is, however, the better indicator of long-term status and of tissue folate stores. Elevated plasma homocysteine concentrations are a strong predictor of inadequate folate status. However, other vitamin deficiencies (e.g. vitamins B_2, B_6 and B_{12}) also increase homocysteine values. Indicators of folate status are summarized in **Table 4.3** (*93,128,129*).

The global prevalence of folate deficiency is uncertain, owing to a lack of data (*130*). Only a few countries have national or even regional biochemical data on folate status. Furthermore, efforts to compare usual dietary intakes with estimated requirements (an alternative means of assessing the likely prevalence of deficiency in a population) are hampered by difficulties in measuring the folate content of foods.

TABLE 4.3
Indicators for assessing folate (vitamin B_9) status at the population level

Indicator	Sample	Population group	Cut-off to define deficiency	Comments
Folate	Serum	Applies to all population groups	<10 nmol/l (4.4 µg/l)	Serum folate is the most widely used indicator of folate status. It is considered to be a sensitive indicator of recent intake, but a less valid indicator of body stores.
Folate	Erythrocytes (RBC)	Applies to all population groups	<305 nmol/l (140 µg/l)	Erythrocyte folate concentrations reflect long-term folate status and tissue folate stores.
Total homocysteine (free and bound)	Plasma	Applies to all population groups	12–16 µmol/l (1.62–2.2 mg/l)	Total plasma homocysteine is a good predictor of folate status: it is increased in cases of inadequate folate status. Not specific because also increased by vitamin B_2, B_6 and B_{12} deficiencies and influenced by gender, race and renal insufficiency.

RBC, red blood cell.
Sources: references (*93, 128, 129*).

Folate deficiency tends to be more prevalent in populations that have a high intake of refined cereals (which are low in folate) and a low intake of leafy greens and fruits (which are high in folate). Dietary surveys in India show that people eating predominantly cereal-based diets only consume about 75 µg folate per day *(131)*. Prior to the introduction of mandatory wheat flour fortification with folic acid in 1998, about 15% of adult women in the United States were believed to have low serum and/or erythrocyte folate levels. Similarly, in Chile, where the consumption of white wheat flour is high, low serum and erythrocyte folate concentrations were common before the fortification of flour with folic acid *(132)*. In contrast, low plasma values are rare in countries such as Guatemala, Mexico and Thailand *(77)* where diets typically contain a higher proportion of fruits and vegetables. For instance, few whole blood samples from the Mexican National Nutrition Survey were low in folate, with the exception of those of children under 4 years of age, in which the prevalence of low blood folate was about 10% *(133)*. Because of the high folate content of certain legumes, fruits and vegetables relative to refined cereals, it is possible that populations in some developing countries consume more folate than those in industrialized countries. Similarly, a study of pregnant women in Germany found that those who are lacto-ovo vegetarians (i.e. milk and egg consumers) or low meat consumers had higher levels of erythrocyte folate than the non-vegetarians; this was attributed to the fact that the lacto-ovo vegetarians were consuming proportionately more folate-rich vegetables than their non-vegetarian counterparts *(134)*.

4.2.2 Risk factors for deficiency

The main sources of dietary folate are leafy green vegetables, fruits, yeast and liver. A low intake of these foods combined with a relatively high intake of refined cereals thus increases the risk for folate deficiency. Malabsorption conditions, infection with *Giardia lamblia*, bacterial overgrowth, genetic disorders (of folic acid metabolism) and chronic alcoholism are also risk factors for folate deficiency (see **Table 1.2**).

4.2.3 Health consequences of deficiency and benefits of intervention

Possible health consequences of a low folate status, which include megaloblastic anaemia, are summarized in Table 1.2. Folic acid has long been included in iron supplements provided to pregnant women in developing countries, despite rather limited evidence from Africa and India that folic acid reduces the risk of megaloblastic anaemia. In fact, there is little evidence to suggest that giving folic acid with iron is any better at preventing anaemia than providing iron alone *(77,135)*.

Randomized trials conducted in China *(136)*, the United States *(137)* and in various other locations have consistently shown that folic acid supplements taken before and during the first 28 days after conception reduce the risk of women giving birth to an infant with a neural tube defect (*138*). Neural tube defects are serious malformations resulting in death or major lifelong disability in survivors; worldwide, an estimated 300 000 or more neonates are affected each year (*139*). Studies have also demonstrated that folic acid supplementation benefits some women who have an abnormal folate metabolism because of a genetic defect that affects their ability to utilize folate (*140*). Moreover, an analysis of data from different trials in which micronutrients were provided during pregnancy found folic acid to be the only micronutrient that was associated with a reduced risk of preterm delivery (*141*).

Several intervention trials have demonstrated that folic acid fortification lowers plasma homocysteine, even in populations with a relatively low prevalence of folate deficiency (*49*). Several lines of evidence indicate that even moderately elevated plasma homocysteine is an independent risk factor for cardiovascular disease (*142*) and stroke (*143*), both leading causes of death in many countries. While there is still some controversy concerning the direction of causality (*144*), a comparison of the results of genetic and prospective epidemiological studies, which would be expected to have different biases, strongly points to a direct causal pathway leading from elevated homocysteine to cardiovascular disease (*145*). Higher plasma homocysteine levels are also associated in industrialized countries with a higher risk of impaired cognitive function in adults (*146*), and many abnormal pregnancy outcomes, including eclampsia and premature delivery, and other birth defects such as orofacial cleft palate and heart defects. However, the evidence for the benefits of supplementation for these conditions is not as strong than that linking supplementation to prevention of neural tube defects (*147*).

The addition of folic acid to enriched grain products in the United States, a practice which, as mentioned above, was introduced in 1998, has since produced a substantial increase in average blood folate levels among women of childbearing age (*148*). This has resulted in the virtual elimination of low serum folate (*149*) and the lowering of plasma homocysteine in the population at large (*49*). The level of folic acid added (140 µg/100 g flour) is unlikely to bring total folate intakes above the Tolerable Upper Intake Level (UL) of 1 000 µg per day in any life stage or gender group (*128*), or to exacerbate or obscure problems caused by vitamin B_{12} deficiency (see section 4.3).

4.3 Vitamin B_{12}

Vitamin B_{12} (cobalamin) is a cofactor in the synthesis of an essential amino acid, methionine. Its metabolic role is closely linked to that of folate in that one of the vitamin B_{12}-dependent enzymes, methionine synthase, is vital to the functioning of the methylation cycle in which 5-methyltetrahydrofolate acts as a source of methyl donor groups which are necessary for cell metabolism and survival. Deficiency of this vitamin can thus impair the utilization of folate and causes neurological deterioration, megaloblastic anaemia, elevated plasma homocysteine and possibly, impaired immune function. In infants and young children it can cause severe developmental delays.

4.3.1 Prevalence of deficiency

Vitamin B_{12} status is usually assessed by measuring concentrations in plasma or serum (**Table 4.4**) (*93,128,129*) Although elevated urinary and plasma methylmalonic acid (MMA) levels are more specific, and often more sensitive, indicators of vitamin B_{12} deficiency, MMA concentrations are more difficult and expensive to measure than those of vitamin B_{12}. Elevated homocysteine is a good predictor of vitamin B_{12} status.

TABLE 4.4
Indicators for assessing vitamin B_{12} (cobalamin) status at the population level

Indicator	Sample	Population group	Cut-off to define deficiency	Comments
Vitamin B_{12}	Serum or plasma	Applies to all population groups	<150 pmol/l (<203 mg/l)	Reflects both recent intake and body stores. Values above the cut-off do not necessarily indicate adequate status. If values are marginal, analysis of serum methylmalonic acid is indicated.
Methylmalonic acid (MMA)	Serum or plasma	Applies to all population groups	>271 nmol/l	Increased when supply of vitamin B_{12} is low. Preferred indicator since increased levels are highly specific to vitamin B_{12} deficiency.
Total homocysteine (free and bound)	Plasma	Applies to all population groups	12–16 mmol/l (1.62–2.2 mg/l)	Total plasma homocysteine is a good predictor of vitamin B_{12} status: it is increased in cases of inadequate folate status. Not specific because also increased by vitamin B_2, B_6 and B_{12} deficiencies and influenced by gender, race and renal insufficiency.

Sources: references (*93,128,129*).

Variability in the plasma levels used to define vitamin B_{12} deficiency (see **Table 4.4**) make the results of the few studies of its prevalence difficult to generalize. Moreover, there is no clear evidence that vitamin B_{12} deficiency varies with countries or regions. In countries where vitamin B_{12} deficiency has been assessed at the national level, low serum vitamin B_{12} concentrations were prevalent, i.e. in Venezuela (11–12% in preschool and school-aged children), Germany (15% in women of reproductive age), the United Kingdom (31% of the elderly) and New Zealand (12% of the elderly). The prevalence was lower in the United States (0–3% in preschool and school-aged children, adults and the elderly) and in Costa Rica (5.3% in lactating women). In smaller studies, a high proportion of low plasma vitamin B_{12} concentrations were found in Kenya (40% in school-aged children), Zimbabwe (24% of the elderly), Israel (21% in adults), and India (46% in adults), while in other countries such as Botswana (preschool-aged children), Thailand (school-aged children) and Japan (adults), <1% of plasma vitamin B_{12} concentrations were low *(130,150–152)*.

4.3.2 Risk factors for deficiency

Vitamin B_{12} is synthesized by microorganisms in the gut of animals and is subsequently absorbed and incorporated into animal tissues. Products from herbivorous animals (i.e. meat, eggs, milk) are thus the only source of the vitamin for humans. Consequently, intakes are very low or close to zero in many population groups that are economically disadvantaged, or among those who avoid animal products for religious or other reasons. There is a high risk of deficiency in strict vegetarians and even lacto-ovo vegetarians (i.e. milk and egg consumers) have lower plasma concentrations of the vitamin compared with meat-consumers *(153)*. Low maternal intake and/or status in the lactating mother will lead to inadequate amounts of vitamin B_{12} in breast milk, and subsequently, deficiency in the infant. Malabsorption syndromes and some inborn errors of metabolism are also risk factors for vitamin B_{12} deficiency.

Gastric atrophy, which occurs with ageing and following prolonged *Helicobacter pylori* infection, results in very poor absorption of vitamin B_{12} from food. However, the crystalline form of the vitamin that is used as a fortificant and in supplements can still be absorbed by most individuals. For this reason, Canada and the United States recommend that their elderly population, more than 20% of which is likely to have some level of vitamin B_{12} deficiency, should consume a substantial part of their recommended vitamin B_{12} intake as fortified foods and/or supplements *(128)*. The prevalence of vitamin B_{12} deficiency due to gastric atrophy may be even higher in developing countries, due to a much earlier age of onset and a higher prevalence of *Helicobacter pylori* infection.

4.3.3 Health consequences of deficiency and benefits of intervention

Moderate to severe vitamin B_{12} deficiency results in megaloblastic anaemia and the demyelination of the central nervous system, and in turn, various neurological disorders. The latter are variably reversible after correction of the deficiency (*154*). When serum vitamin B_{12} concentrations fall below 150 pmol/l, abnormalities in the function of some enzymes may occur with the risk, at lower concentration, of potentially irreversible poor memory and cognitive function, impaired nerve conduction and megaloblastic anaemia in individuals of all ages. In a peri-urban area of Guatemala City, for example, schoolchildren with low plasma vitamin B_{12} performed less well on tests of perception and memory, were less accurate in a reasoning (oddity) task, and had poorer academic performance and adaptability (*155*). Infants fed with breast milk from vitamin B_{12}-deficient mothers exhibited a failure to thrive, poor brain development and, in some cases, mental retardation (*156*).

Several studies, mainly from industrialized nations, have demonstrated the benefits of vitamin B_{12} supplementation in susceptible population groups. For example, vitamin B_{12} supplementation of deficient infants born to strictly vegetarian mothers reduced the incidence of anaemia and tremors, and improved their general development (*156*). Among the elderly, vitamin B_{12} supplementation produced improved symptoms in those with clinical signs of deficiency (*157*). To date, few vitamin B_{12} intervention trials have been carried out in developing countries. A recent supplementation programme involving Kenyan schoolchildren has, however, reported significant reductions in the prevalence of vitamin B_{12} deficiency in those receiving supplements of meat or milk compared with placebo or energy-supplemented groups (*152*).

4.4 Other B vitamins (thiamine, riboflavin, niacin and vitamin B_6)

As the food sources of the various B-complex vitamins are similar, it is not surprising that diets inadequate in one B vitamin are more than likely to be deficient in the others. These water-soluble vitamins are readily destroyed during cooking in water and by heat (although niacin is stable to heat). More significantly, the milling and degerming of cereal grains removes almost all of the thiamine (vitamin B_1), riboflavin (vitamin B_2) and niacin (vitamin B_3), which is the reason why restoration of these particular nutrients to wheat and corn flour has been widely practised for the last 60 years. This strategy has certainly contributed to the virtual elimination of vitamin B deficiencies and their associated diseases (i.e. beriberi and pellagra) in the industrialized countries.

Historically, little attention has been paid to the assessment of thiamine, riboflavin, niacin and vitamin B_6 status. One of the reasons why these B-complex vitamins have been neglected in the past is the lack of reliable information about the consequences of marginal or subclinical deficiencies (see **Table 1.2**). However, evidence is mounting that vitamin B deficiencies are highly prevalent in many developing countries, in particular where diets are low in animal products, fruits and vegetables, and where cereals are milled prior to consumption. Pregnant and lactating women, infants and children are at the highest risk of deficiency. Because the mother's intake and body stores of these vitamins affect the amount she secretes in breast milk, appropriate fortification can provide her with a steady supply during lactation and thereby improve the vitamin B status of her infants and young children.

4.4.1 Thiamine

Thiamine (vitamin B_1) is a cofactor for several key enzymes involved in carbohydrate metabolism and is also directly involved in neural function. It is likely that thiamine deficiency, in its subclinical form, is a significant public health problem in many parts of the world. Severe deficiency causes beriberi, a disease that was once commonplace among populations with a high carbohydrate intake, especially in the form of white rice. As mentioned above, beriberi has been largely eradicated in most industrialized countries, but the disease still occurs in some Asian countries where rice is the staple food. In addition, outbreaks of beriberi are regularly reported in regions suffering social and economic stress brought about by war, famine and other emergency situations.

4.4.1.1 Prevalence of deficiency

The most widely used biochemical indicators of thiamine status are urinary thiamine excretion (UTE), erythrocyte thiamine transketolase activity (ETKA) and the thiamine pyrophosphate effect (TPPE), which is increased in thiamine deficiency (see **Table 4.5**). UTE provides information about the adequacy of dietary intakes of thiamine, but not about the degree of depletion of tissue reserves. Nor is it a very sensitive indicator in cases of subclinical deficiency. Both ETKA and TPPE reflect tissue reserves of thiamine and provide a direct functional evaluation at the cellular level. ETKA is generally regarded as the best single test of thiamine status, despite some reports of poor correlations between this and other measures of thiamine status. Ideally, ETKA should be used in combination with TPPE in order to confirm a diagnosis of thiamine deficiency. In lactating women, the concentration of thiamine in breast milk can be used as an indicator of thiamine deficiency.

Although the lack of reliable biochemical data means that it is not known just how widespread a problem subclinical thiamine deficiency is, thiamine levels in breast milk coupled with infant mortality rates can provide valuable information on the likelihood of the existence of thiamine deficiency in a community. These

TABLE 4.5
Indicators for assessing thiamine (vitamin B_1) status at the population level

Indicator	Sample	Population group	Cut-off to define deficiency		Comments
			Mild	Severe	
Thiamine excretion (µg/g creatinine)	Urine	1–3 years	<175 µg/g	<120 µg/g	Reflects recent intakes. Cut-offs are substantially higher for children. Not a very sensitive indicator of mild deficiency.
		4–6 years	<120 µg/g	<85 µg/g	
		7–9 years	<180 µg/g	<70 µg/g	
		10–12 years	<180 µg/g	<60 µg/g	
		13–15 years	<150 µg/g	<50 µg/g	
		Adults	<65 µg/g	<27 µg/g	
		Pregnancy (second trimester)	<55 µg/g	<27 µg/g	
		Pregnancy (third trimester)	<50 µg/g	<21 µg/g	
Thiamine excretion (µg/24 hours) (UTE)	Urine	Adult	<100 µg/d	<40 µg/d	
Thiamine	Breast milk	Lactating women	<100 µg/l	<50 µg/l	Low levels of thiamine in breast milk combined with an increased infant mortality rate suggest the existence of thiamine deficiency in a community.
Thiamine transketolase activity coefficient (ETKA)	Erythrocytes (RBC)	Can apply to all population groups	≥1.20%	≥1.25%	Generally regarded as the best test of thiamine status, but some studies find poor correlation with other measures. Poor standardization of the test.
Thiamine pyrophosphate effect (TPPE)	Erythrocytes (RBC)	Can apply to all population groups	>15%	>25%	The assay is performed in the absence and in the presence of added thiamine and the result expressed as an activity coefficient, i.e. as the percentage increase in thiamine transketolase activity that is obtained after the addition of thiamine pyrophosphate to the erythrocyte.

RBC, red blood cell.

Source: references (93, 128, 129, 158).

TABLE 4.6
Proposed criteria for assessing the public health severity of thiamine deficiency

Indicator	Severity of public health problem (% of population below the cut-off value defining deficiency, unless otherwise stated)		
	Mild	Moderate	Severe
Clinical signs (clinical cases)	<1 (or ≥1 clinical case)	1–4	≥5
TPPE test >25%	5–19	20–49	≥50
Urinary thiamine (per g creatinine)	5–19	20–49	≥50
Breast milk thiamine <50 µg/l	5–19	20–49	≥50
Dietary intake <0.33 mg/1 000 kcal	5–19	20–49	≥50
Infant mortality between 2nd and 5th month	No decline in mortality rates	Slight peak in mortality rates	Marked peak in mortality rates

TPPE, thiamine pyrophosphate effect.
Source: references (*158*).

and other proposed criteria for classifying thiamine deficiency in relation to its public health severity are shown in **Table 4.6**.

Although far less prevalent than in the past, recent cases of severe thiamine deficiency or beriberi have been reported in Indonesia (*159*) and the Seychelles (*160*). The disease still appears in Japan and in north-eastern parts of Thailand where intakes of raw fish (which contain an anti-thiamine compound, thiaminase) and polished rice are high (*161,162*). Thiamine depletion is also a fairly regular occurrence among displaced populations and in refugees dependent on milled white cereals in countries such as Djibouti, Ethiopia, Guinea, Nepal and Thailand (*158*), which would suggest that refugees, displaced populations and those affected by famines are among those at especially high risk for thiamine deficiency. Sporadic outbreaks of thiamine deficiency have occurred in The Gambia, the number of cases peaking during the rainy season, i.e. a time of food shortages (*163*) and in Cuba during the 1992–1993 epidemic of neuropathy (*164*). Despite the concomitant nature of poor thiamine status and the outbreak of neuropathy in the Cuban outbreak, it is by no means certain that thiamine deficiency was responsible for the wide-scale neuropathy (*165*).

4.4.1.2 Risk factors for deficiency

The main sources of thiamine are wheat germ and yeast extracts, offal from most animals, legumes (i.e. pulses, groundnuts and beans) and green vegetables. A low intake of animal and diary products and legumes, and a high consumption of refined rice and cereals are thus the main risk factors for thiamine deficiency. A diet rich in foods that contain high levels of anti-thiamine compounds is an additional risk factor. The most common thiamine antagonist is thiaminase which is naturally present in some raw fish (*166,167*) and sometimes as a bacterial food contaminant (*168*). Anti-thiamine compounds may also be found in tea, ferns and betel nuts (*169*). Chronic alcohol abuse and genetic disorders are also risk factors for thiamine deficiency (see **Table 1.2**).

4.4.1.3 Health consequences of deficiency and benefits of intervention

There are two distinct forms of severe thiamine deficiency: an oedematous form known as wet beriberi and a non-oedematous neurological form known as dry beriberi. The wet form is associated with potentially fatal heart failure, whereas the dry form tends to be chronic and results in peripheral neuropathy. Many cases of thiamine deficiency present with a mixture of symptoms and thus are properly termed "thiamine deficiency with cardiopathy and peripheral neuropathy" (*158*). Thiamine deficiency in infants is rarely seen today, and is largely confined to infants who are breastfed by thiamine-deficient mothers. In such cases, it is almost always an acute disease, involving oedema and cardiac failure with a high fatality rate.

The Wernicke–Korsakov syndrome is induced by thiamine deficiency and usually manifests as various neurological disorders that are typically associated with impaired cognitive function. It is only observed in chronic alcoholics or in those with a genetic abnormality in transketolase, a thiamine-dependent enzyme.

Several studies have indicated that supplementation can reverse the symptoms of thiamine deficiency. During an outbreak *of beriberi* in The Gambia, for example, the affected groups responded well to thiamine supplementation (*163*).

4.4.2 Riboflavin

Riboflavin (vitamin B_2) is a precursor of various nucleotides, most notably flavin mononucleotide (FMN) and flavin adenine dinucleotide (FAD), which act as coenzymes in various metabolic pathways and in energy production. Riboflavin deficiency rarely occurs in isolation, and is frequently associated with deficiencies in one or more of the other B-complex vitamins.

4.4.2.1 Prevalence of deficiency

The urinary excretion of riboflavin, which is reduced in case of deficiency, has been used in several studies to assess riboflavin status. Urinary riboflavin reflects recent intake of the vitamin, but it is not a particularly good indicator of body stores (**Table 4.7**). A more useful functional test in this respect is the erythrocyte glutathione reductase activity coefficient (EGRAC) (*170*). Erythrocyte flavin nucleotides (FMN + FAD) concentration is, however, probably the best measure of riboflavin status: not only is this less susceptible to short-term fluctuations, but it is also more stable than EGRAC values (*171*).

TABLE 4.7
Indicators for assessing riboflavin (vitamin B_2) status at the population level

Indicator	Sample	Population group	Cut-off to define deficiency		Comments
			Mild	Severe	
Flavin excretion nmol/g creatinine	Urine	Applies to all population groups	<72 nmol/g	<50 nmol/g	Reflects recent intakes. HPLC analysis gives the best determination.
Flavin nucleotides (FMN and FAD)	Erythrocytes (RBC)	Applies to all population groups	<400 nmol/l	<270 nmol/l	Probably the best measure of riboflavin status; less susceptible to short-term fluctuation and more stable than the erythrocyte glutathione reductase activity coefficient. Method involves hydrolysis of FAD to flavin nucleotide. HPLC analysis gives the best determination.
Erythrocyte glutathione reductase activity coefficient (EGRAC)	Erythrocytes (RBC)	Applies to all population groups	>1.2	>1.4	Functional assay that reflects body stores. Not specific as affected by G6PD deficiency and heterozygous β-thalassemia.

HPLC, high performance liquid chromatography; FMN, flavin mononucleotide; FAD, flavin adenine dinucleotide; RBC, red blood cell; G6PD, glucose 6-phosphate deshydrogenase.

Sources: references (*93,128,129*).

In the few studies in which riboflavin status has been assessed at the population level, the prevalence of deficiency is alarmingly high *(172)*. Abnormal riboflavin-dependent enzyme function has been reported in almost all pregnant women in The Gambia *(173)*; in 50% of elderly and 77% of lactating women in Guatemala *(174)*; and in 87% of night-blind women in rural Nepal *(171)*. Furthermore, in a survey in China, urinary riboflavin was low in more than 90% of adults *(175)*.

4.4.2.2 Risk factors for deficiency

The main dietary sources of riboflavin are meat and dairy products; only small amounts are found in grains and seeds. Leafy green vegetables are also a fairly good source of riboflavin and in developing countries tend to be the main source of the vitamin. Deficiency is thus likely to be more prevalent among those whose intake of animal source foods is low. In common with several of the other B-complex vitamins, chronic alcoholism is also a risk factor.

4.4.2.3 Health consequences of deficiency and benefits of intervention

Symptoms of riboflavin deficiency are non-specific. Early symptoms may include weakness, fatigue, mouth pain, burning eyes and itching. More advanced deficiency is characterized by dermatitis with cheilosis and angular stomatitis, brain dysfunction and microcytic anaemia (**Table 1.2**). Riboflavin deficiency also reduces the absorption and utilization of iron for haemoglobin synthesis. It is possible that riboflavin deficiency is a contributory factor in the high prevalence of anaemia worldwide (see *section 3.1.1*), a suggestion which is supported by reports from The Gambia and Guatemala that riboflavin supplementation improved the haemoglobin response to iron supplementation in anaemic subjects *(176,177)*. Almost nothing is known about the effects of milder deficiency, although depletion studies conducted in the United States found evidence of electroencephalogram abnormalities.

4.4.3 Niacin

Niacin (nicotinic acid or vitamin B_3), as a functional group of the coenzymes, nicotinamide adenine dinucleotide (NAD) and its phosphate (NADP), is essential for oxidative processes. Deficiency results in pellagra and is associated with a heavily cereal-based diet that is low in bioavailable niacin, tryptophan (an amino acid) and other micronutrients needed for the synthesis of niacin and tryptophan. Niacin is unique among the vitamins in that at least part of the body's requirement for it can be met through synthesis from an amino acid (tryptophan): the conversion of 60 mg tryptophan (via a niacin derivative) produces 1 mg of niacin.

4.4.3.1 Prevalence of deficiency

There are no direct indicators of niacin status (**Table 4.8**). Assessment is therefore based on the measurement of one or preferably more urinary metabolites of niacin, such as N'-methyl-nicotinamide (NMN) (which reflects recent dietary intake) or the ratio of 2-pyridone:NMN. Provisional criteria proposed by WHO for defining the severity of the public health problem based on these biomarkers are listed in **Table 4.9**.

At present, evaluation of the prevalence of niacin deficiency is almost entirely based on occurrence of clinical signs of deficiency, i.e. pellagra. There is very little biochemical information on niacin status, and thus on the prevalence of subclinical deficiency, from developing countries.

Pellagra was widespread in parts of southern Europe and in the United States during the 19th and early 20th centuries, but fortification of cereal grain products has since all but eradicated the condition from industrialized countries. It is, however, still common in India, and in parts of Africa and China, especially where populations are dependent on maize-based diets. More recently, pellagra has been reported in areas where diets are largely sorghum-based, and where there is a dependence on polished rice. The prevalence of pellagra is also high among displaced populations living in refugee camps based in south and eastern parts of Africa (*178*). For example, up to 6.4% of Mozambican refugees based in Malawi were affected by an outbreak of pellagra (*179*).

4.4.3.2 Risk factors for deficiency

Niacin is widely distributed in plant and animal foods. The main sources are baker's yeast, animal and dairy products, cereals, legumes and leafy green vegetables. Niacin depletion is a risk where diets rely heavily on refined grains or grain products and have little variety. Severe deficiency, pellagra, is predominantly found in people who consume diets that are deficient in bioavailable niacin and low in tryptophan, such as maize- or sorghum-based diets.

In maize, niacin is largely present in a bound form, only 30% of which bioavailable. However, the bioavailability of this bound form of niacin can be improved by hydrolysis with a mild alkali. The soaking of maize in lime water, as is traditionally done in the preparation of *tortillas* in some Latin American countries, releases niacin from niacytin, and thus increases the amount of niacin that can be absorbed. Bound niacin can be also be released by heat: the roasting of coffee beans, for instance, increases the bioavailability of the nicotinic acid content from 20 to 500 mg/kg (*167*). These practices possibly account, at least in part, for the absence of pellagra in Latin America. The regular consumption of milk and rice can also help prevent pellagra; although they are low in niacin, milk and rice are rich in tryptophan.

TABLE 4.8
Indicators for assessing niacin (nicotinic acid) status at the population level[a]

Indicator	Sample	Population group	Cut-off to define deficiency		Comments
			Mild	Severe	
N'-methyl-nicotinamide (NMN)	Urine	Adults	<1.6 mg/g creatinine (<17.5 µmol/24 h)	<0.5 mg/g creatinine (<5.8 µmol/24 h)	Reflects recent dietary intake of niacin.
		Pregnancy (second trimester)	<2.0 mg/g creatinine	<0.6 mg/g creatinine	
		Pregnancy (third trimester)	<2.5 mg/g creatinine	<0.8 mg/g creatinine	
Ratio of 2-pyridone: N'-methyl-nicotinamide	Urine	Applies to all population groups	<0.5	<0.5	Provides a measure of protein adequacy rather than niacin status.
Pyridine nucleotides	Erythrocytes (RBC)	Applies to all population groups	No universally agreed cut-offs at this time		A potentially sensitive indicator of niacin inadequacy.

RBC, red blood cell.
[a] As no direct indicator of niacin status is currently available, it is necessary to measure one or preferably more urinary metabolites of niacin.

Sources: references (93, 128, 129, 178).

TABLE 4.9
Proposed criteria for assessing the public health severity of niacin deficiency

Indicator	Severity of public health problem (% of population below the cut-off value defining deficiency)		
	Mild	Moderate	Severe
Clinical signs (clinical cases)	<1	1–4	≥5
Urinary N′-methyl-nicotinamide ≥0.50 mg/g creatinine	5–19	20–49	≥50
Urinary ratio of 2-pyridone: N′-methyl-nicotinamide <1.0	5–19	20–49	≥50
Dietary intake <5 mg niacin equivalents/day	5–19	20–49	≥50

Source: reference (*178*).

4.4.3.3 Health consequences of deficiency and benefits of intervention

Clinical signs of niacin deficiency, pellagra, develop within 2 to 3 months of consuming a diet inadequate in niacin and/or tryptophan (**Table 1.2**). The most characteristic sign of pellagra is a symmetrically pigmented rash on areas of skin exposed to sunlight. Other manifestations include changes in the mucosa of the digestive tract, leading to oral lesions, vomiting and diarrhoea, and neurological symptoms such as depression, fatigue and loss of memory.

4.4.4 Vitamin B_6

Vitamin B_6 is in fact a group of three naturally-occurring compounds: pyridoxine (PN), pyridoxal (PL) and pyridoxamine (PM). The different forms of vitamin B_6 are phosphorylated and then oxidized to generate pyridoxal 5′-phosphate (PLP), which serves as a carbonyl-reactive coenzyme to various enzymes involved in the metabolism of amino acids. Vitamin B_6 deficiency alone is relatively uncommon, but occurs most often in association with deficiencies of the other B vitamins.

4.4.4.1 Prevalence of deficiency

Although there are several biochemical indicators of vitamin B_6 status (**Table 4.10**), all suffer from limitations of one kind or another. For this reason, vitamin B_6 status is best evaluated by using a combination of indicators. The absence of a suitable single indicator means that vitamin B_6 status has only rarely been assessed at the population level but according to a recent report from Indonesia, low intakes among children are likely to be common; among the children surveyed about 10% of those from urban areas and 40% of those from rural areas exhibited biochemical signs of deficiency (*180*). Moreover, about 40% of lactating mothers in Egypt had low concentrations of vitamin B_6 in breast milk, and both these women and their infants presented abnormal behaviours (*181*).

TABLE 4.10
Indicators for assessing vitamin B_6 (pyridoxine) status at the population level[a]

Indicator	Sample	Population group	Cut-off to define deficiency		Comments
			Mild	Severe	
Pyridoxal 5'-phosphate (PLP)	Plasma	Adults	<20 nmol/l	<10 nmol/l	Probably the best indicator of vitamin B_6 status. Reflects tissue stores. Concentration reported to fall with age.
	Urine	Adults	<3 mmol/day	No universally agreed cut-offs at this time	Reflects recent dietary intake.
Aspartate aminotransferase apoenzyme form: total enzyme	Erythrocytes (RBC)	Adults	>1.6	No universally agreed cut-offs at this time	Measured before and after addition of pyridoxal 5'-phosphate (PLP) to ascertain amounts of apoenzyme. The ratio is increased in cases of vitamin B_6 deficiency. Reflects long-term vitamin B_6 status.
Alanine aminotransferase apoenzyme form: total enzyme	Erythrocytes (RBC)	Adults	>1.25	No universally agreed cut-offs at this time	Measured before and after addition of pyridoxal 5'-phosphate (PLP) to ascertain amounts of apoenzyme. The ratio is increased in cases of vitamin B_6 deficiency. Reflects long-term vitamin B_6 status.
Total homocysteine (free and bond)	Plasma	Adults	12–16 µmol/l	No universally agreed cut-offs at this time	Influenced by vitamin B_6, B_{12}, folate status, gender, race and renal insufficiency.

RBC, red blood cell.
[a] No direct indicator of vitamin B_6 status is currently available; in order to assess vitamin B_6 status it is therefore necessary to measure a combination of indicators.

Sources: references (*93,128,129*).

4.4.4.2 Risk factors for deficiency

Vitamin B_6 is widely distributed in foods, but meats, wholegrain products, vegetables and nuts are especially good sources of the vitamin. Cooking and storage losses range from a few percent to nearly half of the vitamin B_6 originally present. Plants generally contain pyridoxine (PN), the most stable form, while animal products contain the less stable pyridoxal (PL) and the functional PLP form. In common with several of the other B vitamins, low intakes of animal products and a high consumption of refined cereals are the main risk factors for vitamin B_6 deficiency. Similarly, chronic alcoholism is an additional risk factor for deficiency.

4.4.4.3 Health consequences of deficiency and benefits of intervention

Symptoms of severe vitamin B_6 deficiency are non-specific (**Table 1.2**) and include neurological disorders (i.e. epileptic convulsions), skin changes (i.e. dermatitis, glossitis, cheilosis) and possibly anaemia. Vitamin B_6 deficiency is a risk factor for elevated plasma homocysteine (*182*). In trials, vitamin B_6 supplements increased secretion of the vitamin in the breast milk of lactating women (*183*).

4.5 Vitamin C

Vitamin C is a redox system comprised of ascorbic acid and dehydroascorbic acid, and as such acts as an electron donor. Its main metabolic function is the maintenance of collagen formation. It is also an important antioxidant. Although severe vitamin C deficiency (scurvy) is now relatively rare, the prevalence of milder or marginal deficiency is probably quite high.

4.5.1 Prevalence of deficiency

Concentrations of ascorbic acid in blood plasma or serum reflect recent intakes of vitamin C, and in this respect, are more reliable indicators of vitamin C status than ascorbic acid concentrations in erythrocytes (**Table 4.11**). White blood cell (leukocyte) ascorbic acid concentrations are more closely related to tissue stores and probably provide the most sensitive indicator of vitamin C status, but being technically more difficult to measure, are impractical for routine and large-scale population surveys. Criteria for defining the public health significance of vitamin C deficiency, as proposed by WHO, are given in **Table 4.12**.

Despite its near eradication, severe vitamin C deficiency (scurvy) still occurs periodically in displaced populations maintained for long periods of time (i.e. 3–6 months) on food aid and without access to fresh fruit and vegetables (*184*). Outbreaks have been repeatedly reported from refugee camps in the Horn of Africa (i.e. Ethiopia, Kenya, Somalia, Sudan) and Nepal. In the mid-1980s, the prevalence of scurvy in refugee camps in north-west Somalia varied between

TABLE 4.11
Indicators for assessing vitamin C status at the population level

Indicator	Sample	Population group	Cut-off to define deficiency		Comments
			Mild	Severe	
Ascorbic acid	Serum/plasma	Applies to all population groups	<0.3 mg/100 ml	<0.2 mg/100 ml	Reflects recent intake.
Ascorbic acid	Erythrocytes (RBC)	Applies to all population groups	<0.5 mg/100 ml	<0.3 mg/100 ml	Reflects recent intake, but less reliable than serum/plasma ascorbic acid concentration.
Ascorbic acid	Leukocytes	Applies to all population groups	<114 nmol/10^8 cells	<57 nmol/10^8 cells	Reflects body stores. Considered to be the most sensitive indicator of vitamin C status, but as technically complex to measure and interpretation is limited by the absence of standardized reporting procedures, not widely used for population surveys.

RBC, red blood cell.
Sources: references (*129,184,190*).

TABLE 4.12
Proposed criteria for assessing the public health severity of vitamin C deficiency

Indicator	Severity of public health problem (% of population)		
	Mild	Moderate	Severe
Clinical signs (clinical cases)	<1	1–4	≥5
Serum ascorbic acid:			
<0.2 mg/100 ml	10–29	30–49	≥50
<0.3 mg/100 ml	30–49	50–69	≥70

Sources: adapted from references (*184,190*).

7% and 44% (*185*); in eastern Sudan the prevalence rate was 22% (*186*), and in Kassala, Sudan, 15% (*187*). Scurvy has also been observed in selected population groups, such as infants, and in some communities of mine labourers (*188*).

In contrast, the prevalence of mild vitamin C deficiency worldwide is probably fairly high. In the United States, data from the third National Health and Nutrition Examination Survey (NHANES III 1988–1994) have indicated that the prevalence of marginal vitamin C deficiency (defined as less than 0.3 mg ascorbic acid per 100 ml serum) is about 9% in women and 13% in men (*189*).

4.5.2 Risk factors for deficiency

Vitamin C is widely available in foods of both plant and animal origin, but the best sources are fresh fruits and vegetables, and offal. As germination increases vitamin C content, germinated grains and pulses also contain high levels of vitamin C. However, because vitamin C is unstable when exposed to an alkaline environment or to oxygen, light and heat, losses may be substantial during storage and cooking.

Deficiency is usually a result of a low consumption of fresh fruits and vegetables, caused by any one or a combination of factors such as seasonal unavailability, transportation difficulties and/or unaffordable cost. Displaced populations who rely on cooked, fortified rations and who do not have access to fresh fruits and vegetables are at a high risk for deficiency. For these population groups, vitamin C supplementation is recommended, at least until they are able to obtain a more normal diet. Chronic alcoholics, institutionalized elderly and people living on a restricted diet containing little or no fruits and vegetables, are also at risk of vitamin C deficiency. As the vitamin C content of cow's milk is low, infants represent a further subgroup that is potentially high-risk for vitamin C deficiency. There have been a number of reports – across several world regions – of scurvy in infants fed on evaporated cow's milk (*191,192*).

4.5.3 Health consequences of deficiency and benefits of intervention

The clinical symptoms of scurvy include follicular hyperkeratosis, haemorrhagic manifestations, swollen joints, swollen bleeding gums and peripheral oedema, and even death. These symptoms appear within 3–4 months of consuming diets with a very low vitamin C content (<2 mg per day). In infants, manifestations of scurvy include a haemorrhagic syndrome, signs of general irritability, tenderness of the legs and pseudoparalysis involving the lower extremities (see Table 1.2). The adverse effects of mild deficiency are uncertain, but may include poor bone mineralization (due to slower production of collagen), lassitude, fatigue, anorexia, muscular weakness and increased susceptibility to infections.

As vitamin C increases the absorption of non-haem iron from foods, a low intake of vitamin C will exacerbate any iron deficiency problems, especially in individuals who consume only small amounts of meat, fish or poultry. Indeed, anaemia is a frequent manifestation of scurvy. The addition of vitamin C to iron-fortified foods greatly improves the absorption of the iron. In Chile, for example, it was necessary to also add vitamin C to iron-fortified dried milk consumed by young children before any significant improvements in iron status could be detected (40) (see also *section 5.1.2.1*).

4.6 Vitamin D

Vitamin D is one of the most important regulators of calcium and phosphorus homeostasis. It also plays many roles in cell differentiation and in the secretion and metabolism of hormones, including parathyroid hormone and insulin. Vitamin D (calciferol) is synthesized in the skin of most animals, including humans, from its precursor, 7-dehydrocholesterol, by the action of sunlight. This produces a naturally-occurring form of the vitamin known as vitamin D_3. Vitamin D can also be obtained from the diet, either as vitamin D_3 or as a closely-related molecule of plant origin known as vitamin D_2. Since both forms are metabolized by humans in much the same way, from a nutritional perspective, vitamin D_3 and vitamin D_2 can be considered to be equivalent. Vitamin D_3 is metabolized first in the liver to 25-hydroxyvitamin D (25-OH-D_3), and then in the kidney to 1,25-dihydroxyvitamin D (1,25-$(OH)_2$-D_3), which is the biologically active form of the vitamin.

Severe vitamin D deficiency produces the bone disease called rickets in infants and children, and osteomalacia in adults, conditions which are characterized by the failure of the organic matrix of bone to calcify. The global prevalence of vitamin D deficiency is uncertain, but it is likely to be fairly common worldwide, and especially among infants and young children, the elderly and those living at high latitudes where daylight hours are limited in the winter months.

4.6.1 Prevalence of deficiency

In infants and young children, a concentration of 25-OH-D in serum below about 27.5 nmol/l (11 ng/ml) is indicative of a low vitamin D status (**Table 4.13**). An elevated serum concentration of alkaline phosphatase can also indicate vitamin D deficiency; alkaline phosphatase is increased in patients with rickets or osteomalacia but is not specific to either of these conditions. In adults, the combination of low plasma 25-OH-D and elevated parathyroid hormone (PTH) is probably the most reliable indicator of vitamin D deficiency (*193*). In the absence of biochemical data, the existence of rickets in infants and children, and a high fracture risk among the elderly population, would suggest that vitamin D deficiency might be a public health problem.

Breast-fed infants who are not exposed to sunlight are unlikely to obtain enough vitamin D from breast milk beyond the first few months of life, especially if their mother's stores of the vitamin are low. Vitamin D deficiency in infants as a result of low maternal stores and/or infant exposure to sunlight (especially during winter months) has been reported in countries as diverse as China (*194*) and France (*195*). Infants and children on macrobiotic diets tend to have a high prevalence of rickets, due to the low vitamin D content of maternal milk and the absence of fortified cow's milk in their diets (*196*).

Children living in the far northerly latitudes, whose exposure to ultraviolet light is low especially during the winter months, are at high risk for rickets (*197*). Vitamin D deficiency is also common in adults living at higher latitudes: for

TABLE 4.13
Indicators for assessing vitamin D status at the population level

Indicator	Sample	Population group	Cut-off to define deficiency	Comments
25-hydroxyvitamin D (25-OH-D)	Serum	Applies to all population groups	<27.5 nmol/l (<11 ng/ml)	Serum 25-hydroxyvitamin D in combination with parathyroid hormone is a valuable indicator of vitamin D status.
Parathyroid hormone (PTH)	Serum	Applies to all population groups	No universally agreed cut-offs at this time	Serum parathyroid hormone is inversely correlated with serum 25-hydroxyvitamin D and may be a valuable indicator of vitamin D status.
Alkaline phosphatase	Serum	Applies to all population groups	No universally agreed cut-offs at this time	Increased in cases of osteomalacia or rickets.

Sources: references (*93, 129, 193*).

instance, surveys carried out in China after winter in populations living at about 41°N found that 13–48% of adults were deficient in this vitamin, with the highest prevalence occurring in older men (*198*). In Beijing, 45% of adolescent girls were found to be deficient (*199*).

4.6.2 Risk factors for deficiency

Most (about 80%) of the vitamin D in the body is produced in the skin. This process usually supplies all of the vitamin D needed by infants, children and adults. However, above and below latitudes 40°N and 40°S, the intensity of ultraviolet radiation in sunlight is not sufficient to produce adequate amounts of vitamin D in exposed skin during the 3–4 winter months. At the very high latitudes, synthesis can be inadequate for as long as 6 months of the year. Inadequate synthesis in winter is seen as far south as Turkey and Israel; low serum levels of vitamin D are also highly prevalent in the winter in Delhi, India (29°N) (*200*). Vitamin D synthesis in the skin will also be inadequate if the body is consistently covered by clothing, a probable factor in the high prevalence of deficiency among veiled women (e.g. Kuwaiti women) and their breast-fed infants and children (*201*).

In the elderly, dietary requirements for vitamin D are increased because the ability of the skin to synthesize this vitamin decreases with age; at age 65 years, vitamin D synthesis in the skin is about 75% slower than that in younger adults. Dark-skinned individuals synthesize less vitamin D when exposed to ultraviolet light, and are therefore more vulnerable to deficiency at low levels of exposure to ultraviolet light. In the United States, cases of rickets have been reported among black breast-fed children (*202*), and according to the results of a recent national survey, 42% of African-American women had low plasma vitamin D concentrations (*56*).

Being naturally present in relatively few foods, dietary sources of vitamin D usually supply only a small fraction of the daily requirements for the vitamin. Salt-water fish such as herring, salmon, sardines and fish liver oil are the main dietary sources. Small quantities of vitamin D are found in other animal products (e.g. beef, butter), and if hens are fed vitamin D, eggs can provide substantial amounts of the vitamin. Because the consumption of these foods tends to be relatively low, in industrialized countries most dietary vitamin D comes from fortified milk and margarine. Milk only provides small amounts of vitamin D unless it is fortified.

Several studies have shown that the effects of poor vitamin D status are exacerbated by low calcium intakes. This has been demonstrated in adults from India (*200*) and in children from Nigeria (*203*). The Nigerian children with nutritional rickets responded better to calcium, with or without vitamin D, than to vitamin D alone (*203*).

4.6.3 Health consequences of deficiency and benefits of intervention

The clinical features of rickets include bone deformities and changes in the costochondral joints. The lesions are reversible after correction of vitamin D deficiency. In osteomalacia, in which the loss of calcium and phosphorus from bone causes it to lose strength, the main symptoms are muscular weakness and bone pain, but little bone deformity. Osteomalacia contributes to osteoporosis, a condition in which the bone becomes more brittle and porous due to the loss of bone tissue. Vitamin D supplementation reduced seasonal loss of bone tissue in North American women (*204*), and prevented fractures associated with osteoporosis in the elderly.

In many locations, the addition of vitamin D to selected foods has proved to be a prudent public health measure. The vitamin has been added to milk in Canada and the United States since the 1920s, a policy that has been largely responsible for the elimination of vitamin D deficiency rickets in children. However, low intakes of fortified dairy products by some elderly individuals, and by some black populations, are still associated with a much higher risk of vitamin D deficiency among these groups.

4.7 Calcium

Calcium is the most abundant mineral in the body. Most (>99%) of the body's 1000–1200g of calcium is located in the skeleton where it exists as hydroxyapatite. In addition to its role in maintaining the rigidity and strength of the skeleton, calcium is involved in a large number of metabolic processes, including blood clotting, cell adhesion, muscle contraction, hormone and neurotransmitter release, glycogen metabolism, and cell proliferation and differentiation.

Osteoporosis, a disease characterized by reduced bone mass and thus increased skeletal fragility and susceptibility to fractures, is the most significant consequence of a low calcium status. Although an adequacy of calcium is important during the whole life span, it is especially important during childhood and adolescence (as these are periods of rapid skeletal growth), and for postmenopausal women and the elderly whose rate of bone loss is high.

4.7.1 Prevalence of deficiency

Unfortunately there are no practical population level indicators of calcium status (**Table 4.14**). Serum calcium, for example, is regulated by a complex homeostatic mechanism, which makes it an unreliable indicator of calcium status. For this reason, in most countries the prevalence of deficiency is not known. In the absence of reliable biochemical indicators, the best indication of calcium adequacy at present, especially for developing countries, is probably provided by comparing dietary intakes with recommended nutrient intakes (RNIs), despite

TABLE 4.14
Indicators for assessing calcium at the population level

Indicator	Sample	Population group	Cut-off to define deficiency	Comments
Calcium	Serum	Applies to all population groups	No universally agreed cut-offs at this time	Tightly homeostatically regulated and therefore does not reflect calcium status.
Calcium	Dietary intake	Applies to all population groups	No universally agreed cut-offs at this time	Probably the best indicator of calcium adequacy.

[a] At present there are no good biochemical measures for assessing calcium status.
Sources: references (*93,193*).

the variability and uncertainty in the currently recommended intakes for calcium (*93,193*). On the basis of the fact that intakes of dairy products are low, it is thus highly likely that low or very low calcium intakes are very common in developing countries.

Measurements of bone mineral density (BMD) and bone mineral content (BMC) have provided an alternative means of assessing the likely extent of calcium deficiency in some countries. In the United States, for example, it has been estimated that 5–6 million older women and 1–2 million older men have osteoporosis. Other approaches include measuring markers of bone resorption in urine or plasma, which tend to be higher in calcium deficient individuals. Such methods are, however, relatively expensive. All of the above measures are affected by, among many other factors, vitamin D status, level of physical activity and hormone levels, which further complicates the assessment of calcium adequacy at the population level.

4.7.2 Risk factors for deficiency

Intakes of calcium will almost certainly fall below the recommended levels where dairy product intake is low. Dairy products supply 50–80% of dietary calcium in most industrialized countries, while foods of plant origin supply about 25%. The calcium content of, and contribution from, most other foods is usually relatively small. Calcium absorption efficiency is increased by a low calcium status and by a low dietary calcium content. Absorption is homeostatically controlled through regulation by vitamin D. The strongest known inhibitor of calcium absorption is dietary oxalate, followed by the presence of phytates (*193*). Oxalate is not an important factor in most diets (although it is high in spinach, sweet potatoes and beans) but phytates are often consumed in large amounts, for instance, in legumes and wholegrain cereals.

4.7.3 Health consequences of deficiency and benefits of fortification

The numerous metabolic roles of calcium are sustained even when intakes are low, because calcium is withdrawn from the bone should homeostatic mechanisms fail to maintain an adequate calcium status in the extracellular fluid. Thus inadequate calcium intakes lead to decreased bone mineralization and subsequently an increased risk for osteoporosis in adults (**Table 1.2**).

In healthy individuals, bone mineral density increases until about 30 years of age, and thereafter begins to decline. Low intakes during childhood and adolescence can reduce peak bone density and thus increase the risk of osteoporosis in adulthood. The age of onset and severity of osteoporosis depends not only on the duration of inadequate calcium intakes, but also on a number of other factors, such as estrogen levels, vitamin D status and level of physical activity.

Although rickets is usually associated with vitamin D deficiency (see *section 4.6*), rickets has been observed in vitamin D-replete infants who also had low calcium intakes (*203*). In Chinese children aged 5 years from China, Hong Kong Special Administrative Region (Hong Kong SAR), intakes of <250 mg calcium per day were associated with a 14% lower bone mineral content and a 4% reduction in height relative to those consuming twice as much calcium (*205*). Supplementation of Gambian children with 1000 mg calcium per day improved their bone mineralization (*206*). It has been suggested that calcium may confer other benefits, including the prevention of cancer and hypertension, but the role played by calcium in such diseases is unclear at the present time.

4.8 Selenium

Selenium is an essential element and a key constituent of at least 13 selenoproteins. These can be grouped into a number of distinct families, the glutathione peroxidases and the thioredoxin reductases, which are part of the antioxidant defence system of cells, and iodothyronine deiodinase, an enzyme which converts the inactive precursor of thyroxine, tetraiodothyronine (T_4) into the active form, tri-iodothyronine (T_3). In humans, the biological roles of selenium include the protection of tissues against oxidative stress, the maintenance of the body's defence systems against infection, and the modulation of growth and development. Severe deficiency can result in Keshan or Kaschin-Beck disease, which are endemic in several world regions.

4.8.1 Prevalence of deficiency

There are several reliable indicators of selenium status, such as the concentration of selenium in plasma, urine, hair or nails. However, the measurement of selenium in human samples presents a number of technical difficulties, a factor that limits the usefulness of such measures as indicators of status (**Table 4.15**). Indeed, the lack of simple assay techniques for selenium means that currently

TABLE 4.15
Indicators for assessing selenium status at the population level[a]

Indicator	Sample	Population group	Cut-off to define deficiency	Comments
Selenium	Plasma, urine	Applies to all population groups	0.8–1.1 µmol/l	Might reflect recent intake in low selenium environments but levels depend on the chemical form of the ingested selenium. Not appropriate for use in population surveys as technically difficult to measure.
Selenium	Erythrocytes (RBC)	Applies to all population groups	No universally agreed cut-offs at this time	Reflects stores but not appropriate for use in population surveys as technically difficult to measure.
Selenium	Hair, nails	Applies to all population groups	No universally agreed cut-offs at this time	Correlations do exist between dietary intake and hair and nail concentrations. Concentrations are affected by several factors such as frequency of hair washing (shampoos are high in selenium) and hair colour.

RBC, red blood cell.
[a] Selenium status is probably best assessed by means of a combination of indicators.

Sources: references (*93,208*).

there are no suitable biochemical indicators of selenium status that are appropriate for use in population surveys. Information regarding the prevalence of selenium deficiency is thus largely based on clinical observations and limited to the more severe forms, i.e. Keshan or Kaschin-Beck disease.

Selenium deficiency is endemic in some regions of China (*207*), where Keshan disease was first described, and also in parts of Japan, Korea, Scandinavia and Siberia. Endemic deficiency tends to occur in regions characterized by low soil selenium. For example, the distribution of Keshan disease and Kaschin-Beck disease in China reflects the distribution of soils from which selenium is poorly available to rice, maize, wheat and pasture grasses. Fortification of salt and/or fertilizers with selenium is crucial in these parts of the world.

4.8.2 Risk factors for deficiency

Usual diets in most countries satisfy selenium requirements. As indicated in the previous section, deficiency occurs only where the soil, and consequently the foods produced on those soils, is low in available selenium. Worldwide, the selenium content of animal products and that of cereals and plants, varies widely (at least 10-fold) depending on soil selenium content (*209*). The selenium content of foods of plant origin ranges from less than 0.1 µg/g to more than 0.8 µg/g, while the amount in animal products ranges from 0.1 to 1.5 µg/g (*210*). Where animal feeds are enriched with selenium, such as in the United States, the selenium content of animal products may be much higher. Concentrations of less than 10 ng/g in the case of grain and less than 3 ng/g in the case of water-soluble soil selenium have been proposed as indexes to define selenium-deficient areas (*93*).

In industrialized countries, meat provides about half of the dietary selenium. It is also a good source in areas of low soil selenium because animals absorb more of this nutrient when their intake is low. A low intake of animal source foods is thus likely to increase the risk of selenium deficiency. It is generally assumed that the bioavailability of selenium from the diet is high.

4.8.3 Health consequences of deficiency and benefits of intervention

Keshan disease is a cardiomyopathy associated with a low selenium intake and low levels of selenium in blood and hair. Reports of its occurrence across a wide zone of mainland China first appeared in the mainstream scientific literature in the 1930s. It has since also been observed in some areas of the southern Siberia. Symptoms include cardiac insufficiency and arrhythmias, congestive heart failure and heart enlargement (*211*), which are responsive to supplementation with sodium selenite. Because some features of Keshan disease cannot be explained by selenium deficiency alone, other contributing factors have been suggested, in particular, infection with the cocksackie virus (*212*).

The selenium deficiency syndrome known as Kaschin-Beck or Urov disease is found in parts of China and Siberia, and in Japan and Korea. This is a disease of cartilage tissue that occurs in pre-adolescent and adolescent children, causing osteoarthropathy, joint problems and growth stunting. Like Keshan disease, additional causal factors have been proposed to account for the etiology of Keschin-Beck disease, including exposure to mycotoxins from *Fusarium* mould (*213*), mineral imbalances and iodine deficiency (*214*).

Low intakes of selenium have been linked to a reduced conversion of the thyroid hormone, T_4 to T_3. The metabolic interrelations between selenium and iodine are such that deficiencies in one can sometimes exacerbate problems with the other. In the Democratic Republic of Congo, for instance, combined selenium and iodine deficiencies were shown to contribute to endemic myxoedematous cretinism. Administration of selenium alone appeared to aggravate this disease; by restoring selenium-dependent deiodinase activity, the synthesis and use of thyroxine (T_4) and iodine is increased, thereby exacerbating the iodine deficiency (*215*). Low selenium intakes have also been associated by some researchers with an increased incidence of cancer, in particular, oesophageal cancer and also with cardiovascular disease (*216*).

In areas of endemic selenium deficiency, fortification with selenium has been shown to rapidly increase plasma glutathione peroxidase levels and urinary selenium. For example, when selenium was added to fertilizers in Finland in 1984, plasma selenium levels doubled by 1991 and glutathione peroxidase activity was normalized (*217*). In addition, according to the results of large-scale survey (over 1 million people) selenium fortification of table salt has significantly reduced the prevalence of Keshan disease in China (*218*).

4.9 Fluoride

Unlike the other micronutrients considered in these guidelines, fluoride is not generally considered to be an essential nutrient according to the strict definition of the term (see Chapter 2: *section 2.1.1*). Nevertheless, fluoride is undoubtedly protective against tooth decay.

4.9.1 Prevalence of dental caries

There are no universally agreed methods for assessing fluoride status and no generally accepted criteria with which to define deficiency. However, concentrations in urine have sometimes been used as an indicator of fluoride status (**Table 4.16**).

The prevalence of dental caries is 40–60% lower in those areas of the United States where water is fluoridated compared with those where it is not. However, the increased use of fluoridated toothpaste and supplements by infants and

TABLE 4.16
Indicators for assessing fluoride status at the population level[a]

Indicator	Sample	Population group	Cut-off to define deficiency	Comments
Fluoride	Urine	Applies to all population groups	<0.5 mg/l	No universally agreed criteria for defining deficiency. The following cut-offs for urinary fluoridine are, however, sometimes used: adequate, 0.5–1.0 mg/l; deficient, <0.5 mg/l; excessive >1.5 mg/l.

[a] At present there are no universally agreed methods for assessing fluoride status.
Source: reference (*193*).

young children has made it difficult to differentiate between the beneficial effects of a fluoridated water supply and that of other sources of the mineral.

4.9.2 Risk factors for low intakes

Fluoride intake from most natural water supplies will be relatively low; a low fluoride content of water is thus the main risk factor for a low intake of this mineral. In Canada and the United States, for instance, water sources typically contain less than 0.4 mg/l, which compares with concentrations of 0.7–1.2 mg/l in fluoridated supplies. Moreover, the fluoride content of breast milk is low and foods contain well below 0.05 mg per 100 g, with exception of those prepared with fluoridated water and infant formulas.

4.9.3 Health consequences of low intakes and benefits of intervention

If ingested in water or foods, fluoride will become incorporated into the mineral of growing teeth and thus make them more resistant to decay. Continued exposure of the tooth surfaces to fluoride throughout life is also beneficial because it reduces the ability of bacteria to cause decay and promotes the remineralization of decayed areas. For these reasons, the addition of fluoride to public water supplies, or to salt or milk, can be an effective public health strategy for dental caries prevention (*219*). This practice does not increase the risk of osteoporosis for older individuals in the population (*220*), and according to the results of some studies, might even lower the risk (*221,222*).

Excessive fluoride intake carries a risk of enamel fluorosis, especially during the first 8 years of life. In severe cases of this condition, the enamel of the tooth becomes stained and pitted; in milder forms the enamel acquires opaque lines or patches. Enamel fluorosis does not occur at fluoride intakes ≤0.10 mg/kg body weight per day (*193*). In adults, excessive fluoride intake can result in skeletal fluorosis, with symptoms that include bone pain, and in more severe cases, muscle calcification and crippling. Mild skeletal fluorosis only occurs at fluoride intakes that are in excess of 10 mg/day for more than 10 years. Symptoms of skeletal fluorosis are rarely seen in communities where the fluoride content of water supplies is below 20 ppm (20 mg/l).

4.10 Multiple micronutrient deficiencies

4.10.1 Prevalence and risk factors

Based on what is known about the prevalence of deficiencies in individual micronutrients, it is probable that multiple micronutrient deficiencies are common in several parts of the world and in certain population groups. Micronutrient deficiencies are more likely to coexist in individuals who consume diets that are poor in nutritional quality, or who have higher nutrient requirements due to high growth rates and/or the presence of bacterial infections or parasites. In particular, a diet that is low in animal source foods typically results in low intakes of bioavailable iron and zinc, calcium, retinol (pre-formed vitamin A), vitamin B_2 (riboflavin), vitamin B_6 and vitamin B_{12}. Often, poor quality diets also lack fresh fruits and vegetables, which means that intakes of vitamin C (ascorbic acid), β-carotene (provitamin A) and folate will also be inadequate. The milling of cereals removes several nutrients, notably, iron and zinc, various B vitamins (i.e. thiamine, riboflavin, niacin) and folate. Individuals who rely heavily on refined cereals are thus at increased risk of deficiency of all of these micronutrients. The breast milk of undernourished lactating women consuming a limited range of foods and with multiple micronutrient deficiencies, is most likely to be low in concentrations of vitamin A (retinol), the B vitamins, iodine and selenium. If the micronutrient content of breast milk is inadequate for optimal infant development, maternal supplementation may be required until adequate fortification programmes can be launched.

4.10.2 Health consequences and benefits of intervention

As several previous subsections have indicated, a deficiency in one micronutrient can impair the utilization of another. Conversely, improving an individual's status in one micronutrient, or even several micronutrients simultaneously in the case of multiple deficiencies, can have wider benefits. For example, iron deficiency may cause vitamin A to be trapped in the liver; several studies have shown that iron supplementation alone can increase serum retinol concentrations markedly (*85*). Goitre is more resistant to improvement by iodine supplementation in the presence of iron deficiency, and iron supplementation of deficient children improves their rate of goitre response to iodine supplements or iodine fortified salt (*87*). Similarly, the addition of vitamin A to iron supplements increases blood haemoglobin by a substantial amount in vitamin A-depleted, anaemic populations (*99*) and can help to further increase iron stores (*223*). Deficiencies of vitamin B_{12}, folate, vitamin B_2 (riboflavin) and several other micronutrients can also contribute to anaemia (*77*). As vitamin C (from foods or added as a fortificant) improves the absorption of non-haem iron from food and many iron fortificants, it too is frequently added as well as iron as a fortificant.

In the past, interventions have targeted deficiencies in iron, vitamin A and iodine, in part because these can be detected more easily and more is known about their adverse effects. Typically, separate programmes were developed for each nutrient. In more recent years, it has become increasingly apparent that there are many reasons why multiple micronutrient fortification may be more appropriate and should be considered. In addition to treating and preventing iron, vitamin A and iodine deficiencies, fortification affords a good opportunity to control other micronutrient deficiencies that are likely to coexist in many populations.

PART III

Fortificants: physical characteristics, selection and use with specific food vehicles

Introduction

By providing a critical review of the fortificants that are currently available for fortification purposes, Part III of these guidelines is intended to assist programme managers in their choice of firstly, a suitable food vehicle and secondly, a compatible fortificant. Having established – through the application of appropriate criteria – that the nature of the public health risk posed by a micronutrient deficiency justifies intervention in the form of food fortification, the selection of a suitable combination of food vehicle and fortificant(s), or more specifically, the chemical form of the micronutrient(s) that will added to the chosen food vehicle, is fundamental to any food fortification programme. Subsequent chapters (Part IV) cover other important aspects of food fortification programme planning, including how to calculate how much fortificant to add to the chosen food vehicle in order to achieve a predetermined public health benefit (Chapter 7), monitoring and impact evaluation (Chapters 8 and 9), marketing (Chapter 10) and regulatory issues (Chapter 11).

In practice, the selection of a food vehicle–fortificant combination is governed by range of factors, both technological and regulatory. Foods such as cereals, oils, dairy products, beverages and various condiments such as salt, sauces (e.g. soy sauce) and sugar are particularly well suited to mandatory mass fortification. These foods share some or all of the following characteristics:

- They are consumed by a large proportion of the population, including (or especially) the population groups at greatest risk of deficiency.

- They are consumed on a regular basis, in adequate and relatively consistent amounts.

- They can be centrally processed (central processing is preferable for a number of reasons, but primarily because the fewer the number of locations where fortificants are added, the easier it is to implement quality control measures; monitoring and enforcement procedures are also likely to be more effective).

- Allow a nutrient premix to be added relatively easily using low-cost technology, and in such a way so as to ensure an even distribution within batches of the product.

- Are used relatively soon after production and purchase. Foods that are purchased and used within a short period of time of processing tend to have better vitamin retention, and fewer sensorial changes due to the need for only a small overage[1].

The choice of fortificant compound is often a compromise between reasonable cost, bioavailability from the diet, and the acceptance of any sensory changes. When selecting the most appropriate chemical form of a given micronutrient, the main considerations and concerns are thus:

- *Sensory problems.* Fortificants must not cause unacceptable sensory problems (e.g. colour, flavour, odour or texture) at the level of intended fortification, or segregate out from the food matrix, and they must be stable within given limits. If additional packaging is needed to improve stability of the added fortificant, it is helpful if this does not add significantly to the cost of the product and make it unaffordable to the consumer.

- *Interactions.* The likelihood or potential for interactions between the added micronutrient and the food vehicle, and with other nutrients (either added or naturally present), in particular any interactions that might interfere with the metabolic utilization of the fortificant, needs to be assessed and checked prior to the implementation of a fortification programme.

- *Cost.* The cost of fortification must not affect the affordability of the food nor its competitivity with the unfortified alternative.

- *Bioavailability.* The fortificant must be sufficiently well absorbed from the food vehicle and be able to improve the micronutrient status of the target population.

Safety is also an important consideration. The level of consumption that is required for fortification to be effective must be compatible with a healthy diet.

The following two chapters consider the above factors in relation to specific micronutrients or micronutrient groups. Chapter 5 deals with iron, vitamin A and iodine; Chapter 6 covers some of the other micronutrients (such as zinc, folate and the other B vitamins, vitamin D and calcium) for which the severity of the public health problem of deficiencies is less well known but is believed to be significant. The discussion is limited to those fortificants and food vehicles that currently are the most widely used, or that have potential for wider application. Details of publications and articles containing more in-depth information about the fortification of foods with specific nutrients are provided in the attached further reading list.

---

[1] Overage is the term used to describe the extra amount of micronutrient that is added to a food vehicle to compensate for losses during production, storage, distribution and selling.

CHAPTER 5
Iron, vitamin A and iodine

5.1 Iron

5.1.1 Choice of iron fortificant

Technically, iron is the most challenging micronutrient to add to foods, because the iron compounds that have the best bioavailability tend to be those that interact most strongly with food constituents to produce undesirable organoleptic changes. When selecting a suitable iron compound as a food fortificant, the overall objective is to find the one that has the greatest absorbability, i.e. the highest relative bioavailability[1] (RBV) compared with ferrous sulfate, yet at the same time does not cause unacceptable changes to the sensory properties (i.e. taste, colour, texture) of the food vehicle. Cost is usually another important consideration.

A wide variety of iron compounds are currently used as food fortificants (**Table 5.1**). These can be broadly divided into three categories: (*224–226*)

— water soluble;

— poorly water soluble but soluble in dilute acid;

— water insoluble and poorly soluble in dilute acid.

5.1.1.1 Water-soluble compounds

Being highly soluble in gastric juices, the water-soluble iron compounds have the highest relative bioavailabilities of all the iron fortificants and for this reason are, more often than not, the preferred choice. However, these compounds are also the most likely to have adverse effects on the organoleptic qualities of foods, in particular, on the colour and flavour. During prolonged storage, the presence of fortificant iron in certain foods can cause rancidity and subsequent off-flavours. Moreover, in the case of multiple fortification, free iron, produced from the degradation of iron compounds present in the food, can oxidize some of the vitamins supplied in the same fortificant mixture.

---

[1] Relative bioavailability is a measure which scores the absorbability of a nutrient by comparing its absorbability to that of a reference nutrient that is considered as having the most efficient absorbability.

TABLE 5.1
Key characteristics of iron compounds commonly used for food fortification purpose: solubility, bioavailability and cost

Compound	Iron content (%)	Relative bioavailability[a]	Relative cost[b] (per mg iron)
Water soluble			
Ferrous sulfate. 7H$_2$O	20	100	1.0
Ferrous sulfate, dried	33	100	1.0
Ferrous gluconate	12	89	6.7
Ferrous lactate	19	67	7.5
Ferrous bisglycinate	20	>100[c]	17.6
Ferric ammonium citrate	17	51	4.4
Sodium iron EDTA	13	>100[c]	16.7
Poorly water soluble, soluble in dilute acid			
Ferrous fumarate	33	100	2.2
Ferrous succinate	33	92	9.7
Ferric saccharate	10	74	8.1
Water insoluble, poorly soluble in dilute acid			
Ferric orthophosphate	29	25–32	4.0
Ferric pyrophosphate	25	21–74	4.7
Elemental iron	–	–	–
H-reduced	96	13–148[d]	0.5
Atomized	96	(24)	0.4
CO-reduced	97	(12–32)	<1.0
Electrolytic	97	75	0.8
Carbonyl	99	5–20	2.2
Encapsulated forms			
Ferrous sulfate	16	100	10.8
Ferrous fumarate	16	100	17.4

EDTA, ethylenediamineteraacetate; H-reduced, hydrogen reduced; CO-reduced, carbon monoxide reduced.
[a] Relative to hydrated ferrous sulfate (FeSO$_4$.7H$_2$O), in adult humans. Values in parenthesis are derived from studies in rats.
[b] Relative to dried ferrous sulfate. Per mg of iron, the cost of hydrated and dry ferrous sulfate is similar.
[c] Absorption is two-three times better than that from ferrous sulfate if the phytate content of food vehicle is high.
[d] The high value refers to a very small particle size which has only been used in experimental studies.

Sources: adapted from references (*224–226*), with additional data supplied by P. Lohmann (cost data) and T. Walczky (ferrous lactate, H-reduced elemental iron).

The water-soluble forms of iron are especially suited to fortifying cereal flours that have a relatively fast turnover, i.e. one month in warm, humid climates and up to 3 months in dry, cold climates. Water-soluble iron compounds are also useful for dry foods, such as pasta and milk powder, as well as dried milk-based infant formulas. Encapsulated forms, i.e. iron compounds that have been coated to physically separate the iron from the other food components, can be used for slowing down or preventing sensory changes.

Ferrous sulfate is by far the most frequently used water-soluble iron fortificant, principally because it is the cheapest. It has been widely used to fortify flour (see *section 5.1.5.1*). However, depending on its physical characteristics, the climate and the fat content of the flour to which it is added, ferrous sulfate can cause rancidity, and therefore its suitability as a fortificant needs to be evaluated in trials before use.

5.1.1.2 Iron compounds that are poorly soluble in water but soluble in dilute acid

Compounds that fall into the second category of iron fortificants (see **Table 5.1**) are also reasonably well absorbed from food, as they are soluble in the gastric acids produced in the stomach of normal healthy adults and adolescents. Some concern has been raised about absorption in infants who may secrete less acid but further research is needed in this area before any firm conclusions can be drawn. In most people, however, with the possible exception of individuals who suffer from a lack of gastric acid due to medical problems, iron absorption from these compounds is likely to be similar to that from water-soluble iron compounds. Poorly water-soluble iron compounds, such as ferrous fumarate, have the advantage of causing fewer sensory problems in foods than the water-soluble compounds, and are generally next in line for consideration, especially if more water-soluble forms cause unacceptable organoleptic changes in the chosen food vehicle.

Ferrous fumarate and ferric saccharate are the most commonly used iron compounds in this group, and in adults are as bioavailable as ferrous sulfate. The former is frequently used to fortify infant cereals and the latter, chocolate drink powders. Ferrous fumarate is used to fortify maize flour in Venezuela and wheat flour in Central America, where it has also been proposed as a potential fortificant for maize masa. Ferrous fumarate can be used in an encapsulated form to limit sensory changes.

5.1.1.3 Iron compounds that are insoluble in water and poorly soluble in dilute acid

Relative to ferrous sulfate, the absorption of iron from water-insoluble compounds ranges from approximately 20% up to 75%. Despite their reduced absorbability, water-insoluble iron compounds have been widely used by the food industry as fortificants because they have far less effect on the sensory properties of foods (at the levels currently used) and because they are cheaper than the more soluble compounds. However, they are generally regarded as the last resort option, especially in settings where the diet of the target population is high in iron absorption inhibitors. If it is necessary to use a water-insoluble iron fortificant, it should ideally have an absorption equivalent to at least 50% that of ferrous sulfate (as measured in rat or human assays), and twice as much would need to be added in order to compensate for the reduced absorption rate.

Within this category of iron fortificants, the ferric phosphate compounds – ferric orthophosphate and ferric pyrophosphate – are used to fortify rice, and some infant cereals and chocolate-containing foods. They have a modest iron bioavailability: the relative bioavailability of ferric pyrophosphate is reported to be 21–74%, and that of ferric orthophosphate, 25–32%. However, the relative bioavailability of the ferric phosphates may change during the processing of a food (227,228).

Elemental iron powders are used in a number of countries to fortify cereals, but the bioavailabilities of the different forms of elemental iron that are currently available (**Table 5.1**) are not well established (229). The solubility of elemental iron is very dependent on the size, shape and surface area of the iron particles (characteristics which are governed by the manufacturing process[1]), as well as the composition of the meals in which it is consumed.

According to the conclusions of the Sharing United States Technology to Aid Improvement of Nutrition (SUSTAIN) Task Force, only electrolytic iron powders (diameter <45 microns or 325 mesh) have been proven to be sufficiently bioavailable to humans (229). At the time of the meeting of the Task Force, the only electrolytic iron powders to have been tested were those manufactured by OMG Americas under the trade name "Glidden 131"[2]. More recent data indicate that carbonyl iron and some hydrogen-reduced (H-reduced) iron powders have comparable bioavailability to electrolytic iron. Atomized iron and carbon monoxide-reduced (CO-reduced) iron are not recommended at the present time because of their lower bioavailability. (Atomized iron is a reduced-iron powder that has been processed by striking a stream of molten iron with high-pressure water jets.) Elemental iron with a large particle size (diameter >149 microns or 100 mesh) is probably too insoluble in the intestine and is therefore not generally recommended for use as a food fortificant. Further testing of the bioavailability of various elemental iron powders is ongoing (42).

5.1.2 Methods used to increase the amount of iron absorbed from fortificants

The bioavailability of iron from fortificants is dependent not only on the solubility of the fortificant as discussed above, but also on the composition of the

---

[1] For more details, please refer to the *Handbook of powder metal technologies and applications (230)*.
[2] At the time of writing, Glidden 131 was still available.

diet, in particular, on the proportion of inhibitors of iron absorption in the diet, notably iron-binding phytates and certain phenolic compounds. The addition of ascorbic acid (vitamin C) or sodium ethylenediaminetetraacetic acid (sodium EDTA or Na_2EDTA) and the removal of phytates, all of which reduce the effect of the inhibitors, can be effective ways of increasing the total amount of iron absorbed from iron-fortified foods.

5.1.2.1 Ascorbic acid

The addition of ascorbic acid causes a substantial increase in the amount of iron absorbed from most iron compounds (40,224). Ascorbic acid addition to iron-fortified foods is thus a widely adopted practice throughout the food industry, especially for processed foods. This option is, however, not recommended for staples and condiments because of stability issues (see *section 5.1.5.1*). For example, Chile fortifies milk powder delivered through its public health programme with both iron and ascorbic acid (as well as some other micronutrients) to control anaemia in infants and young children.

In most studies, the co-addition of ascorbic acid and iron in a 2:1 molar ratio (6:1 weight ratio) increased iron absorption from foods 2- to 3-fold in adults and children (224). This ratio of ascorbic acid to iron is thus recommended for most foods; a higher ascorbic acid:iron molar ratio (4:1) can be used for high-phytate foods. The main problem with using ascorbic acid as a food additive is that substantial amounts can be lost during food storage and preparation. This means that, relative to some of the alternatives, it can be an expensive option.

5.1.2.2 Sodium EDTA

Sodium EDTA is a permitted food additive in many countries, and unlike ascorbic acid, is stable during processing and storage. At low pH (i.e. in the stomach), sodium EDTA acts as a chelating agent, and as such prevents iron from binding to phytic acid or phenolic compounds, which would otherwise inhibit iron absorption (231). Its addition enhances the absorption of both food iron and soluble iron fortificants (232), but not that of the relatively insoluble iron compounds such as ferrous fumarate (233), ferric pyrophosphate (232) or elemental iron (234).

In the case of foods fortified with soluble iron compounds, such as ferrous sulfate, the addition of sodium EDTA in a molar ratio of Na_2EDTA:iron of between 0.5 and 1.0 (between 3.3:1 and 6.6:1 weight ratio) is recommended. Under these circumstances iron absorption is increased by up to 2–3 times (224).

5.1.2.3 Dephytinize cereals and legumes

The phytic acid content of cereals, pulses and legumes can be substantially reduced by several methods (*224*), some of which are particularly suitable for ensuring adequate iron absorption from cereal-based complementary foods or soy-based infant formulas. However, the molar ratio of phytic acid:iron needs to be decreased to at least 1:1, or even to less than 0.5:1, in order to achieve a meaningful increase in iron absorption.

Milling removes about 90% of the phytic acid from cereal grains, but the remaining 10% is still strongly inhibitory. The action of phytases (enzymes) is usually necessary in order to achieve complete phytate degradation. Naturally-occurring cereal phytases can be activated by traditional processes, such as soaking, germination and fermentation. At the industrial level, it is possible to completely degrade phytic acid in complementary food mixtures of cereals and legumes by adding exogenous phytases or by adding whole wheat or whole rye as a source of phytases, these being naturally high in phytases (*224,235–237*). Because of the risk of bacterial contamination, it is better to add the phytases under factory conditions, but as yet, this practice has not been adopted commercially.

5.1.3 Novel iron fortificants

In recent years, considerable effort has been devoted to the development and testing of alternative iron fortificants, in particular, fortificants that provide better protection against iron absorption inhibitors than those currently available. Among those at an experimental stage are sodium iron EDTA (NaFeEDTA), ferrous bisglycinate and various encapsulated and micronized iron compounds. In recent years, NaFeEDTA has been selected as the iron compound to fortify government-led soy sauce fortification and wheat flour fortification programs in China, and fish sauce fortification in Vietnam.

5.1.3.1 Sodium iron EDTA

In high-phytate foods, the absorption of iron from NaFeEDTA is 2–3 times greater than that from either ferrous sulfate or ferrous fumarate. In foods with a low phytate content, however, iron absorption is similar (*231,232*). In addition to better absorption from high-phytate fortified foods, NaFeEDTA offers a number of other advantages: it does not promote lipid oxidation in stored cereals, or the formation of precipitates in foods that are high in free peptides, such as soy sauce and fish sauce. On the down side, it is expensive, and because it is slowly soluble in water, it may cause colour changes in some foods.

The Joint FAO/WHO Expert Committee on Food Additives has approved the use of NaFeEDTA at 0.2 mg Fe/kg body weight per day (*238*). Nevertheless, the use of Na_2EDTA plus ferrous sulfate (or possibly other soluble iron compounds) rather than NaFeEDTA might yet prove to be the better option for high-phytate foods. In most settings, the choice will depend on the relative costs of, and accessibility to, the EDTA compounds, the acceptability of sensory changes in the food, and current legislation.

5.1.3.2 Ferrous bisglycinate

Ferrous bisglycinate is an iron–amino acid chelate in which the iron is protected from the action of absorption inhibitors by being bound to the amino acid, glycine. Absorption from this form of iron has been reported to be 2–3 times better than that from ferrous sulfate in a high-phytate cereal and in whole maize. In contrast, a closely-related compound, ferric trisglycinate, is not well absorbed from maize (*239,240*).

Ferrous bisglycinate seems to be particularly well suited to the fortification of liquid whole milk and other dairy products where use of ferrous sulfate leads to rancid off-flavours. However, ferrous bisglycinate can also cause rancidity by oxidizing fats in food, which can be a problem in cereal flours and weaning cereals unless an antioxidant is added as well. Furthermore, the bisglycinate is much more expensive than many other iron compounds.

5.1.3.3 Encapsulated ferrous sulfate and ferrous fumarate

Several iron compounds are available commercially in encapsulated form, namely ferrous sulfate and ferrous fumarate, and are currently used in dry infant formulas and in infant cereals, predominantly in industrialized countries. In future, use of encapsulated forms of iron compounds may extend to developing countries, although their cost may be a problem. Encapsulation increases costs 3- to 5-fold, which when expressed in terms of iron amounts, is equivalent to a 10-fold increase in cost relative to the use of dried ferrous sulfate (**Table 5.1**).

As previously indicated, the main purpose of encapsulation is to separate the iron from the other food components, thereby mitigating sensory changes. In double fortified salt (i.e. salt fortified with iodine and iron), encapsulation of iron has been shown to help prevent iodine losses and to slow down colour changes.

When developing encapsulated iron fortificants, it is important to select a coating that provides an adequate balance between stability and bioavailability. Iron compounds are usually encapsulated with hydrogenated vegetable oils, but mono- and diglycerides, maltodextrins and ethyl cellulose, have also been used. Because of the different methods of manufacture, and because different capsule materials and thicknesses are possible, it is imperative to confirm bioavailability, at least in rat assays, before widespread use as a fortificant. Tests have shown that encapsulation of ferrous sulfate and ferrous fumarate does not alter iron bioavailability to rats. In addition, dual fortification of salt with encapsulated iron has been found to be efficacious in humans (see section 1.3.2.3) (*44*).

5.1.3.4 Micronized ferric pyrophosphate

Just as the bioavailability of elemental iron powders is increased by reducing their particle size, so too can that of insoluble iron salts, such as ferric pyrophosphate. Micronizing insoluble iron salts to an extremely small submicron particle size cannot, however, be achieved by physical grinding, only by a chemical process.

A micronized form of ferric pyrophosphate (diameter, 0.5 microns) has been developed recently for use as a food fortificant. It is available in both liquid and dried forms. In order to make it dispersible in liquids, the particles of ferric pyrophosphate are coated with emulsifiers. Relative to ordinary ferric pyrophosphate (mean particle size of around 8 microns), iron absorption by adult humans is improved by 2–4 four times in milk products (*241*). Its principal advantage is that, being insoluble in water, it is unlikely to cause many sensory problems, although this remains to be tested adequately. Currently it is added to liquid milk and yoghurt products in Japan, but its more widespread use in the foreseeable future is prohibited by its very high cost.

5.1.4 Sensory changes

In the case of iron fortificants, the two most common problems are increased rancidity due to oxidation of unsaturated lipids and unwanted colour changes. The latter typically include a green or bluish colouration in cereals, a greying of chocolate and cocoa, and darkening of salt to yellow or red/brown.

Sensory changes are highly variable and not always predictable. Just because an iron fortificant does not cause adverse sensory changes to a food product in one situation, does not necessarily mean that the same fortificant will not cause a problem with the same food product in another situation. Thus, having selected a potential iron fortificant, it is essential that its effects on the sensory properties of the food to which it is to be added are determined prior to use.

5.1.5 Experience with iron fortification of specific foods

Iron fortification is already widely practised in many parts of the world. For example, more than 20 countries in Latin America have implemented mass iron fortification programmes, most of which involve the fortification of wheat or maize flours (*237*). Elsewhere, other frequently used food vehicles include cereal-based complementary foods, fish sauce, soy sauce and milk. Salt has also been fortified with iron in efficacy trials. Products derived from cereal flours (e.g. bread, cereal snacks and breakfast cereals) are also useful food vehicles, but the amount of iron provided via this route will depend on the quantity of food

TABLE 5.2
Suggested iron fortificants for specific food vehicles

Food vehicle	Fortificant
Low extraction (white) wheat flour or degermed corn flour	Dry ferrous sulfate
	Ferrous fumarate
	Electrolytic iron (×2 amount)
	Encapsulated ferrous sulfate
	Encapsulated ferrous fumarate
High extraction wheat flour, corn flour, corn masa flour	Sodium iron EDTA
	Ferrous fumarate (×2 amount)
	Encapsulated ferrous sulfate (×2 amount)
	Encapsulated ferrous fumarate (×2 amount)
Pasta	Dry ferrous sulfate
Rice[a]	Ferric pyrophosphate (×2 amount)
Dry milk	Ferrous sulfate plus ascorbic acid
Fluid milk	Ferric ammonium citrate
	Ferrous bisglycinate
	Micronized ferric pyrophosphate
Cocoa products	Ferrous fumarate plus ascorbic acid
	Ferric pyrophosphate (×2 amount) plus ascorbic acid
Salt[a]	Encapsulated ferrous sulfate
	Ferric pyrophosphate (×2 amount)
Sugar[a]	Sodium iron EDTA
Soy sauce, fish sauce	Sodium iron EDTA
	Ferrous sulfate plus citric acid
Juice, soft drinks	Ferrous bisglycinate, ferrous lactate
	Micronized ferric pyrophosphate
Bouillon cubes[a]	Micronized ferric pyrophosphate
Cereal-based complementary foods[b]	Ferrous sulfate
	Encapsulated ferrous sulfate
	Ferrous fumarate
	Electrolytic iron (×2 amount)
	All with ascorbic acid (≥2:1 molar ratio of ascorbic acid: Fe)
Breakfast cereals	Electrolytic iron (×2 amount)

EDTA, ethylenediaminetetraacetic acid.
[a] Technical problems, specifically sensory changes and/or segregation, still exist with the iron fortification of these food vehicles.
[b] Recent evidence has indicated that infants may only absorb ferrous fumarate 25% as well as adults, so concentrations of poorly soluble iron compounds in complementary foods may need to be adjusted to allow for this.

eaten and on the level of fortification. Iron compounds suitable for the fortification of specific food vehicles are listed in **Table 5.2**.

5.1.5.1 Wheat flour

The nutritional usefulness of iron fortification of wheat flour has recently been confirmed in an efficacy study in Thailand (242). In that study the relative efficacy of electrolytic iron as compared to ferrous sulfate was about 70% in women consuming fortified wheat flour cookies, compared to 50% for H-reduced iron. Based on this evidence, adding double the amount of electrolytic iron or H-reduced iron as compared to ferrous sulfate, should give an equivalent efficacy to ferrous sulfate.

Ferrous sulfate and elemental iron powders have traditionally been used to fortify wheat and other cereal flours. Electrolytic iron remains the preferred elemental iron fortificant, however H-reduced iron could also be considered. In addition, recent evidence from rat studies suggests that carbonyl iron may be as good as electrolytic iron as a fortificant, however human efficacy studies are still necessary to confirm this.

Although ferrous sulfate has been successfully used for many years in Chile (where fortified flour is consumed within 6–8 weeks of purchase), and ferrous fumarate has been employed in Venezuela and throughout Central America, in other countries the addition of these iron compounds to wheat flours has caused rancidity. This problem could be overcome by using encapsulated forms to improve stability. Ferrous sulfate, and to a lesser extent ferrous fumarate, are also suitable fortificants for pasta, which, because of its low moisture content, is less susceptible than wheat flour to the development of rancidity.

Although potentially useful for some high-phytate flours, NaFeEDTA has not been used widely in any large-scale iron fortification programmes because of reports that it interferes with the bread fermentation process (*243*). However, China is currently introducing NaFeEDTA to fortify wheat in several provinces, and so far there have been no recorded problems. Although ascorbic acid is often added to iron-fortified foods in order to enhance absorption (see *section 5.1.2.1*), its usefulness in this respect in bread flours is limited by the fact that it is destroyed by the action of heat during baking. Ascorbic acid is nevertheless frequently added to flours, not so much to enhance iron absorption, but rather as a raising agent.

In its guidelines on iron fortification of cereal-based staples, the SUSTAIN Task Force (*42*) recommended the use of ferrous sulfate in preference, followed by ferrous fumarate, and lastly electrolytic iron (but at twice the iron concentration of the other iron compounds). In order to ensure the successful fortification of wheat flour and wheat flour products, it may be necessary for individual countries to adopt different strategies to take account of differences in climate, wheat flour quality, processing methods and storage conditions, as well as differences in the main uses of flour (i.e. to make bread or other foods).

5.1.5.2 Maize

In general, maize flours are equally, if not more difficult, to fortify with iron than wheat flours. Lime-treated (nixtamalized) corn masa, a staple used to make tortillas in much of Latin America, goes rancid when soluble iron compounds, such as ferrous sulfate, are added to it. Further colour and texture changes occur during the preparation of tortillas. The difficulties are further compounded by the fact that iron absorption from corn masa is strongly inhibited by its high phytate and high calcium content. For these reasons, iron fortification of maize flours has not been widely adopted, except in a number of Latin American countries where the consumption of maize is high. In Venezuela, for example, ferrous fumarate mixed with elemental iron is used to fortify maize flours.

In view of its highly inhibitory nature (especially if it is not degermed), the Pan American Health Organization (PAHO) recently recommended the use of either NaFeEDTA or ferrous fumarate (at twice the amount) for maize flour fortification (*237*). These recommendations have yet to be put into practice. Whether or not they are appropriate for maize meal that is used to prepare porridge also needs to be evaluated. For maize flours that are not high in phytic acid (e.g. degermed) and are not lime-treated, the same iron compounds as those recommended for the fortification of white wheat flour can be considered (*237*).

5.1.5.3 Cereal-based complementary foods

Complementary foods (i.e. foods intended for infants during the weaning period) are usually based on dry cereals and consumed as a porridge or gruel with milk or water. Alternatively, they are based on blends of cereals and legumes, which again can be made into a porridge or gruel with water. The addition of ferrous sulfate, ferrous bisglycinate and other soluble iron compounds to these products can cause rancidity, and sometimes colour changes as well, particularly if the porridges are fed with fruits. To overcome such problems, one option would be to use encapsulated forms, such as ferrous sulfate. Although encapsulation helps to prevent fat oxidation during storage, the capsule is removed by hot milk or water, and off-colours may still develop in the presence of some fruits and vegetables.

Another option is to use a less soluble iron fortificant, such as ferrous fumarate or electrolytic iron (but at a higher concentration), both of which are commonly used to fortify complementary foods. Ferric pyrophosphate is another possibility, although it is rarely used in practice. If ferric pyrophosphate were to be used to fortify complementary foods, it too should be added at twice the concentration (relative to ferrous sulfate). Recent evidence has indicated that ferrous fumarate may be less well absorbed in children than in adults (absorption of iron from ferrous fumarate by children may only be 25% of that by adults) and so its use as a fortificant, or at least its level of addition, may need to be re-evaluated (*244*).

In order to enhance iron absorption, ascorbic acid is usually added together with the iron compound to complementary foods whenever possible (see section

5.1.2.1). Ideally, ascorbic acid and iron should be added in at least a 2:1 molar ratio (ascorbic acid:iron). Dry complementary foods should also be packaged in such as way as to minimize ascorbic acid degradation during storage. As described above (see *section 5.1.2.3*), another useful way of optimizing iron absorption from cereal-based foods is to degrade any phytic acid present with naturally-occurring cereal phytases (i.e. activate those already in the food by soaking, germinating or fermenting) or by adding microbial phytases during manufacture. However, the addition of phytases to processed foods has yet to be attempted on a commercial scale.

5.1.5.4 Dairy products

Dried whole milk powders and dried or ready-to-feed milk-based infant formulas can be successfully fortified with ferrous sulfate (together with ascorbic acid to enhance absorption). In Chile, for example, ascorbic acid (700 mg/kg) and iron (100 mg as ferrous sulfate/kg) are routinely added to dried milk powders consumed by infants. In the case of soy formulas, it has been found necessary to use ferrous sulfate encapsulated with maltodextrin in order to prevent unwanted colour changes (i.e. darkening).

Ferrous sulfate, and many other soluble iron compounds, cannot be used to fortify liquid whole milk and other dairy products because they cause rancidity and off-flavours. Ferric ammonium citrate (*245*), ferrous bisglycinate and micronized ferric pyrophosphate are generally more suitable for this purpose. Iron fortificants are best added after the milk has been homogenized and the fat internalized in micelles, so as to help protect against oxidation. Ferrous bisglycinate is widely used to fortify whole milk and dairy products in Brazil and Italy; micronized ferric pyrophosphate is added to dairy products in Japan (see also *section 5.1.3.4*).

5.1.5.5 Rice

The fortification of rice grains presents a number of technical challenges. It can be achieved, as is done in the United States, by coating the grain with an appropriate formulation. Alternatively, a rice-based extruded grain that contains a high concentration of iron can be mixed with normal rice grains (usually at a ratio of 1:200). Ferric pyrophosphate, added at a two-fold higher level, and micronized, ferric pyrophosphate (0.5 micron) have recently been recommended for adding to extruded artificial rice grains (*246*).

Technical difficulties, combined with cultural preferences for specific types of rice, mean that mass fortification of rice, although desirable, remains problematic. The fact that in most of the big rice-producing countries, production takes place in thousands of small mills, also creates problems for mass rice fortification. Not only are smaller mills sensitive to small increases in costs, the sheer number of them makes it difficult to maintain adequate quality control programmes. Although the extruded grains have found some application in targeted food fortification programmes, such as school feeding programmes, much more research and development is required before mass rice fortification programmes can be implemented on a wider scale.

5.1.5.6 Cocoa products

As cocoa is naturally high in phenolic compounds, the addition of ferrous sulfate and other water-soluble iron compounds tends to cause colour changes in cocoa-based products (*247*). Ferrous fumarate is a useful alternative for some products, but grey or blue/grey colours are still a problem for chocolate drinks, especially if boiling water is used to make up the drink (*227*). Furthermore, the currently available encapsulated iron compounds are not useful for chocolate drink fortification as the capsules are removed by heat either during product manufacture or during preparation of the drink.

Ferric pyrophosphate, ferric saccharate or ferric orthophosphate are usually used to fortify cocoa products as these tend to produce fewer off-colours. However, relative to ferrous sulfate, larger amounts of these iron compounds would need to be added to allow for their lower absorption. Ascorbic acid addition is also required (in at least a 2:1 molar ratio) in order to offset the inhibitory effects of cocoa phenolics on iron absorption (*227,248*).

5.1.5.7 Soy sauce and fish sauce

Sodium iron EDTA has proved to be a useful fortificant for both fish sauce and soy sauce (see also *section 1.3.1*). Studies have demonstrated that absorption of iron by human subjects fed NaFeEDTA-fortified fish or soy sauce added to rice meals is similar to that from the same meals to which ferrous sulfate-fortified sauces had been added (*249*). The iron status of iron-deficient Vietnamese women improved significantly following regular intakes of NaFeEDTA-fortified fish sauce over a period of 6 months (*28*) (see also *section 1.3.1.1*). Similarly, in trials conducted in China, NaFeEDTA soy sauce, providing 20 mg iron per day, significantly improved the iron status of anaemic adolescents (*250*). Large-scale effectiveness studies of soy sauce fortification with NaFeEDTA are currently underway in both Viet Nam and China.

Until very recently, NaFeEDTA has been the preferred iron fortificant for soy and fish sauces because most of the potential alternatives (i.e. other soluble iron compounds) cause peptide precipitation during storage. However, latterly ferrous sulfate stabilized with citric acid has been successfully used to fortify fish sauce in Thailand, and may offer a less expensive alternative to NaFeEDTA.

5.1.5.8 Salt

The success of salt iodization programmes (see *section 5.3.2.1*) has led several countries to consider using salt as a vehicle for iron fortification. In practice, this means the double fortification of salt, i.e. with iron and iodine. Promising approaches that are already being tested include the addition of encapsulated ferrous fumarate, encapsulated ferrous sulfate (see *section 1.3.2.3*) or ferric pyrophosphate (at twice the concentration). Encapsulation is necessary as ferrous sulfate, ferrous fumarate and other soluble iron compounds very quickly cause a yellow or red/brown discoloration in the moist, low quality salt that is currently used in many developing countries. The main disadvantage of the encapsulation options is the increase in the price of the fortified product, which can be by as much as 30%.

5.1.6 Safety issues

Concern has been raised about increased iron intakes, particularly in terms of the potential effects on infection rates and on the risk of cardiovascular disease and cancer. Much of this concern, however, relates to the use of pharmaceutical iron supplements and not to fortified foods.

A recent review of intervention studies with iron-fortified milk or cereals, concluded that iron fortification did not increase infectious morbidity in children under 18 months of age (*251*). Studies in Chile (*252*), Hungary (*253*) and South Africa (*254*) reported that iron added to milk formula had no influence on infectious outcome. Only one study, conducted in a poor community in Chile, reported an increase in episodes of diarrhoea in young infants fed iron-fortified formula (*255*). On balance, studies have indicated that iron fortification of milk formula is safe (*251*).

It has been suggested that higher levels of iron intake and elevated body stores are potential risk factors for both coronary heart disease (CHD) and cancer. Results from studies carried out over the last 10 years to test this hypothesis are, however, inconclusive. The association between serum ferritin and risk of CHD has been examined in at least 12 studies, but a meta-analysis of such evidence failed to establish a strong relationship between the two (*256*). Inflammatory response is an important risk factor for CHD and also increases serum ferritin, which might explain why an association between the risk of CHD and increased serum ferritin is sometimes observed.

Possible links between cancer and iron intake or iron status have been the subject of only a few studies, but are largely unsubstantiated. It has been hypothesized that the presence of unabsorbed fortificant iron in the body, much of which reaches the colon, leads to free radical generation that damages the colon mucosa (*257*). However, iron is highly insoluble at the pH of the colon, and although unabsorbed ferrous sulfate can increase free radical generation in the stool (*257*), there is no evidence to suggest that the free radicals survive long enough to cause tissue damage. The finding that serum transferrin was higher in men who developed colon cancer (*258*) was not confirmed when the follow-up was extended to 17 years.

Summary: iron fortification

- For most food vehicles, the recommended iron fortificants, in order of preference, are: ferrous sulfate, ferrous fumarate, encapsulated ferrous sulfate or fumarate, electrolytic iron (at twice the amount), and ferric pyrophosphate (at twice the amount).

- The co-addition of ascorbic acid in a 2:1 molar ratio is recommended in order to enhance iron absorption. This applies to infant foods and market-driven foods. In the case of high phytic acid foods, the molar ratio (ascorbic acid:iron) can be increased to 4:1.

- NaFeEDTA is recommended for the mass fortification of high-phytate cereal flours and for sauces with a high peptide content (e.g. fish sauce, soy sauce).

- For liquid milk products, ferrous bisglycinate, micronized ferric pyrophosphate and ferric ammonium citrate are the most appropriate fortificants.

5.2 Vitamin A and β-carotene

5.2.1 Choice of vitamin A fortificant

The choice of a vitamin A fortificant is largely governed by the characteristics of the food vehicle, as well as various technological, regulatory and religious considerations. As preformed vitamin A (retinol) is an unstable compound, in commercial preparations it is esterified, usually with palmitic or acetic acid, to the more stable corresponding esters. Retinyl acetate and retinyl palmitates, along with provitamin A (β-carotene), are thus the main commercial forms of vitamin A that are available for use as food fortificants. The intense orange colour of β-carotene makes it unsuitable for use as a fortificant in many foods, but it is widely used to give an orange-yellow colour to margarines and beverages.

Since vitamin A is fat-soluble, it is easily added to fat-based or oily foods. When the food vehicle is either dry or a water-based liquid, an encapsulated form of the vitamin is needed. Based on this distinction, vitamin A fortificants can be divided into two categories:

- Oily forms that can be incorporated directly into fat-based foods or emulsified into water-based ones (e.g. milk).

- Dry forms that can be dry mixed into foods or dispersed in water, depending on whether they are cold water dispersible or non-cold water dispersible.

TABLE 5.3

Commercially available forms of vitamin A, their characteristics and their main applications

Product	Characteristics	Application(s)
Oily vitamin A acetate	Retinol ester of acetic acid which may be stabilized with antioxidants	Fortification of fat-based foods, especially margarine and dairy products
Oily vitamin A palmitate	Retinol ester of palmitic acid which may be stabilized with antioxidants	Fortification of fat-based foods, especially margarine and dairy products
Oily vitamin A palmitate or acetate with vitamin D_3	Retinol ester and cholecalciferol mix, stabilized with antioxidants	Fortification of fat-based foods, especially margarine and dairy products where the combination of both vitamins is required
Dry vitamin A palmitate or acetate	Vitamin A embedded in a water-soluble matrix (e.g. gelatin, gum acacia, starch) and stabilized with antioxidants	Fortification of dry food products, (i.e. flour and dry milk, beverage powders) and fortification of water-based foods
Dry vitamin A palmitate or acetate with vitamin D_3	Vitamin A and vitamin D_3 embedded in a water-soluble matrix (e.g. gelatin, gum acacia, starch) and stabilized with antioxidants	Fortification of dry food products, (i.e. flour and dry milk, beverage powders) and fortification of water-based foods

Source: Hector Cori, personal communication, 2004.

Pure vitamin A and β-carotene in solution are unstable when exposed to ultraviolet light, oxygen or air. Thus all forms of vitamin A – oily or dried – are protected with antioxidants to prolong their shelf-life. The use of airtight packaging provides further protection. For example, the loss of vitamin A in sealed cans of oil is minimal, but losses from fortified cereals, fortified sugar or oil can be as high as 40%, depending on ambient conditions and storage times (*259–261*). Opaque packaging is indispensable for maintaining stability in vitamin A-fortified oils.

The characteristics and applications of the various forms of vitamin A are listed in **Table 5.3**. Each formulation includes stabilizers, and each is compatible with existing food regulations (e.g. contain permitted antioxidants) and/or religious requirements (e.g. Kosher, Halal). The fat-soluble forms of retinol are about one half to one third as expensive as the dry forms. Appropriate vitamin A fortificants for specific foods are given in **Table 5.4**.

5.2.2 Experience with vitamin A fortification of specific foods

Of the food vehicles suitable for mass fortification, margarine is the one that is most frequently associated with vitamin A. In both industrialized and

TABLE 5.4
Vitamin A fortificants and their suitability as fortificants for specific food vehicles

Food vehicle	Form of vitamin A	Stability
Cereal flours	Retinyl acetate or retinyl palmitate (dry stabilized forms)	Fair
Fats and oils	β-carotene and retinyl acetate or retinyl palmitate (oil-soluble)	Good
Sugar	Retinyl palmitate (water dispersible forms)	Fair
Milk powder	Retinyl acetate or palmitate (dry water dispersible forms)	Good
Liquid milk	Retinyl acetate (preferred) or palmitate (oily form, emulsified)	Good/fair depending on packaging
Infant formula	Retinyl palmitate (water dispersible beadlets)	Good
Spreads	Retinyl acetate or palmitate (oily form)	Good

Source: Hector Cori, personal communication, 2004.

developing countries, vegetable oils are also used, and, in recent years, cereal flours have increasingly been fortified with vitamin A in several parts of the world. In parts of Central America, sugar is often the preferred food vehicle for vitamin A. The amount and forms of vitamin A used in a selection of food fortification programmes are detailed in **Table 5.5**. It is estimated that about 90% of fortificant vitamin A will usually be absorbed (262).

5.2.2.1 Oils and margarine

There are two reasons why margarines and oils are the ideal foods for vitamin A fortification. Not only is the oil-soluble form of the vitamin the cheapest available, but the oil protects the vitamin A from oxidation during storage and so facilitates absorption of the vitamin (264). The vitamin A fortification of margarines has a relatively long history, having been introduced in some countries as early as the 1920s, following the realization that the replacement of butter with margarine in the diet was causing widespread xerophthalmia in children (265). Vitamin A fortification of margarine in Newfoundland, Canada, for example, resulted in a marked improvement in vitamin A status (266). Likewise, in India, a hydrogenated oil (vanaspati), which is used as an alternative to ghee, has been fortified with vitamin A since 1953 (267).

Although the technology for adding vitamin A to oils is simple and inexpensive, and oils are widely used, the fortification of oils with this vitamin is relatively rare, at least compared with that of margarines. The fortification of oils is thus a potentially useful means of expanding the present range of vitamin A-fortified foods. Stability may be a problem in some settings; experimental studies have shown that when vitamin A is added to soybean oil in sealed cans, the

TABLE 5.5
Examples of vitamin A fortification programmes

Food item	Country or programme	Amount of retinol added (mg/kg)	Form of vitamin A added	Amount of food consumed (g/day)	Contribution to recommended daily intake (%)
Margarine	Philippines	25	Retinyl palmitate (oil)	24 (preschool-aged children)	150[a]
Margarine	Various	1–15	Retinyl palmitate (oil)	15	2–40[a]
Vegetable oil (PL–480)	US Food Aid	18	Retinyl palmitate (oil)	16	50[a]
Hydrogenated fat	India, Pakistan	7.5	Retinyl palmitate (oil)	0.3–17	0.4–21[a]
Maize flour	Venezuela	2.7	Retinyl palmitate (dry)	80	30
Wheat flour	Philippines	4.5	Retinyl palmitate (dry)	40 (bread)	19[a]
Wheat flour	US Food Aid	6.6–7.9	Retinyl palmitate (dry)	75	80–100[a]
Sugar	Guatemala	15	Retinyl palmitate (dry)	30–120 (average, 60) (adults)	45–180 (adults)
				20–30 (young children)	30 (<3 years)

[a] Assuming no losses during shipping, storage or food preparation. Unless otherwise stated, the contribution to the recommended nutrient intake (RNI) is based on an RNI for an adult male, which is 600 µg/day.

Source: adapted from reference (263).

vitamin was stable for up to 9 months. However, although less than 15% of the vitamin A was lost during boiling or pressure cooking of rice or beans, about 60% was lost when the oil was reused several times for frying (*260*).

There has been little systematic evaluation of the effectiveness of margarine and oil fortification, although historical data from Europe suggest that it has been effective in controlling vitamin A deficiency. In the Philippines, consumption of "Star margarine", which is fortified with 25 mg vitamin A/kg plus 3.5 mg β-carotene/kg, significantly reduced the prevalence of low serum retinol. PL-480 vegetable oil, which is distributed in emergency feeding programmes, is intended to provide about 50% of the recommended daily intake of vitamin A for an adult male (assuming a daily intake of 16 g per person) (see **Table 5.5**). The stability of vitamin A in previously unopened pails of PL-480 oil is excellent, although up to 30% losses can occur in opened pails after 30 days of storage. Vitamin A retention in the oil is also good, with only a 10% loss after 30 minutes of heating (*268*).

5.2.2.2 Cereals products and flours

Wholegrain cereals and flours contain negligible, if any, amounts of intrinsic vitamin A. Flours are, nevertheless, potentially good vehicles for vitamin A fortification, because dry forms of vitamin A can easily be mixed in with other additives. Despite this, cereal flours are not fortified with vitamin A in most industrialized countries, because, for historical reasons, margarines are the preferred vehicle and, furthermore, because vitamin A deficiency is no longer a significant problem. The United States Title II Food Aid Program has been fortifying wheat-soy and corn-soy blends with vitamin A for about 30 years; working on the assumption that the recipients are likely to be highly dependent on these fortified foods for their vitamin A needs, it adds sufficient amounts to provide 100% of the recommended daily intake of this particular vitamin (*269*). However, between 30% and 50% of the vitamin A that is added to the blended cereals is lost in shipping and storage (*268,270*).

Wheat flour is fortified with 4.5 mg retinol/kg in some mills in the Philippines, a practice which provides an average concentration in bread of 2.2 µg retinol/g (**Table 5.5**). This supplies about 33% of the recommended daily intake for vitamin A for school-age children. At this level of fortification, retinol liver stores in deficient children were significantly increased at the end of a 30-week efficacy trial (*33*) (see also *section 1.3.1.2*).

Pre-cooked maize flour has been fortified with vitamin A in Venezuela since 1993 (**Table 5.5**). A fortification level of 2.7 mg/kg and an intake of 80 g flour/day supplies about 40% of an average family's recommended intake (*271*). However, the impact of maize fortification on the vitamin A status of the general population is not known.

5.2.2.3 Sugar

In the 1970s, vitamin A fortification of sugar was implemented in Costa Rica and Guatemala, because it was the only centrally processed food vehicle that was consumed in adequate amounts by the poorer segments of the population. Such programmes ceased for a time during the 1980s but are again functioning Guatemala, and also in El Salvador, Honduras and Nicaragua where they receive strong support from the sugar industry (*272*). An early evaluation of vitamin A fortification of sugar in Guatemala showed that it is an effective strategy for improving vitamin A status and for increasing the amount of the vitamin in breast milk of lactating mothers (*273*) (see also *section 1.3.2.4*). Fortified sugar in Guatemala provides children with about one third of their recommended intake of vitamin A (*274*) (**Table 5.5**). Sugar fortification is now being implemented in other parts of the world, such as Zambia.

Large quantities of sugar are used in a wide range of commercial foods, such as confectionery and soft drinks. Retinol in fortified unrefined sugar survives the baking process but is lost during soft-drink production (in fortified unrefined sugar only one third of the initial level remains after 2 weeks of storage). Depending on the level of soft drink production, these losses can have important cost implications and it may be appropriate for the soft drink sector to be exempt from having to use fortified sugar (*275*).

5.2.2.4 Rice

Given that rice is an important staple in many countries where the prevalence of vitamin A deficiency is high, vitamin A fortification of rice has the potential to be an effective public health strategy for the elimination of VAD. However, as is the case with iron, for technical reasons, rice fortification with vitamin A is still at an experimental stage. Again, the predominance of small-scale mills in the rice-producing countries hinders the implementation of fortification programmes using rice as the chosen food vehicle.

5.2.2.5 Other foods and beverages

Other foods that have been fortified successfully with preformed or provitamin A include:

— dry milk;

— complementary foods for infants and young children;

— biscuits and beverages, which are sold commercially or used in school feeding programmes such as those implemented in Indonesia, Mexico and other countries in Central America (*276*), (*277*), Peru (*278*) and South Africa (*34*);

— instant noodles (in Thailand), the vitamin A (and elemental iron[1]) being supplied in the spices that are provided in a separate sachet (*279*);

— yoghurt (worldwide) (*280*).

5.2.3 Safety issues

Adverse physiological effects have been associated with both acute hypervitaminosis A and chronic high intake. The routine consumption of large amounts of vitamin A over a period of time can result in a variety of toxic symptoms including liver damage, bone abnormalities and joint pain, alopecia, headaches, vomiting and skin desquamation (*93*).

For long-term daily intakes, the United States Institute of Medicine's Food and Nutrition Board (IOM/FNB) have defined Tolerable Upper Intake Levels (ULs) for vitamin A, as follows (*91*):

— 600 µg/day for children <3 years,

— 900 µg/day for children 4–8 years,

— 1700 µg/day for children 9–13 years,

— 2800 µg/day for adolescents,

— 3000 µg/day for both women at risk of becoming pregnant and adult men.

The UL for children, i.e. the highest level of daily vitamin A intake that is likely to pose no risk of adverse health effects, is a factor of 10 lower than the level of intake at which any toxic effect has been observed in this age group.

The ULs as defined by the United States Food and Nutrition Board are based on data obtained from healthy populations in developed countries. They may not apply, nor are intended to do so, to communities of malnourished individuals that receive vitamin A prophylactically, either periodically or through fortification, as a means of preventing vitamin A deficiency. A recent review has indicated that the risk of excessive vitamin A consumption from fortified foods in women and young children is likely to be negligible (*281*), but that it is nevertheless a matter that deserves attention as many foods are increasingly being fortified with vitamin A.

β-Carotene and other provitamin A carotenoids are less of a concern in terms of potential toxicity, not being active forms of the vitamin and because at high doses they are absorbed less efficiently (*91*). Furthermore, the synthesis of vitamin A from β-carotene and other provitamin A carotenoids is strictly regulated in the body. Hypervitaminosis A has never been reported as a result of provitamin A supplementation.

---

[1] Elemental iron is used because more soluble iron compounds would give the spices a black colour.

Summary: vitamin A fortification

■ A variety of oily and dry forms of the retinol esters, retinyl acetate and retinyl palmitate, are available for food fortification purposes. The dry forms are usually gelatin-, starch- or gum-coated and all forms contain antioxidants.

■ Absorption of all forms is good (around 90%) but losses of vitamin A during processing, storage and food preparation may be high.

■ Vitamin A fortification of margarine and sugar has been shown to be efficacious. Vegetable oils and cereal flours are also considered to be useful fortification vehicles.

■ Adverse health effects have been associated with acute and chronic high intakes of retinol (mainly through supplementation) but not with high intakes of the pro-vitamin A carotenoids.

TABLE 5.6

Iodine fortificants: chemical composition and iodine content

Fortificant	Formula	Iodine content (%)
Calcium iodide	CaI_2	86.5
Calcium iodate	$Ca(IO_3)_2.6H_2O$	65.0
Potassium iodide	KI	76.5
Potassium iodate	KIO_3	59.5
Sodium iodide	$NaI.2H_2O$	68.0
Sodium iodate	$NaIO_3$	64.0

5.3 Iodine

5.3.1 Choice of iodine fortificant

There are two chemical forms of iodine that are suitable for use as food fortificants, namely, iodate and iodide. They are usually added as the potassium salt, but sometimes as the calcium or sodium salt (**Table 5.6**).

Potassium iodide has been used as an additive in bread and salt for about 80 years, and potassium iodate for about 50 years. Iodates are less soluble in water than the iodides, more resistant to oxidation and evaporation, and being more stable under adverse climatic conditions, do not require the co-addition of stabilizers. Although more expensive, potassium iodate is thus preferred to potassium iodide, especially in hot and humid climates, and is recommended as an additive for many foods, including salt (*282,283*). For historical reasons, however, countries in Europe and North America still use potassium iodide, while most countries with tropical climates use potassium iodate. Losses of iodine because of iodide oxidation are increased by moisture, humidity, exposure to heat and sunlight, or by impurities in the salt to which it is added.

5.3.2 Experience with iodine fortification of specific foods

5.3.2.1 Salt

Salt is the most widely used food vehicle for iodine fortificants. Indeed, universal salt iodization (USI), that is, the iodization of all salt for human (food industry and household) and livestock consumption, is the strategy recommended by WHO for the control of iodine deficiency disorders (284). The choice of this strategy is based on the following factors:

— salt is one of the few commodities consumed by everyone;

— salt consumption is fairly stable throughout the year;

— salt production is usually limited to a few geographical areas;

— salt iodization technology is easy to implement and available at reasonable cost throughout the developing world (0.2–0.3 US cents/kg, or 1 US cent per person/year);

— the addition of iodine to salt does not affect its colour, taste or odour;

— the quality of iodized salt can be monitored at the production, retail and household levels.

The mining of solid rock deposits is the main source of salt in Australia, Europe and North America. Elsewhere, i.e. in Africa, Asia and South America, solar evaporation of either sea water, lake or underground brines is the main source. After extraction, crude salt is refined so that its purity increases from 85–95% NaCl to 99% NaCl. Specifications for the physical characteristics and chemical composition required for food grade salt are laid down in the Codex Alimentarius (285).

Iodine is usually added to salt after the salt has been refined and dried, by one of two main techniques. In the wet method, a solution of potassium iodate (KIO_3) is either dripped or sprayed at a uniform rate onto salt passing by on a conveyor belt. The technique is particularly cost-effective. For instance, in Switzerland, a single conveyor belt and sprayer produces enough salt for 6 million people at a cost of 1 US$ per 100 kg salt or 7 US cents per person per year (286). The alternative method, the dry method, involves sprinkling potassium iodide powder (KI) or potassium iodate (KIO_3) over the dry salt. This technique is more demanding, in that it requires a salt made of small homogenous crystals and the thorough mixing of the salt after addition of the iodine compound to ensure an even distribution of iodine. Poor mixing is a major cause of inappropriate salt iodization. Technical information on the salt iodization process is available elsewhere (287).

The stability of iodine in salt depends on the water content, acidity and purity of the salt to which it is added. In order to reduce iodine losses during storage, the iodized salt must be as pure and as dry as possible, and it must be appropriately packaged. Iodine tends to migrate from the top to the bottom of a container when the water content is too high. It will evaporate if the acidity is too high. Losses also tend to occur when packaging with impervious linings is used; as the packaging becomes damp, the iodide migrates from the salt to the fabric, and then evaporates. This is less likely to happen with potassium iodate because the iodates are less soluble and more resistant to oxidation. Types of packaging that help to prevent iodine losses include high density polyethylene bags that are either laminated with low density polyethylene or lined with a continuous film that is resistant to puncture. In a multi-country study of iodine losses from salt, high humidity combined with porous packing (such as jute bags), caused a 30–80% loss of iodine over a period of 6 months (288).

Because salt iodization is cheap and easy to implement, great strides in salt iodization programmes have been made in a relatively short period of time (**Table 5.7**). During the 10-year period, 1989 to 1999, the proportion of households consuming iodized salt increased from 10% to 68% and by 1999, of 130 countries affected by iodine deficiency, 98 had in place legislation requiring the iodization of salt (284). Several factors have limited progress towards the goal of USI; these include difficulties in enforcing legislation on iodized salt; problems caused by having a high number of small-scale salt producers and the absence of an operational monitoring system. The existence of pockets of populations living in remote areas that cannot easily access iodized salt is another factor which can hinder the effective implementation of salt iodization programmes and their sustainability in some countries. In order to assist countries

TABLE 5.7

Progress towards universal salt iodization in WHO regions, status as of 1999

WHO region	Coverage (% of households)	No. of countries with legislation on iodized salt
Africa	63	34
Americas	90	17
South-East Asia	70	7
Europe	27	20
Eastern Mediterranean	66	14
Western Pacific	76	6
Total	68	98

Sources: adapted from references (284,289).

develop and sustain effective salt iodization programmes, several international organizations, including WHO, have jointly established a mechanism for strengthening national capacity in activities that support salt iodization, in particular, quality assurance and monitoring. The work of the International Resource Laboratory for Iodine network (IRLI), which includes training and technology transfer and information sharing, is outlined in more detail in **Annex B**.

5.3.2.2 Bread

From a technical point of view, bread is a good vehicle for iodine and has been shown to be an effective way of ensuring a constant supply of dietary iodine. It has been used in a few European countries where bread is a staple food, such as Russia (*290,291*), and in Tasmania. The main carrier for iodine in the Netherlands is the salt added to bread, i.e. baker's salt, which has been enriched with iodine since 1942. In recent years, the potassium iodide content of Dutch baker's salt has been increased.

5.3.2.3 Water

Because water is consumed daily, it too has the potential to be a useful vehicle for iodine fortification. Its major limitation, compared with salt, is that sources of drinking water are so numerous and ubiquitous that iodization would be difficult to control. Moreover, iodine has limited stability in water (no longer than 24 hours) such that continuous daily dosing of the water supply would be necessary. Although the use of water as a vehicle for iodine fortification is technically more difficult than the use of salt, there are certain conditions where water iodization could be a suitable method for the correction of iodine deficiency.

The simplest way of fortifying water with iodine is to add a concentrated iodine solution (as potassium iodide or iodate) in a dropwise fashion until a specified concentration in the water contained in a given vessel is reached. This method is widely used in schools in northern Thailand (*292*). Alternatively, in the case of hand pumps and open wells, iodine in porous polymer containers can be introduced into the water supply. The porous containers allow the slow release of potassium iodide solution into the water supply. However, such containers have a limited shelf-life and must be changed every year. Such practices have been successful in several parts of the world; in Africa, in the Central African Republic, Mali (*293*) and Sudan (*294*), in Asia, in the central Asian republics, Malaysia (*295*) and Thailand and in Europe, in Italy (Sicily). In most settings, the limiting factor, especially in terms of cost-effectiveness, is that the whole population and the livestock need to use the iodized water supply point to benefit from iodization (*296*). A third option, which is suitable for piped water supplies, is to divert some of the piped water through a canister packed with iodine crystals, and then reintroduce this iodized water back into the main water supply. The direct addition of an iodine solution to freshwater supplies has also been attempted. For instance, a 5% potassium iodate solution was introduced into the single river which supplied water to an isolated population in China for a period of 12–24 days (297). The result was an improvement in urinary iodine of children, and a relatively stable increase in soil iodine.

A review of the efficacy and cost-effectiveness of the different procedures used to iodize water concluded that while efficacious for the most part, there is no doubt that the cost, and the monitoring systems needed, are more problematic than those required for iodized salt (296).

5.3.2.4 Milk

Iodine-enriched milk has been instrumental in the control of iodine deficiency in several countries. However, this has been largely a consequence of the use of iodophors by the dairy industry rather than the result of a deliberate addition of iodine to milk. Iodine-enriched milk has become a major adventitious source of iodine in many countries in northern Europe, as well as in the United Kingdom (298) and the United States. Use of iodized bread in Tasmania was discontinued when other sources of iodine, notably milk (consequent to the use of iodophors by the dairy industry), became available.

5.3.2.5 Other vehicles

The feasibility of using sugar as a vehicle for iodine fortification has been assessed in pilot studies in Sudan (299), and that of fish sauce in south-east Asia where it is a major source of dietary sodium (i.e. salt). Besides fortifying table salt (300). Finland fortifies its animal fodders and as a result the iodine content of foods derived from animal sources has increased.

5.3.3 Safety issues

Iodine fortification is generally very safe. Iodine has been added to salt and bread for more than 50 years without any notable toxic effects (301). At its fifty-third meeting in 1999, the Joint FAO/WHO Expert Committee on Food Additives concluded that potassium iodate and potassium iodide could continue to be used to fortify salt for the prevention and control of iodine deficiency disorders (238). Because the synthesis and release of thyroid hormones is usually well regulated, through mechanisms that enable the body to adjust to a wide range of iodine intakes, intakes of up to 1 mg (1000 µg) per day are tolerated by most people.

Nevertheless, an acute, excessive increase in iodine intake can increase the risk of iodine toxicity in susceptible individuals, that is, those who have had chronic iodine deficiency. This condition is known as iodine-induced hyperthyroidism (IIH) and it is the most common complication of iodine prophylaxis. Outbreaks have been associated with almost all iodine supplementation programmes *(302)*; it tends to occur in the early phase of programme implementation and mainly affects the elderly who have long-standing thyroid nodules. IIH is, however, usually transitory in nature and its incidence rate reverts to normal levels after 1–10 years of intervention.

Outbreaks of IIH, which were subsequently attributed to the sudden introduction of excessively iodized salt in populations who had been severely iodine deficient for very long periods, have recently been reported from the Democratic Republic of the Congo *(303)* and Zimbabwe *(304)*. Such reports would appear to indicate that IIH could occur if salt is excessively iodized *(305)*. If an outbreak of IIH was to occur following the introduction of iodized salt, it would be expected to follow a similar pattern to that observed during iodine supplementation programmes, that is, manifest early on in the history of the programme and predominantly among the elderly. IIH prevention requires the monitoring of salt iodization levels and the iodine status of the population, coupled with proper training of health staff in the identification and treatment of IIH *(306)*.

Iodine-induced thyroiditis is another condition that can be aggravated or even induced by increasing iodine intakes *(307)*. To date, there have been no large-scale investigations of the impact of iodine intervention programmes on iodine-induced thyroiditis.

Summary: iodine fortification

- Universal salt iodization, that is, the iodization of all salt for both human and animal consumption, is the strategy recommended by WHO to correct iodine deficiency.

- Potassium iodate is preferred to potassium iodide for salt iodization because it is more stable.

- The benefits of correcting iodine deficiency far outweigh the potential risks of fortification. Iodine-induced hyperthroidism and other potential adverse effects can be almost entirely avoided by adequate and sustained quality assurance and monitoring of iodine fortification.

CHAPTER 6
Zinc, folate and other B vitamins, vitamin C, vitamin D, calcium, selenium and fluoride

6.1 Zinc

6.1.1 Choice of zinc fortificant

Zinc compounds that are suitable for use as food fortificants include the sulfate, chloride, gluconate, oxide and the stearate. All of these compounds are either white or colourless, but have varying water solubilities; some have an unpleasant taste when added to certain foods. Although it is only poorly water soluble, zinc oxide is the cheapest of the zinc fortificants and therefore tends to be the preferred choice. Recent studies have shown that the absorption of zinc from cereal products fortified with zinc oxide is as good as that from those fortified with the more soluble zinc sulfate (*308,309*), presumably because the oxide is soluble in gastric acid. However, zinc absorption from the oxide may be poor in individuals with low stomach acid secretion.

6.1.2 The bioavailability of zinc

Zinc absorption from food is dependent on the amount of zinc consumed and the ratio of phytate to zinc in the meal being consumed. According to recent estimates by the International Zinc Nutrition Consultative Group (IZiNCG), when zinc intake is just adequate to meet the physiological requirements for absorbed zinc, in adult men about 27% of the zinc content is absorbed from diets having a phytate:zinc molar ratio of less than 18, which drops to about 19% when the phytate:zinc molar ratio is greater than 18 (i.e. high phytate). The corresponding zinc absorption rates for adult women are 35% and 26%, respectively (*109*). When zinc intake is greater than the critical level needed to meet requirements, the fractional absorption becomes progressively less, although the net absorption of zinc increases slightly. In one study involving healthy, well-nourished adults from the United States, zinc absorption from the sulfate (or the oxide) added to a low-phytate bread meal was about 14% (total zinc content, 3.1–3.7 mg per meal) compared with around 6% from the same fortificants added to a high-phytate wheat porridge meal (total zinc content, 2.7–3.1 mg per meal) (*309*).

6.1.3 Methods used to increase zinc absorption from fortificants

In light of the above findings, and given the similarities to iron (see *section 5.1.2*), it is reasonable to assume that reducing the phytic acid content of food will increase the absorption of zinc from fortificants, at least in the case of adults (*310*). Whether the same applies to infants and young children is uncertain. A lower extraction rate will result in a reduced phytate content of cereals but also a reduced zinc content, so the net effect on zinc supply tends to be minimal. Alternatively, the phytate content can be reduced by activating the phytases that are naturally present in most phytate-containing foods (through germination, fermentation and/or soaking) or by adding microbial or fungal phytases. Including sources of animal protein in the diet has also been shown to be an effective way of improving zinc absorption from high-phytate diets (*93*).

Absorption enhancers equivalent to ascorbic acid for iron, do not exist for zinc. However, according to the results of one study conducted in adult women, the addition of NaFeEDTA as a fortificant can increase zinc absorption from the diet, in this case from about 20% to 35%; 1% of the additional amount of zinc absorbed was excreted in the urine (*311*). This finding has yet to be confirmed in other studies. However, if, as reports suggest, the addition of Na_2EDTA or NaFeEDTA to cereal flours inhibits the action of yeast during the bread-making process, these compounds would be of limited use, at least in cereal flours.

6.1.4 Experience with zinc fortification of specific foods

Hitherto, fortification with zinc has been fairly limited, and is generally confined to infant formula milks (with zinc sulfate), complementary foods and ready-to-eat breakfast cereals (in the United States). In Indonesia it is mandatory to add zinc to wheat noodles. More recently, several Latin American countries have expressed some interest in fortifying cereal flours with zinc.

Several studies have demonstrated the benefits of zinc supplementation on the growth rate of children (see *section 4.1.3*). However, very few trials have assessed the efficacy or effectiveness of zinc fortification. Although the addition of zinc oxide to breakfast cereals increased plasma zinc concentrations in preschool-aged children in the United States, there was no evidence of concomitant increases in growth rates or in food intake (*312*). However, in Turkey, zinc fortification of bread did increase the growth rates of schoolchildren who initially had low plasma zinc (*313*).

Little is known about the effects of added zinc on the sensory properties of foods. The fortification of wheat flour with relatively high levels of zinc (as zinc acetate) did not affect the baking or organoleptic properties of the bread dough (*313*). Likewise, the addition of 60 or 100 mg zinc/kg wheat flour (as zinc sulfate or zinc oxide) did not change the acceptability of bread (*314*). Encapsulation of zinc compounds is possible but has not been considered to date. This would, however, be a convenient way to mask the unpleasant taste of some zinc compounds.

6.2 Folate and other B vitamins

The B-complex vitamins are considered as a group in this chapter, as not only do they share some similar characteristics when used as food fortificants but they also tend to be added to the same foods. Members of the group of B vitamins covered here include folate/folic acid (vitamin B_9), thiamine (vitamin B_1), riboflavin (vitamin B_2), niacin, pyridoxine (vitamin B_6) and vitamin B_{12} (cobalamin).

6.2.1 Choice of vitamin B fortificants

The characteristics of the vitamin B compounds that are suitable for adding to foods are summarized in **Table 6.1**. In general, the B vitamins are relatively stable, with thiamine being the most labile to heat. Synthetic folate, i.e. folic acid (in the form of pteroyl monoglutamic acid) is moderately heat stable (*315*), but is susceptible to the effects of oxidizing and reducing agents (*316*).

Some fortificant loss is inevitable, the degree of loss being dependent on factors such as the temperature used during food processing or preparation, the moisture content, extrusion temperatures and pressures, the presence of other micronutrients (in the premix and in the fortified food), the nature of the packaging, and the anticipated shelf-life of the fortified product. Vitamin recoveries in bread made from fortified flour range from about 70% to 95% for niacin, and from 75% to 90% for thiamine and pyridoxine. About 70% of any added thiamine, pyridoxine and niacin is retained when enriched flour is used to prepare pasta, even after drying and cooking. On this basis, and assuming that any added B vitamins are 100% absorbed, in flour an overage of approximately 20–30% is thus usually sufficient to provide the desired amount in food products such as breads and cereals.

Folic acid has a light yellow colour, which does not carry over to fortified foods because it is added at such low levels, typically between 1.5 and 2.4 ppm. There is some loss of the vitamin on exposure to light, and during cooking and baking. The biggest losses tend to occur from biscuits and pasta, but even these are probably no more than 20%. As folic acid concentrations in foods are difficult to measure, reported levels in fortified flour and baked products are often subject to considerable assay error.

TABLE 6.1
Vitamin B fortificants: physical characteristics and stability

Vitamin	Fortificant compound	Physical characteristics	Stability
Thiamine (B_1)	Thiamine hydrochloride	More soluble in water than the mononitrate form. White or almost white	Both salts are stable to oxygen in the absence of light and moisture but are unstable in neutral or alkaline solutions and in the presence of sulfites.
	Thiamine mononitrate	White or almost white	Losses during leavening and baking are estimated to be 15–20%. Available in a coated form. The mononitrate is preferred for dry products.
Riboflavin (B_2)	Riboflavin	Relatively water insoluble. Yellow	Very unstable in light. Rapid loss from milk on exposure to light but stable in white bread.
	Sodium salt of riboflavin 5′-phosphate	Soluble in water. Yellow	
Niacin	Niacin (nicotinic acid)	Soluble in alkali, sparingly soluble in water. White	Very stable to oxygen, heat and light, both in the dry state and in aqueous solution.
	Niacinamide (nicotinamide)	Water soluble. White	
Pyridoxine (B_6)	Pyridoxine hydrochloride	Water soluble. White or almost white	Stable in oxygen and heat, but relatively sensitive to UV light. Available in a coated form.
Folic acid (B_9)	Pteroyl monoglutamic acid	Sparingly soluble in water, soluble in dilute acid and alkali. Yellow-orange	Moderately stable to heat. Stable in solution at neutral pH but increasingly unstable at higher or lower pH. Unstable in UV light.
Vitamin B_{12} (cobalamin)	Cyanocobalamin	Pure vitamin B_{12} is sparingly soluble in water; the diluted forms are however completely soluble. Dark red, often supplied diluted on a carrier (0.1%)	Relatively stable to oxygen and heat in neutral and acid Solution, but unstable in alkali and strong acids, in strong light, and in alkaline solutions at >100°C.

6.2.2 Experience with vitamin B fortification of specific foods

There is a long history of experience of adding B vitamins to cereals (including wheat and maize flours) and rice grains, in both industrialized and developing countries. The benefits of restoration of thiamine, riboflavin and niacin in cereals and flours, 65–80% of which are removed by milling, have long been recognized. Indeed, the enrichment of flours and cereals has made, and continues to make, a major contribution to meeting the recommended intake of these vitamins even in the industrialized countries (*317*). The amount of niacin added to wheat flour typically ranges from 15 to 70 mg/kg (*178*); thiamine (vitamin B_1) addition levels range from 1.5 to 11 mg/kg, and those for vitamin B_{12}, from 1.3 to 4 mg/kg (*318*).

About 75% of the folate in whole wheat is also lost during milling, but folic acid has been included in cereal fortification programmes only relatively recently. In 1998, it became mandatory to fortify grain products with folic acid in the United States, the rationale being that it would lower the prevalence of neural tube defect births. The required fortification level is 154 µg/100 g flour (Mandate 21 CFR 137.165). According to one assessment the impact of this measure has been a 26% reduction in the incidence of neural tube defects (*48*). Mandatory folate acid fortification has also quite rapidly lowered the prevalence of low plasma folate concentrations in adults from around 22% to almost zero, and reduced the prevalence of elevated plasma homocysteine by about 50% (*49*). In addition to the United States, some 30 countries now add folic acid to flour, including Canada (150 µg/100 g), Chile (220 µg/100 g wheat flour), Costa Rica (180 µg/100 g), Dominican Republic (180 µg/100 g), El Salvador (180 µg/100 g), Guatemala (180 µg/100g), Honduras (180 µg/100g), Indonesia (200 µg/100 g wheat flour), Mexico (200 µg/100 g wheat flour), Nicaragua (180 µg/100 g) and Panama (180 µg/100 g) (*318*).

The B-complex vitamins are added directly to flour as single nutrients or as a premix (which usually also contains iron), or they are diluted with a small amount of flour at the mill before being added to the bulk. In the case of ready-to-eat breakfast cereals, the B vitamins can either be added to the dry mix prior to extrusion or other processes, or a vitamin solution or suspension can be sprayed onto the cereals after they have been toasted. Riboflavin has a strong yellow colour and slightly bitter taste, but at the levels that are typically added to white flour any colour or taste problems are likely to be minimal. Coated forms of the water-soluble vitamins, such as thiamine and vitamin B_6, are available if off-flavours or other problems arise (**Table 6.1**).

6.2.3 Safety concerns

6.2.3.1 Thiamine, riboflavin and vitamin B_6

As toxicity is not a problem, the United States Food and Nutrition Board has not defined upper intake limits (ULs) for thiamine and riboflavin. In the case of vitamin B_6, sensory neuropathy has been linked to high intakes of supplements but according to the findings of the United States Food and Nutrition Board, "No adverse effects associated with vitamin B_6 from food have been reported. This does not mean that there is no potential for adverse effects resulting from high intakes. Because data on the adverse effects of vitamin B_6 are limited, caution may be warranted". A UL of 100 mg for adults and 30–40 mg for children has thus been set (128). These levels are very unlikely to be obtained from fortified foods.

6.2.3.2 Niacin (nicotinic acid and niacinamide)

Vasodilation or flushing (i.e. a burning or itching sensation in the face, arms and chest) has been observed as a first adverse effect in patients given high doses of nicotinic acid for the treatment of hyperlipidemia. Based on such evidence, the United States Food and Nutrition Board has defined a UL of 35 mg/day for nicotinic acid (128). Intakes of niacinamide have, however, not been associated with flushing effects.

Bearing in mind the different characteristics of the two forms of niacin, the Scientific Committee for Food in the European Union has proposed a UL for nicotinic acid of 10 mg/day and a separate, much higher, UL for niacinamide of 900 mg/day (319). The latter thus poses no safety limitations in common food fortification practice.

6.2.3.3 Folic acid fortificants

The consumption of folic acid in amounts normally found in fortified foods has not been associated with adverse health effects. However, there has been some concern that high folic acid intakes could mask or exacerbate neurological problems, such as pernicious anaemia, in people with low intakes of vitamin B_{12} (128). This has led to a reluctance to fortify with folic acid in some countries. This concern is particularly pertinent to those individuals who derive folic acid from both supplements and a range of fortified foods, as it is the case in many industrialized countries. In this situation, some people may exceed the UL for folic acid, which has been set at 1 mg/day (128)(129 old 110). An obvious solution to this potential problem is to fortify foods with both vitamin B_{12} and folic acid.

To avoid any possible risk of adverse effects, folic acid fortification programmes should be designed so as to limit regular daily intakes to a maximum of 1 mg. In addition, measures which require folic acid-containing supplements and fortified foods to also contain vitamin B_{12} could be considered, especially in the case of products consumed by older citizens who are at greater risk of vitamin B_{12} deficiency and its associated conditions, in particular, pernicious anaemia.

6.3 Vitamin C (ascorbic acid)

6.3.1 Choice of vitamin C fortificant

Ascorbic acid and ascorbyl palmitate are often added to oils, fats, soft drinks and various other foods as a way of improving the stability of other added micronutrients (e.g. vitamin A) or as an iron absorption enhancer (see *section 5.1.2.1*). However, ascorbic acid is itself relatively unstable in the presence of oxygen, metals, humidity and/or high temperatures. To retain vitamin C integrity (especially during storage), foods must therefore be appropriately packaged, or the ascorbic acid encapsulated.

6.3.2 Experience with vitamin C fortification of specific foods

As a general rule, foods that are not cooked are better vehicles for vitamin C fortification. Blended foods, such as those used for feeding programmes in emergency situations, were often fortified with vitamin C as this was believed to be the most efficient way of delivering this nutrient to populations likely to be deficient. However, a trial with PL-480 cereals found that although almost all of the encapsulated fortificant ascorbic acid was retained during transit from the United States to Africa, it was rapidly destroyed when the cereal product was cooked for 10 minutes (*270*). On the other hand, the addition of vitamin C to commercially processed foods such as dry milk, infant formulas, cereal-based complementary foods, chocolate drink powders and beverages has been found to be successful in increasing intakes of this nutrient. As sugar helps to protect the ascorbic acid in soft drinks, sugar has been proposed as a possible vehicle for the vitamin (*184*).

6.4 Vitamin D

6.4.1 Choice of vitamin D fortificant

Either vitamin D_2 (ergocalciferol) or D_3 (cholecalciferol) can be added to foods. The two forms have similar biological activities and both are very sensitive to oxygen and moisture, and both interact with minerals. A dry stabilized form of vitamin D, which contains an antioxidant (usually tocopherol) that protects activity even in the presence of minerals, is generally used for most commercial applications.

6.4.2 Experience with vitamin D fortification of specific foods

Milk and other dairy products, including dried milk powder and evaporated milk, are often fortified with vitamin D. Many countries also fortify margarines with this vitamin.

Low exposure to sunlight is a risk factor for vitamin D deficiency and can be a problem among those who live in the more northerly or southerly latitudes where UV radiation levels are lower during the winter months, and among women who, for cultural reasons, spend a large proportion of their time indoors or covered with clothing. In such situations, vitamin D fortification of milk and margarine have been found to be useful strategies for increasing intakes; the goal is to supply up to 200 IU/day in the total diet.

6.5 Calcium

Compared with other micronutrients, calcium is required in relatively large amounts. A heightened awareness of the need to increase intakes of calcium for osteoporosis prevention has meant that calcium fortification has attracted a good deal of interest in recent years.

6.5.1 Choice of calcium fortificants

Calcium salts suitable for use as food fortificants are listed in **Table 6.2**. Bioavailable forms recommended for the fortification of infant formulas and complementary foods include the carbonate (it can liberate CO_2 in acid systems), the chloride, the citrate and the citrate malate, the gluconate, the glycerophosphate, the lactate, the mono-, di- and tribasic phosphates, the orthophosphate, the hydroxide and the oxide (*320*). All of these salts are either white or colourless. Most are bland although the citrate has a tart flavour, the hydroxide is slightly bitter, and high concentrations of the chloride and the lactate can be unpleasant. The cost of calcium carbonate is very low, usually less than that of flour.

As the daily amount of calcium required is several thousand times higher than that of most other micronutrients, it tends to be added separately (as opposed to part of a premix). The calcium content of commercially available salts ranges from 9% (the gluconate) to 71% (the oxide) (**Table 6.2**). Salts with lower concentrations will have to be added in larger amounts, a factor that may affect the final choice of fortificant.

There is little reason to believe that low solubility is a major constraint to the bioavailability of fortificant calcium. In general, absorption of added calcium is similar to that naturally present in foods, which ranges from about 10% to 30%. However, high levels of calcium inhibit the absorption of iron from foods and so this too is something that needs to be taken into consideration when deciding how much calcium to add. The co-addition of ascorbic acid can help overcome the inhibitory effect of calcium on iron absorption.

6.5.2 Experience with calcium fortification

Wheat flour was first fortified with calcium in the United Kingdom in 1943 in order to restore the calcium lost during milling. Today, it is compulsory to add 940–1560 mg calcium carbonate/kg to white and brown (but not wholegrain)

TABLE 6.2
Calcium fortificants: physical characteristics

Compound	Calcium content (%)	Colour	Taste	Odour	Solubility (mmol/l)
Carbonate	40	Colourless	Soapy, lemony	Odourless	0.153
Chloride	36	Colourless	Salty, bitter	–	6712
Sulfate	29	Varies	–	–	15.3
Hydroxyapatite	40	–	–	–	0.08
Calcium phosphate dibasic	30	White	Sandy, bland	–	1.84
Calcium phosphate monobasic	17	Colourless	Sandy, bland	–	71.4
Calcium phosphate tribasic	38	White	Sandy, bland	Odourless	0.064
Calcium pyrophosphate	31	Colourless	–	–	Insoluble
Glycerophosphate	19	White	Almost tasteless	Odourless	95.2
Acetate	25	Colourless	–	–	2364
Lactate	13	White	Neutral	Almost odourless	0.13
Citrate	24	Colourless	Tart, clean	Odourless	1.49
Citrate malate	23	Colourless	–	–	80.0
Gluconate	9	White	Bland	Odourless	73.6
Hydroxide	54	Colourless	Slightly bitter	Odourless	25.0
Oxide	71	Colourless	–	–	23.3

Source: adapted from reference (*320*).

flours milled in the United Kingdom. In the United States, the addition of calcium to flour has been optional since the early 1940s. Calcium sulfate, carbonate, chloride, phosphate, acetate or lactate are all suitable for fortification of wheat flours, but the oxide and hydroxide may require alterations in the pH of the dough for successful bread-making (*321*).

The range of foods that are fortified with calcium has steadily grown over the years as it became increasingly clear that intakes were low in many populations. The more soluble calcium salts, such as the citrate malate or the gluconate, are generally used to fortify juices and other beverages. Tribasic calcium phosphate, and sometimes calcium carbonate or lactate, is used to fortify milk, to which gums (e.g. carrageenan, guar gum) must also be added to prevent the calcium salt from sedimenting. Yoghurt and cottage cheese can also be fortified with these calcium compounds. In industrialized nations and in some Asian countries, soya beverages are marketed as a replacement for cow's milk in which case these too should be fortified with calcium. Stabilizers such as sodium hexametaphosphate or potassium citrate can improve the quality of soya beverages fortified with calcium gluconate or lactogluconate.

The addition of calcium salts to some foods can cause undesirable changes in colour, texture and stability by increasing the cross-linking of proteins, pectins and gums. Calcium fortificants can also darken the colour of chocolate beverages.

6.6. Selenium

6.6.1 Choice of fortificant

For food fortification purposes, the sodium salts are generally considered to be the most suitable source of selenium. The selenite is a white, water-soluble compound, from which absorption is about 50%. It is readily reduced to unabsorbable elemental selenium by reducing agents, such as ascorbic acid and sulfur dioxide. Sodium selenate is colourless, and is less soluble in water and more stable than the selenite, especially in the presence of copper and iron. It has the better absorption (nearly 100% from the fortificant alone or 50–80% depending on the food vehicle to which it has been added), and also increases the activity of the enzyme, glutathione peroxidase, more effectively. When tested in milk-based infant formulas, more selenium was absorbed from the selenate (97% versus 73%), but as more selenium was excreted in the urine with the selenate (36% versus 10%), the net retention of selenium appears to be similar regardless of which chemical form is used (*322*). The relative retention of selenium from other fortified foods, including salt, has not been investigated. Organic forms of selenium, such as selenomethionine, are absorbed as well as the selenate, but remain longer in the body and thus theoretically pose a higher risk of toxicity. They have not been widely used for food fortification for this reason.

6.6.2 Experience with selenium fortification of selected foods

In regions of China where selenium deficiency is endemic, salt has been fortified with sodium selenite (15 mg/kg) since 1983. This measure increased average daily selenium intakes from 11 µg to 80 µg and has effectively reduced the prevalence of Keshan disease (see also *section 4.8.3*).

Sodium selenate is currently used to fortify a range of foods in various parts of the world. In Finland, for example, sodium selenate is added to fertilizers applied in areas having low soil selenium; measurable increases in the selenium content of milk, meat and cereals grown on these soils were observed within 6 months (*217*). Sodium selenate is an ingredient in some sports drinks (around 10 µg/l) and in the United States is used to fortify infant foods. Until 1985, bread supplied about half of the selenium intake for the United Kingdom population, but after 1985, when European wheat was replaced by Canadian wheat this dropped to about 20%.

6.7 Fluoride

6.7.1 Choice of fortificant

There are a number of ways in which fluoride intakes can be increased: fluoride can be added to water supplies at the point of supply or added to toothpaste. Hexa-fluoro-silicate acid (HUSIAC) is the most commonly used fluoride compound for large-scale water fortification. It is added as a concentrated aqueous solution. The fluoridation of salt and the enrichment of milk with fluoride are alternative options that have been used in some parts of the world.

6.7.2 Experience of fluoridation

The introduction of a salt fluoridation programme in Jamaica was associated with a large reduction in dental decay in children, when assessed after 7 years (*323*). However, a smaller trial in Hungary indicated that residence during early infancy in an area where salt was fluoridated was not associated with a reduced risk of later caries (*324*). In Costa Rica, a national fluoride salt fortification programme, requiring the addition of 225–275 mg fluoride/kg salt, became mandatory in 1989. There then followed a very substantial and progressive reduction in tooth decay, and in 1999, based on measurements of urinary fluorine excretion rates, the level of fluoride in salt was lowered to 175–225 mg/kg (*325*). However, it is possible that other sources of fluoride (i.e. toothpaste) may have contributed to the observed reduction in the prevalence of tooth decay in Costa Rica.

Where it is impractical or unacceptable to fluoridate water or salt, the addition of fluoride to milk is an alternative approach for preventing dental caries. Generally speaking, the level of fluoridation is best governed by the usual volume of milk consumed by young children. Guidelines for fluoride fortification of milk and milk products are available elsewhere (*326*).

A recent evaluation of the feasibility of adding fluoride to school milk in the United Kingdom concluded that fortification was both feasible and desirable (*327*). In rural Chile, preschool-aged children received 0.25–0.75 mg fluoride per day in fortified, powdered milk for a period of 4 years. The rate of decayed, missing and filled teeth declined substantially compared with a control community, and the percentage of children who remained caries-free doubled (*328*). Favourable results have also been reported from Beijing, in children who consumed 0.5 mg fluoride in milk each day at kindergarten and 0.6 mg fluoride in milk at home on weekend days (*329*). Similarly, in Scotland schoolchildren who consumed 1.5 mg fluoride daily in 200 ml milk had a significantly lower prevalence of caries than a control group after 5 years (*330*). However, these results were not replicated in a more recent study conducted in another region of the United Kingdom (*331*).

PART IV

Implementing effective and sustainable food fortification programmes

Introduction

As the preceding chapters have demonstrated, food fortification has a long history of successful practice. Notable successes have been in achieved in the case of the iodization of salt, the fortification of flour with various B vitamins, and the fortification of margarines with vitamin A. It would, however, be something of an overstatement to say that these past successes have been the result of formal, scientifically-rigorous evaluations of the nutritional status and needs of the target population. In many cases, decisions about how much fortificant to add to a chosen food vehicle were based on what was known to be technically possible at the time, and governed by budgetary limits.

With a view to putting fortification programme planning on a sounder footing, this section of the present Guidelines sets out a systematic and methodological approach to designing and planning a food fortification programme. The key elements are as follows:

— defining and setting nutritional goals (i.e. framing decisions about how much micronutrient(s) to add to which foods);

— programme monitoring and evaluation (i.e. establishing procedures which check that fortified foods contain the intended amount of micronutrient(s) and that they are being consumed by the target population in adequate amounts);

— communicating and marketing fortification programmes (i.e. informing the target population about the benefits of fortification so that they chose to consume fortified foods).

In order to be able to correct a micronutrient deficiency in a population, which is after all the ultimate goal of any fortification programme, it is necessary to first ascertain the extent of the deficiency and then the increase in intake that is needed to satisfy the daily requirement for that micronutrient. Chapter 7 explains the application of the Estimated Average Requirement (EAR) cut-point method to the problem of calculating the level of micronutrient additions that is needed to bring the prevalence of low intakes among a target population to an acceptably small level. This is the WHO recommended method and is applicable to all micronutrients covered in these Guidelines, with the exception of iron (for which an alternative methodology is described). The information needs for such computations, e.g. data on food and nutrient intake distributions, are also outlined. Having estimated the ideal level of micronutrient addition required to achieve a given nutritional goal, programme planners are then advised to consider whether this level of fortification is feasible given current technology and any safety or cost constraints that may be operating, or whether, additional measures (e.g. supplementation), may be a better way of reaching nutritional targets, at least for some population subgroups. Technological, cost and safety limits are thus defined and a series of examples are provided to show how these can be used to shape the final decision about fortification levels appropriate to a given situation.

The primary objective of monitoring and evaluation activities is to ascertain whether or not a fortification programme is achieving its nutritional goals once it has been implemented. These are critical to the success of any fortification programme and should be viewed as an integral part of overall programme design. Monitoring and evaluation activities take place at a number of levels. The main purpose of monitoring is to track the operational performance (or implementation efficiency) of a programme. Only after monitoring has established that a fortified product of the desired quality is available and accessible to the target population in adequate amounts, can the impact of the intervention be evaluated. To date, relatively few fortification programmes have been properly evaluated, partly because impact evaluation is widely perceived to be both a complex and costly exercise. The methodologies outlined in Chapter 8 aim to demystify the process of evaluating the impact of fortification programmes. Chapter 9 explores the potential usefulness of the application of cost-effectiveness and cost–benefit analysis techniques to food fortification interventions, something that is also in its infancy. The examples given clearly demonstrate that fortification has the potential to be a particularly cost-effective solution to the problem of micronutrient malnutrition in many settings.

In order to ensure that fortified foods are consumed in adequate amounts by those who require them most, all fortification programmes will need to be supported by the right mix of educational and social marketing activities. Like monitoring and evaluation, this third key element should also be thought about at the design and planning stages of a fortification programme. Chapter 10 outlines the communication needs of all the various parties involved in the running of fortification programmes, not just the consumer, and provides guidance on how messages might be framed to best meet these needs. An understanding of the regulatory environment is also essential, and therefore these Guidelines conclude with an overview of the mechanisms for regulating fortification through national food laws. Reference to the international context is made wherever relevant.

CHAPTER 7
Defining and setting programme goals

7.1 Information needs

In order to be able to design a successful fortification programme that achieves its nutritional objectives, it is necessary to have first gathered some background information and nutritional data, in particular:

- biochemical/chemical data on nutritional status (i.e. data on the scale and severity of specific nutrient deficiencies in different population groups; see Part II);
- data on dietary patterns (i.e. the composition of the usual diet);
- detailed information on dietary intakes of micronutrients of interest (i.e. the distribution of usual intakes of specific micronutrients in a population).

This information is required to confirm the need and provide a rationale for a fortification programme. Having established the need for an intervention, the same information and data can then be used to identify and prioritize the target population groups, decide which micronutrients (and in what amounts) should be added to which foods, and to identify and understand any constraints (e.g. safety, cost, technological) that may impact on the amounts of nutrients that can be added to given foods. Specific data needs are outlined in greater detail below, whereas related issues of a more general nature, but equally important with regards to the planning stages of fortification programmes, are reviewed in **Box 7.1**.

7.1.1 Biochemical and clinical evidence of specific micronutrient deficiencies

Part II of these Guidelines describes how it is possible to classify the severity of a public health problem caused by specific micronutrient deficiencies using various biochemical and clinical indicators and criteria. Where clinical or biochemical data indicate a high prevalence of deficiency of a specific nutrient, this is usually regarded as being good evidence that the diet is not supplying enough of that particular micronutrient and that fortification is warranted. The more severe and widespread the deficiency, the greater the need for intervention.

> **BOX 7.1**
>
> **Planning and designing a fortification programme: preliminary considerations**
>
> - The decision to implement a micronutrient fortification programme requires documented evidence that the micronutrient content of the diet is insufficient or that fortification will produce a health benefit. The objective is to lower the prevalence of micronutrient deficiencies in the population and to optimize health.
>
> - In some situations, an insufficient intake of micronutrients is not the only risk factor for micronutrient deficiency. Other factors can play a substantial role, including, for example, the presence of infections and parasites (which, among other things, can contribute to high rates of anaemia). In these situations, it is important to determine whether fortification is a cost-effective strategy compared with other interventions (e.g. the control of infections and parasites).
>
> - The need for a fortification programme should always be examined in the broader context of all the possible options for controlling micronutrient deficiency. It may be that, overall, a combination of interventions (i.e. fortification plus other interventions) provides the most cost-effective option. For instance, supplementation plus fortification might be a better way to ensure that specific population groups (e.g. pregnant women and young children who are often the most vulnerable groups) are protected against micronutrient deficiencies than fortification alone.
>
> - Health authorities looking to initiate a micronutrient fortification programme should not do so without first collecting food intake data, supported by ancillary information such as biochemical data on nutritional status. This information is necessary to justify the programme, to make an informed judgement about the types and amounts of specific nutrients to include, and to understand which foods would make suitable vehicles for fortification. Given the long-term effort and investment required to implement and sustain fortification programmes, and the need to ensure that the outcome is intakes that are adequate and not excessive, it is essential to make this initial investment in the collection of adequate food intake data. Trained nutritionists will be needed for detailed programme planning, as well as for the subsequent monitoring and evaluation stages, the aim of which is to see how the programme has affected the nutrient intakes and nutritional status of the recipients.

In terms of providing reliable information on micronutrient status at the population level, biochemical and clinical data do, however, have a number of limitations. Firstly, available resources are usually such that only a relatively small number of individuals are tested or observed, and those that are sampled are not always representative of all relevant population subgroups. Secondly, some biochemical data are difficult to interpret because of confounding factors, such as the presence of infections, or interactions among micronutrient deficiencies (see **Tables 3.1, 3.4, 3.6, 4.1, 4.3–4.5, 4.7, 4.8, 4.10, 4.11, 4.13–16**). Biochemical indicators of iron status are especially prone to problems of this nature (**Table 3.1**). It is especially important to recognize situations where non-dietary factors, such as parasitic infections, are likely to be a major cause of observed micronutrient deficiencies; this will be reflected in a greater severity and prevalence of deficiencies than would be predicted from dietary data. Under such circumstances, other public health measures – in addition to fortification – may be needed to reduce the burden of MNM.

A third limitation is a lack of data, either because of the absence of a suitable biomarker of deficiency or simply because, to date, little investigation has taken place. This means that the prevalence of many deficiencies suspected of being relatively common (e.g. riboflavin (vitamin B_2), vitamin B_{12}, zinc and calcium) is not well known (**Table 1.2**). In some cases, however, evidence of a deficiency in one micronutrient predicts the existence of deficiencies in others. For example, a high prevalence of anaemia and vitamin A deficiency is often accompanied by zinc, vitamin B_{12} and riboflavin (vitamin B_2) deficiencies, because the underlying problem in all cases is an inadequate intake of animal source foods (see Chapter 4).

7.1.2 Dietary patterns

Knowledge of the usual foods consumed can be a useful supplement to biochemical and clinical evidence of micronutrient deficiencies, and in the absence of the latter can help pinpoint which micronutrients are most likely to be lacking in the diet. For example, animal source foods are the major source of vitamins A and D, thiamin (vitamin B_1), riboflavin (vitamin B_2), iron, zinc and calcium, and are the *only* source of vitamin B_{12}. They also provide an important amount of fat, the presence of which in the diet improves the absorption of fat-soluble vitamins. Populations with a low intake of animal source foods are thus likely to experience deficiencies in some or all of these nutrients.

It is common for the intake of animal source foods to be low in disadvantaged populations; sometimes these foods are avoided because of religious or other beliefs. Another widespread problem, particularly among refugees and displaced populations, is inadequate consumption of fruits and vegetables and consequently low intakes of vitamin C (ascorbic acid) and folate. In locations where phytate or polyphenol intakes are high, the risk of iron and zinc deficiencies increases because the bioavailability of both of these minerals from foods is reduced in the presence of these compounds.

At the population level, food balance sheets, such as those produced by the Food and Agriculture Organization of the United Nations (FAO), can provide some useful information about usual dietary patterns and also on the average consumption of certain foods that are rich in micronutrients or in absorption inhibitors, which in turn can be used to predict probable micronutrient deficiencies. Their main limitation is that, in providing information on the average intake by the general population, they do not reflect the distribution of intakes by population subgroups.

7.1.3 Usual dietary intakes

As they are the basis of decisions about which micronutrients to add to which foods and in what amounts, the possession of quantitative food and nutrient intake data is a prerequisite for any food fortification programme. Food intake data are also needed for predicting the probable impact of potential fortification interventions. Food and nutrient intake information should be available for, or collected from, different population groups (e.g. those differing in socioeconomic status, ethnicity or religious beliefs) and from different physiological status groups (e.g. children, women).

In reality, there is usually a wide range of food and nutrient intakes within any given population subgroup. As is explained in more detail later in the chapter, it is this range or the distribution of usual intakes that is of primary interest and which forms the basis for both the planning and the evaluation of food fortification interventions (see sections 7.2 and 7.3).

7.2 Defining nutritional goals: basic concepts

The main goal of a fortification programme is to correct inadequate micronutrient intakes through the fortification of foods, thereby preventing, or reducing, the severity and prevalence of micronutrient deficiencies. Interventions of this nature can involve either fortifying a single food product (e.g. the iodization of salt) or the fortification of several foods.

In practice, food fortification programmes are devised so as to achieve a level of fortification such that, when the programme is in place, the probability of the nutrient intake being inadequate in a given population – either insufficient or excessive – is acceptably low.

> The dietary goal of fortification is formally defined in these Guidelines as follows: to provide most (97.5%) of individuals in the population group(s) at greatest risk of deficiency with an adequate intake of specific micronutrients, without causing a risk of excessive intakes in this or other groups.

7.2.1 The EAR cut-point method

The approach recommended in these WHO Guidelines for setting fortificant levels in foods is the *Estimated Average Requirement (EAR)*[1] *cut-point method*. This approach was proposed some years ago, and is described in detail in a report by the United States Food and Nutrition Board of the Institute of Medicine (FNB/IOM) on dietary reference intakes *(333)*.

As its starting point, the EAR cut-point method assumes that the proportion of a population with intakes below the EAR for a given nutrient corresponds to the proportion having an inadequate intake of that nutrient (see **Figure 7.1**). The EAR cut-point approach requires a decision to be made about the acceptable prevalence of inadequate (and excessive) intakes (often taken to be 2–3% for reasons which are explained more fully below: see section 7.3.1). Then by combining information on the range of usual intakes of a population subgroup with information on the nutrient requirements for that subgroup (i.e. the EAR), it is possible to derive a level of food fortification that will give an intake distribution such that usual nutrient intakes meet the requirements of all but a small specified proportion of the subgroup. In other words, the method allows its users to find the additional intake of micronutrients that would shift the distribution of intakes upwards so that only a small proportion of the population group is at risk of having an inadequate intake. Here the term "subgroup" refers to various age, gender and physiological status groups of the population (e.g. pregnant or lactating women). The EAR cut-point methodology is outlined in greater detail in section 7.3 and is illustrated by means of a worked example.

The EAR cut-point method is a simplified, easier to use version of the probability method, which requires calculating the probability of inadequacy of intake for each individual in a population subgroup, averaging the probabilities, and then using this average as an estimate of the prevalence of inadequacy *(333)*. These two approaches, the EAR cut-point method and the probability method, give similar results as long as the assumptions underlying them are met. For the probability method, there should be little or no correlation between intake and requirements, which is assumed to be true for all nutrients but energy. In the case of the EAR cut-point method, the variation in intake of a nutrient by a population group should be greater than the variation in the requirement for this nutrient (also assumed to be true for most nutrients and most groups), and the distribution of requirements must be symmetrical (believed to be true for all nutrients except iron). Thus for most applications and nutrients, either method is appropriate, with the exception of iron for which only the probability method is valid (see section 7.3.3.1).

---

[1] The Estimated Average Requirement (EAR) for a micronutrient is defined as the average daily intake that is estimated to meet the requirements of half of the healthy individuals in a particular life stage and gender subgroup *(332)*.

FIGURE 7.1

An example of a usual intake distribution in which the median intake is at the RNI or RDA (the formerly-used approach)

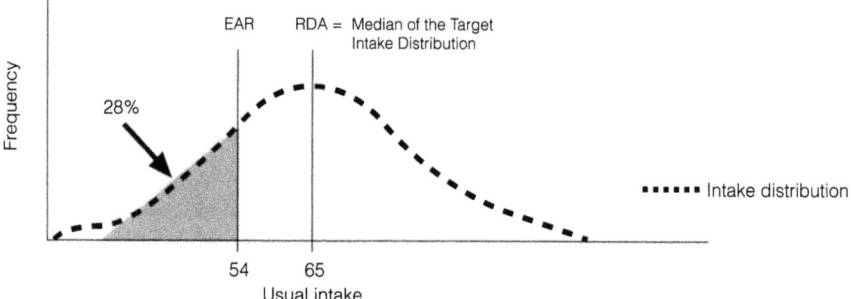

Source: adapted from reference (*333*), with the permission of the United States National Academy Press.

The EAR cut-point approach is different from the past practice of using the Recommended Nutrient Intake (or Recommended Dietary Allowance) of a nutrient as the desirable or "target" intake. For reasons that are explained more fully below, the latter approach is valid for deriving the desired nutritional intake of an individual, but not that of a population.

7.2.2 Dietary reference values: Estimated Average Requirements, Recommended Nutrient Intakes and upper limits

7.2.2.1 Recommended Nutrient Intakes

Dietary requirements for specific micronutrients, aimed at minimizing the risk of nutrient deficit or excess, have been specified by various national and international bodies, including FAO and WHO. The Recommended Nutrient Intake (RNI) is defined by FAO/WHO as the daily dietary intake level that is sufficient to meet the nutrient requirement of almost all (i.e. 97–98%) healthy individuals in a particular age, gender and physiological status group (*93*). For most nutrients, the RNI is set at about 2 standard deviations higher than the average amount required by a population group (i.e. the EAR), in order that the requirements of almost every person in the group are met. The standard deviation (or coefficient of variation)[1] of the requirement for each nutrient varies with age, gender and physiological status but for most nutrients and subgroups is between 10% and 20%.

Table 7.1 lists published FAO/WHO RNI values for all micronutrients covered by these Guidelines for selected age and gender groups (*93*). The

---

[1] The coefficient of variation is the standard deviation divided by the mean, expressed as a percentage.

TABLE 7.1
FAO/WHO Recommended Nutrient Intakes (RNIs) for selected population subgroups

Nutrient (unit)	1–3 years	4–6 years	19–50 years, female	Pregnant women, second trimester	Lactating women, 0–3 months	19–50 years, male
Vitamin A (µg RE)[a]	400	450	500	800	850	600
Vitamin D (µg)[b]	5	5	5	5	5	5
Vitamin E (mg α-tocopherol)	5.0	5.0	7.5	7.5	7.5	10.0
Vitamin C (mg)	30	30	45	55	70	45
Thiamine (vitamin B_1) (mg)	0.5	0.6	1.1	1.4	1.5	1.2
Riboflavin (vitamin B_2) (mg)	0.5	0.6	1.1	1.4	1.6	1.3
Niacin (vitamin B_3) (mg NE)	6	8	14	18	17	16
Vitamin B_6 (mg)	0.5	0.6	1.3	1.9	2.0	1.3
Folate (µg DFE)[c]	150	200	400	600	500	400
Vitamin B_{12} (µg)	0.9	1.2	2.4	2.6	2.8	2.4
Iron (mg)[d]						
■ 15% bioavailability	3.9	4.2	19.6	>50.0	10.0	9.1
■ 10% bioavailability	5.8	6.3	29.4	>50.0	15.0	13.7
■ 5% bioavailability	11.6	12.6	58.8	>50.0	30.0	27.4
Zinc (mg)[e]						
■ High bioavailability	2.4	2.9	3.0	4.2	5.8	4.2
■ Moderate bioavailability	4.1	4.8	4.9	7.0	9.5	7.0
■ Low bioavailability	8.3	9.6	9.8	14.0	19.0	14.0
Calcium (mg)	500	600	1000	1000	1000	1000
Selenium (µg)	17	22	26	28	35	34
Iodine (µg)	90	90	150	200	200	150

[a] 1 RE = 1 µg retinol = 12 µg β-carotene or 24 µg other provitamin A carotenoids. In oil, the conversion factor for vitamin A (retinol): β-carotene is 1:2. The corresponding conversion factor for synthetic β-carotene is uncertain, but a factor of 1:6 is generally considered to be reasonable. 1 µg RE = 3.33 IU vitamin A.
[b] In the absence of adequate exposure to sunlight, as calciferol (1 µg calciferol = 40 IU vitamin D).
[c] 1 DFE = Dietary folate equivalent = 1 µg food folate = 0.6 µg folic acid from fortified foods, which means that 1 µg folic acid = 1.7 DFE.
[d] The RNI depends on the composition of the diet. For a diet rich in vitamin C and animal protein, the bioavailability of iron is 15%; for diets rich in cereals but including sources of vitamin C, bioavailability is 10%, and for diets low in vitamin C and animal protein, bioavailability is reduced to 5%.
[e] The RNI depends on the composition of the diet. The bioavailability of zinc is high from diets rich in animal protein, moderate from diets rich in legumes and pulses or diets that include fermented cereals, and low from diets poor in animal protein or zinc-rich plant foods.

Source: reference (93), which also provides values for other age and gender groups. T.

> **BOX 7.2**
>
> **FAO/WHO RNIs: comparisons with dietary reference values defined by other bodies**
>
> 1. Food and Nutrition Board, Institute of Medicine (FNB/IOM), United States of America
>
> The FAO/WHO RNI is conceptually equivalent to the *Recommended Dietary Allowance* (RDA), one of the four levels of dietary reference intakes used in Canada and the United States of America. The other three values are the *Estimated Average Requirement* (EAR), the *Adequate Intake* (AI), and the *Tolerable Upper Level* (UL)[1].
>
> 2. Department of Health, United Kingdom
>
> The FAO/WHO RNI is conceptually similar to the Reference Nutrient Intake (RNI), one of the four dietary reference values used in the United Kingdom (*334*). The others are the *Estimated Average Requirement*, the *Lower Reference Nutrient Intake* (a concept that is unique to the United Kingdom) and the *Safe Intake*, which is conceptually similar to the Adequate Intake as defined by the United States FNB/IOM.
>
> 3. Scientific Committee for Foods, Commission of the European Community
>
> The European Community currently uses three reference values: the *Population Requirement Intake* (PRI), which is conceptually equivalent to FAO/WHO RNI, the *Average Requirement* (AR) and the *Lower Threshold Intake* (LTI) (*335*).

FAO/WHO RNI values are broadly similar to dietary reference values defined by other national and international bodies. Various dietary reference values in common usage, and their equivalence, are summarized in **Box 7.2**.

For the majority of micronutrients, the highest recommended intakes are for adult males, the notable exception being iron. Nevertheless, this population subgroup usually has the lowest risk of micronutrient deficiencies due to its higher food intake and its lower micronutrient requirements per unit body weight. Individuals at most risk of not meeting their RNIs are infants, young children and women of reproductive age, especially pregnant and lactating women. Some of these groups (e.g. pregnant or lactating women) may even have higher requirements for specific nutrients than do adult men.

7.2.2.2 Calculating Estimated Average Requirements from Recommended Nutrient Intakes

Although they form the basis of most RNIs (which are usually set at 2 standard deviations above the corresponding EAR for any given population subgroup),

---

[1] For further information relating to the work and publications of the Food and Nutrition Board, please refer to the web site of the National Academies Press (http://www.nap.edu).

FAO/WHO do not routinely publish EAR values. However, the FAO/WHO RNIs, or equivalent recommendations made by other countries or regions, can be easily converted into EARs by the application of appropriate conversion factors. The conversion factors, which are presented for the micronutrients covered by these Guidelines in **Annex C**, are the equivalent of subtracting 2 standard deviations from the RNI. For example, the standard deviation of the requirement for vitamin A by 1-3-year-old children is 20%; dividing the relevant RNI (400 µg RE) by 1.4 (i.e. $1 + (2 \times 0.2)$) gives an EAR of 286 µg RE. The EARs corresponding to RNIs given in **Table 7.1**, and calculated in this way, are listed in **Table 7.2**.

7.2.2.3 Upper levels of intake

The most appropriate reference value for determining whether or not the micronutrient intakes of population subgroups are safe, i.e. do not reach levels at which there is any risk of excessive intake, is the Tolerable Upper Intake Level (UL). The UL is the highest average intake that will not pose a risk of adverse health effects for virtually anyone in the population. The risk of adverse effects increases at intakes above the UL. The risks of excessive intakes are described in detail by FAO/WHO (*93*), and the United States FNB/IOM (*332,333*).

Like EARs and RNIs, ULs vary by age and gender but tend to be lower for young children and pregnant women. ULs for a range of micronutrients are given in **Table 7.3**. For those micronutrients for which FAO/WHO have not recommended a UL (i.e. iron, folate, fluoride and iodine), the values given in the table are based on recommendations of either the United States FNB/IOM or the Scientific Committee for Food of the European Community.

7.3 Using the EAR cut-point method to set goals and to evaluate the impact and safety of fortification

In reality, there is usually a wide range of intakes of a nutrient within a population subgroup. This range of usual intakes must be measured and used as the basis for planning and evaluation. As previously mentioned, the goal of fortification is to shift the distribution of usual nutrient intakes of a target population upwards so that only a small proportion of the population is at risk of having an inadequate intake, but not so far that those who consume larger amounts of the food vehicle will be at risk of an excessive intake. The median of the new usual intake distribution is referred to as the "target median intake". It thus follows that one of the first decisions that will need to be made when planning fortification interventions is what is an acceptable prevalence of inadequacy, both for low as well as for high intakes.

TABLE 7.2
Estimated Average Requirements (calculated values) based on FAO/WHO Recommended Nutrient Intakes

Nutrient (unit)	1–3 years	4–6 years	19–50 years, female	Pregnant women, second trimester	Lactating women, 0–3 months	19–50 years, male
Vitamin A (µg RE)[a]	286	321	357	571	607	429
Vitamin D (µg)[b]	5	5	5	5	5	5
Vitamin E (mg α-tocopherol)	4	4	6	6	6	8
Vitamin C (mg)	25	25	37	46	58	37
Thiamine (vitamin B$_1$) (mg)	0.4	0.5	0.9	1.2	1.3	1.0
Riboflavin (vitamin B$_2$) (mg)	0.4	0.5	0.9	1.2	1.3	1.1
Niacin (vitamin B$_3$) (mg NE)	5	6	11	14	13	12
Vitamin B$_6$ (mg)	0.4	0.5	1.1	1.6	1.7	1.1
Folate (µg DFE)[c]	120	160	320	480	400	320
Vitamin B$_{12}$ (µg)	0.7	1.0	2.0	2.2	2.3	2.0
Iron (mg)[d]						
■ 15% bioavailability	3.9[e]	4.2[e]	19.6[e]	>40.0	7.8	7.2
■ 10% bioavailability	5.8[e]	6.3[e]	29.4[e]	>40.0	11.7	10.8
■ 5% bioavailability	11.6[e]	12.6[e]	58.8[e]	>40.0	23.4	21.6
Zinc (mg)[f]						
■ High bioavailability	2.0	2.4	2.5	3.5	4.8	3.5
■ Moderate bioavailability	3.4	4.0	4.1	5.8	7.9	5.8
■ Low bioavailability	6.9	8.0	8.2	11.7	15.8	11.7
Calcium (mg)	417	500	833	833	833	833
Selenium (µg)	14	17	22	23	29	28
Iodine (µg)	64	64	107	143	143	107

[a] 1 RE = 1 µg retinol = 12 µg β-carotene or 24 µg other provitamin A carotenoids. In oil, the conversion factor for vitamin A (retinol): β-carotene is 1 : 2. The corresponding conversion factor for synthetic β-carotene is uncertain, but a factor of 1 : 6 is generally considered to be reasonable. 1 µg RE = 3.33 IU vitamin A.
[b] In the absence of adequate exposure to sunlight, as calciferol. 1 µg calciferol = 40 IU vitamin D.
[c] 1 DFE = Dietary folate equivalent = 1 µg food folate = 0.6 µg folic acid from fortified foods, which means that 1 µg folic acid = 1.7 DFE.
[d] The RNI and thus the calculated EAR depends on the composition of the diet. For a diet rich in vitamin C and animal protein, the bioavailability of iron is 15%; for diets rich in cereals but including sources of vitamin C, bioavailability is 10%, and for diets low in vitamin C and animal protein, bioavailability is reduced to 5%.
[e] EARs cannot be calculated from RNIs for these age groups because of the skewed distribution of requirements for iron by young children and menstruating women. Instead, the corresponding RNI values are given.
[f] The RNI and thus the calculated EAR depends on the composition of the diet. The bioavailability of zinc is high from diets rich in animal protein, moderate from diets rich in legumes and pulses or diets that include fermented cereals, and low from diets poor in animal protein or zinc-rich plant foods.

Source: calculated from FAO/WHO RNIs, using the factors given in Annex C of these Guidelines.

TABLE 7.3
Tolerable Upper Intake Levels (ULs)

Nutrient (unit)[a]	1–3 years	4–8 years	9–13 years	19–70 years
Vitamin A (µg RE)[b]	600	900	1700	3000
Vitamin D (µg)[c]	50	50	50	50
Vitamin E (mg α-tocopherol)	200	300	600	1000
Vitamin C (mg)	400	650	1200	1000[d]
Niacin (vitamin B_3)(mg NE)[e]	10	15	20	35
Vitamin B_6 (mg)	30	40	60	100
Folic acid (µg DFE)[f]	300	400	600	1000
Choline (mg)	1000	1000	2000	3500
Iron (mg)	40	40	40	45
Zinc (mg)	7	12	23	45[g]
Copper (mg)	1	3	5	10
Calcium (mg)	2500	2500	2500	3000[h]
Phosphorus (mg)	3000	3000	4000	4000
Manganese (mg)	2	3	6	11
Molybdenum (µg)	300	600	1100	2000
Selenium (µg)	90	150	280	400
Iodine (µg)	200	300	600	1100
Fluoride (µg)	1300	2200	10000	10000

[a] Although no UL is specified for arsenic, silicon and vanadium, there is no justification for adding these substances to foods.
[b] Refers to preformed vitamin A only (i.e. esters of retinol). 1 µg RE = 3.33 IU vitamin A.
[c] As calciferol, where 1 µg calciferol = 40 IU vitamin D.
[d] The United States Food and Nutrition Board of the Institute of Medicine recommends a UL of 2000 mg vitamin C/day for adults.
[e] Based on the flushing effects of nicotinic acid. If niacinamide is used as the fortificant, the UL would be much higher. A UL for adults of 900 mg niacinamide/day has been recommended by the European Commission (319).
[f] Refers to folic acid derived from fortified foods, or supplemental folic acid.
[g] The United States Food and Nutrition Board of the Institute of Medicine recommends a UL of 40 mg zinc/day for adults (91).
[h] The United States Food and Nutrition Board of the Institute of Medicine recommends a UL of 2500 mg calcium/day for adults (193).

Sources: adapted from references (91,93). FAO/WHO have only recommended ULs for vitamins A, B_3 (niacin), B_6, C, D and E, calcium, selenium and zinc for adults. The remaining values are those recommended by the United States Food and Nutrition Board of the Institute of Medicine.

7.3.1 Deciding on an acceptable prevalence of low intakes

Three different ways of planning an intake distribution for a hypothetical nutrient, which has an EAR of 54 and an RDA of 65, are compared below (**Figures 7.1–7.3**). For simplicity, the intake distributions shown in these examples are normally distributed, although in reality, intake distributions are usually slightly skewed.

FIGURE 7.2
An example of a usual intake distribution in which only 2.5% of the group have intakes below the RNI (or RDA)

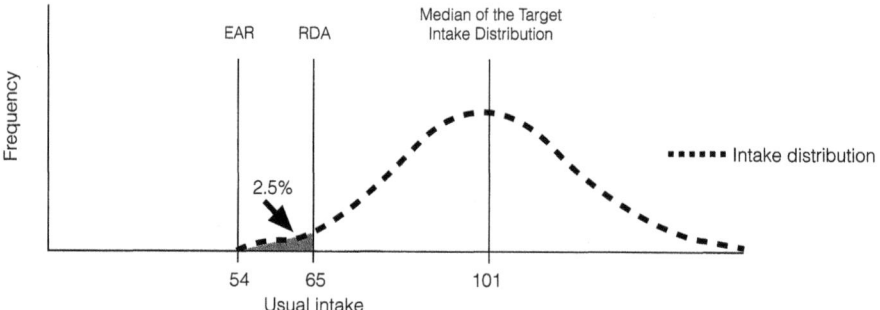

Source: adapted from reference (*333*), with the permission of the United States National Academy Press.

FIGURE 7.3
An example of a usual intake distribution in which 2.5% of the group have intakes below the EAR (the recommended approach)

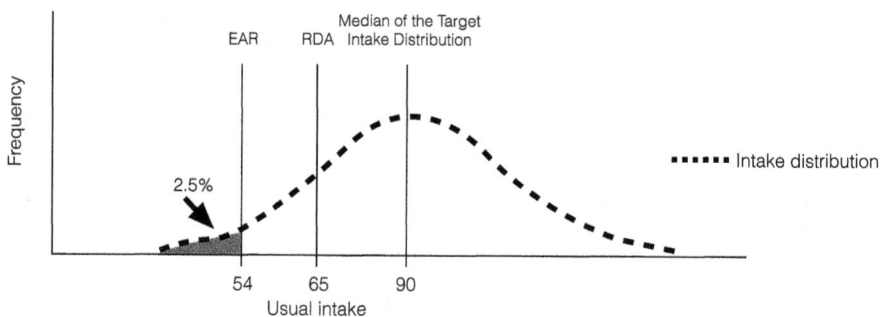

Source: adapted from reference (*333*), with the permission of the United States National Academy Press.

Scenario 1

Until relatively recently, nutritionists used the RNI as the basis for dietary planning and evaluation, and had as their optimum goal a population intake distribution in which the mean or median nutrient intakes for population subgroups met the relevant RNI (or its North American equivalent, the RDA). Assuming that the nutrient intakes are normally distributed, it is clear from **Figure 7.1** that according to this scenario, half of the population subgroup would have intakes that were below the RNI or RDA, while the intakes of the other half would be higher than the RNI (or RDA). More importantly, a relatively large percentage of the population subgroup would have usual intakes below the EAR (28% in this example). A target median intake set at the RNI is now generally considered to result in an unacceptably high prevalence of inadequate low intakes.

Scenario 2

An approach that plans for the usual intakes of all but 2.5% of the group to be above the RNI (or RDA) is equally unacceptable. For this to happen, the target median intake of the group would need to be set at a very high level, that is to say, at almost twice the RNI (or RDA). Virtually no intakes would be below the EAR (**Figure 7.2**). Adopting this approach increases the risk of exceeding the UL (if there is one), and may also result in adverse effects on the organoleptic properties of foods (due to the relatively high levels of added fortificants). On balance, such an approach is widely regarded as being unrealistic, costly, inefficient and potentially risky.

Scenario 3

The recommended strategy is thus to shift the usual distribution of intakes upwards so that the intake of each nutrient is at least at the EAR for all except 2–3% of the target population group (**Figure 7.3**). In this example, if the micronutrient interventions are planned so that only 2–3% of the group have an intake less than the EAR, the target median intake would have to be about 1.5 times the RNI (or RDA) and approximately 20% of the population group would have intakes below the RNI (or RDA). In other words, the program would be satisfactory when most individuals of the population (97–98%) satisfy the EAR, which may be similar to saying that most individuals of the population satisfy 80% of RNI.

7.3.2 Calculating the magnitude of micronutrient additions

This is the section of the Guidelines in which the application of the EAR cut-point method to the calculation of fortification levels (i.e. the amount of fortificant required to bring about the desired upwards shift in the distribution of usual intakes) is explained in greater detail. There are four steps: the first involves examining the prevalence of inadequate intakes of each nutrient in specific population groups. Having identified which population subgroups have the highest prevalence of inadequate intakes (step 2) and estimated the usual consumption of the chosen food vehicle by this group (step 3), the final step is to calculate the reduction in the prevalence of inadequate intakes (i.e. the proportion below the EAR) and the risk of excessive intakes (i.e. the proportion above the UL) that would be expected to occur at different levels of fortification. The methodology is illustrated with reference to a hypothetical case in which wheat flour is to be fortified with vitamin A.

Step 1. Observe the usual distribution of nutrient intakes in specific population subgroups

As mentioned in section 7.1.3, programme planning requires quantitative dietary intake data, initially for evaluating the current level of nutrient intakes in a population subgroup. This information is also necessary for estimating the amount of micronutrient that would need to be supplied by a micronutrient-delivery programme, and for predicting the impact of adding different amounts of micronutrients to different foods.

It is not necessary to conduct large surveys, although intake data should be collected from a stratified, representative sample of the whole target area. Ideally, all population subgroups should be represented. Collecting information from about 200 individuals in each population subgroup with the highest risk of deficiency (e.g. preschool-aged children and reproductive-age women in the lowest rural income group) and the highest risk of excess (e.g. men in the highest urban income group in the case of staple foods), and any other groups that are locally relevant, should provide sufficient valid information. It is helpful to select population subgroups with similar age ranges as those for which EARs are defined (see **Table 7.2**). Pregnant and lactating women should usually be treated as separate population subgroups.

Quantitative food intake data is usually obtained by 24-hour recall survey techniques or a combination of weighed/measured food intakes and recall, depending on what is locally possible. The distribution of usual intakes obtained in this way will be unrealistically wide, reflecting the fact that individuals may eat atypically small or large amounts on the day their intake was measured. By collecting at least 2 (preferably non-consecutive) days worth of food intake data for each individual, it is possible to estimate the day-to-day or intra-individual variability in intake, and adjust the distribution accordingly. For more detailed information about the statistical techniques that are available for reducing day-to-day variability in dietary intake data, readers are referred to relevant texts on this subject *(332,333,336,337)*[1]. If two days of dietary data per person are not available, or cannot be collected for what is felt to be a representative sample of the target population groups, it will then be necessary to use an estimate of day-to-day variability obtained elsewhere, but preferably one that has been obtained from a similar population. A study of the variability in nutrient intakes in a population in Malawi has recently been published and may be useful in this regard *(338)*.

Allowing for day-to-day variation usually has the effect of narrowing the intake distribution, so that fewer individuals will be below the EAR (and above

---

[1] The statistical method for reducing variability in intake data described by the Food and Nutrition Board of the Institute of Medicine *(332)* is also readable at the following web site: http://www.nap.edu/catalog/9956.html).

the UL). If some form of adjustment for variability is not made, the prevalence of inadequacies could be incorrectly estimated because the distribution does not reflect the usual intakes of the individuals in the group.

Having collated information on the quantities of various foods consumed, local, regional or international food composition tables can then be used to convert such data into amounts of nutrients consumed. If local information is not adequate, there are several international and regional databases that have been established expressly for this purpose. The United Nations group, INFOODS[1], is a repository of databases of this type and also serves as a resource for organizations and individuals interested in food composition data. The INFOODS web site provides links to various software programmes, for example, the *WorldFood Dietary Assessment System*[2], which can be used to calculate nutrient intakes from one-day dietary information. The results, i.e. the distribution of usual intake, for each nutrient and for each population group, are displayed as percentiles.

Example

Analysis of quantitative food intake survey data, according to the methodology outlined above, reveals that in adult women the distribution of vitamin A intakes is such that the median consumption is 240 µg RE per day. 5% of adult women have intakes that are less than 120 µg RE per day and 25% have vitamin A intakes that are below 200 µg RE per day. See **Table 7.4**.

Step 2. Identify the population subgroups at greatest risk of inadequate intakes of specific micronutrients

Certain subgroups of the population (usually children and women) tend to be at higher risk of having an inadequate intake of specific nutrients. On completion of step 1, it will be evident which subgroups have the highest prevalence of inadequate intakes for which nutrients. It is important to identify which population groups are at greatest risk so that a micronutrient-delivery programme can target these groups.

---

[1] INFOODS is the acronym of the International Network of Food Data Systems, which was established in 1984, on the recommendation of an international group convened under the auspices of the United Nations University. Its goal is to stimulate and coordinate efforts to improve the quality and availability of food analysis data worldwide and to make sure that accurate and reliable food composition data are readily accessible by all. Further information can be obtained from the web site: http://www.fao.org/infoods (accessed 15 March 2005).

[2] Software links can be accessed via the web site: http://www.fao.org/infoods/software_en.stm, (accessed 15 March 2005).

TABLE 7.4
Predicting the effect on the intake distributions of adult women of fortifying wheat flour with different levels of vitamin A[a]

Percentile	Distribution of usual wheat consumption (g/day)	Distribution of vitamin A intake from all sources (μg/day)			Vitamin A intake in relation to the EAR and the UL		
		Before fortification	After fortification at a level of 3 mg/kg	After fortification at a level of 5 mg/kg	Before fortification	After fortification at a level of 3 mg/kg	After fortification at a level of 5 mg/kg
Group at risk of deficiency							
5	30	120	210	270	–	–	–
10	45	160	295	385	–	–	*
25	120	200	560	800	–	*	*
50	180	240	780	1140	–	*	*
Group at risk of excess							
75	240	600	1320	1800	*	*	*
90	300	1000	1900	2500	*	*	*
95	360	1250	2330	3050	*	*	+
Resulting prevalence of inadequacy and risk of toxicity							
Proportion of women with intakes below the EAR (%)					65	15	8
Proportion of women with intakes above the UL (%)					0	2	6

–, intake is below the EAR; *, intake is above the EAR but below the UL; +, intake above the UL.
[a] For vitamin A an EAR of 357 μg/day is assumed. This is derived from the FAO/WHO RNI for this vitamin of 500 μg/day, to which a conversion factor of 1.4 has been applied (see **Annex C**). The UL is 3000 μg/day. If β-carotene were used rather than preformed vitamin A (retinol), there would be no UL.

Example

In this example, 65% of adult women were found to have inadequate intakes of vitamin A, i.e. intakes that were below the EAR for this vitamin (357 µg/day). The proportion of women who were at risk of exceeding the UL (3 000 µg/d) was very small (**Table 7.4**).

Step 3. Measure the usual amount of the intended food vehicle(s) that is consumed by the population subgroup at greatest risk of inadequate or excessive intakes

It is important that food vehicle consumption estimates are obtained not just for those subgroups that have been found to have the highest prevalence of inadequate intakes in step 2, but also for those subgroups with the highest levels of consumption (i.e. those at greatest risk of excessive intakes). This information will be used to predict the effects of different levels of fortification on the total intake of the nutrient (see step 4).

Example

Hypothetical values for the usual consumption of wheat by adult women, across the percentiles of vitamin A intake, are included in **Table 7.4**. The median consumption of wheat is 180 g/day. Ideally, the intake of the proposed food vehicle needs to be higher in the population groups with the highest prevalence of inadequate intakes, and lower in the relatively well-nourished groups. This would minimize the risk of the vitamin A intakes of the high wheat consumers becoming excessive. Unfortunately, in countries in which wheat flour tends to be consumed in larger amounts by wealthier (i.e. better-nourished) individuals, this is unlikely to be the case. Although Table 7.4 presents the case for adult women, it is important to point out here that the adult males are usually the group that have the highest consumption of staple foods.

Step 4. Simulate the effect of adding different levels of nutrient(s) to the food vehicle

Simulating the effect of micronutrient additions (by recalculating the distribution of vitamin A intakes but this time assuming that the wheat flour contains an additional 3 or 5 mg/kg vitamin A) helps to identify the most appropriate level of fortification for a given food vehicle, i.e. a level that prevents deficiency in a population at risk, yet avoids a high proportion of very high intakes.

> **Example**
>
> The data in **Table 7.4** show the effect of fortifying all wheat flour with vitamin A (as retinol), at a level of 3 and 5 mg/kg, on the distribution of total vitamin A intakes in adult women, the population subgroup identified as being at high risk of vitamin A deficiency. Prior to fortification, the prevalence of inadequate intakes in this group was 65% (see step 2).
>
> At a fortification level of 3 mg/kg of wheat, the prevalence of inadequate intakes (that is, the proportion of the group with intakes below the EAR of 357 µg/day) would fall from the pre-fortification level of about 65% (50–75%) to 15% (10–25%). In other words, as a result of fortification, about 50% of adult women have moved from having an inadequate to an adequate vitamin A intake. If the fortification level is increased to 5 mg/kg of wheat, only 8% of women would have an inadequate intake. However, at the 5 mg/kg fortification level, the highest 6% of wheat consumers would have a total vitamin A intake that might exceed the UL of 3000 µg/day.
>
> Given that calculation does not consider vitamin A intake by adult males,, it may be better to select the 3 mg/kg fortification level and then find another food vehicle to fortify or another delivery mechanism to meet the shortfall in vitamin A intake in the 15% of women whose intake remains unsatisfied through the consumption of fortified wheat flour. Decisions of this nature can only be made on the basis of local information, and with due consideration of the potential risks associated with excessive intakes of vitamin A (see section 7.5).

Step 4 would need to be repeated in order to determine the appropriate fortification level for wheat flour with vitamin A for any other at-risk population groups identified in step 2. Steps 3 and 4 would then be repeated for any other nutrients being considered for the fortification programme, in which case the corresponding EARs and current nutrient intake distribution data would be needed.

7.3.3 Adaptations to the EAR cut-point methodology for specific nutrients
7.3.3.1 Iron

The EAR cut-point approach cannot be used to estimate the prevalence of inadequate iron intakes in some population subgroups, notably children, menstruating adolescents and adult women, on account of the fact that their requirements for iron are not normally distributed (*see section 7.2.1*). The requirements of menstruating adolescents and adult women are not normally distributed largely because of the skewed distribution of their iron losses, and of menstrual losses in particular (*91*). Assuming for present purposes that a coefficient of variation (CV) greater than 40% indicates a skewed distribution, then the population groups with skewed requirements for iron are as follows (based on data from the United States FNB/IOM (*91*):

- children, aged 1–3 years (CV = 67%);
- children, aged 4–8 years (CV = 75%);
- menstruating adolescents, aged 14–18 years (CV = 45%);
- menstruating women (CV = 63%).

For the other population groups, the CV of the distribution of iron requirements is 30% or less.

For those groups with skewed requirements, an alternative approach to the EAR cut-point method must be used, namely a full probability approach. **Table 7.5** gives the probability of an iron intake being inadequate at a given range of usual iron intake for the population subgroups of interest, i.e. young children and menstruating females. Using these values, it is possible to calculate the prevalence of inadequate intakes in a population subgroup from estimates of the percentage of the group with intakes in a given intake range (note that the bioavailability of iron from the usual diet must also be known). For each intake range, a prevalence of inadequacy is obtained by multiplying the percentage of the group with intakes in that range by the probability of inadequacy. Summing the prevalences of inadequacy in each intake range provides an estimate of the total prevalence of inadequacy for the population group of interest.

To illustrate the application of the probability method (using the data in Table 7.5), the prevalence of inadequate iron intakes in a population of adult menstruating women, consuming a diet from which the iron bioavailability is 5%, is calculated in **Table 7.6**. For instance, according to Table 7.5, the women in the lowest iron intake range (i.e. less than 15 mg per day) have a probability of inadequacy of 1.0, which means that all the women in this group have iron intakes that are less than their requirements. Given that 2% of women in the population have intakes in this range, these women contribute 2% to the total prevalence of inadequacy in that population group. Similarly, those women whose iron intake is in the range 23.6–25.7 mg per day will have a probability of an inadequacy of 0.65. If 20% of the women have intakes in this range, the prevalence of inadequacy among women with intakes in this range is 20 × 0.65 or 13% (**Table 7.6**). When similar calculations are performed for each of the other intake ranges, and then summed, an overall prevalence of inadequacy for the group of 66.6% is obtained. In other words, in this example, two thirds of the population of women have intakes that are likely to be below their requirements. Note that such calculations are easily performed with a spreadsheet or a statistical programming language.

TABLE 7.5
Probability of inadequate iron intakes in selected population subgroups at different ranges of usual intake (mg/day)

Probability of inadequacy[a]	Usual intake of children aged 1–3 years consuming a diet from which the bioavailability of iron is			Usual intake of children aged 4–8 years consuming a diet from which the bioavailability of iron is			Usual intake of females aged 14–18 years consuming a diet from which the bioavailability of iron is			Usual intake of menstruating women consuming a diet from which the bioavailability of iron is		
	5%	10%	15%	5%	10%	15%	5%	10%	15%	5%	10%	15%
1.00	<3.6	<1.8	<1.3	<4.8	<2.4	<1.6	<16.2	<8.1	<5.4	<15.0	<7.5	<5.0
0.96	3.6–4.5	1.8–2.3	1.3–1.5	4.8–5.9	2.4–3.0	1.6–2.0	16.2–17.7	8.1–8.8	5.4–5.9	15.0–16.7	7.5–8.4	5.0–5.6
0.93	4.5–5.5	2.3–2.8	1.5–1.8	5.9–7.4	3.0–3.7	2.0–2.4	17.7–19.6	8.8–9.8	5.9–6.5	16.7–18.7	8.4–9.4	5.6–6.2
0.85	5.5–7.1	2.8–3.6	1.8–2.4	7.4–9.5	3.7–4.8	2.4–3.2	19.7–22.1	9.8–11.1	6.5–7.4	18.7–21.4	9.4–10.7	6.2–7.1
0.75	7.1–8.3	3.6–4.2	2.4–2.8	9.5–11.3	4.8–5.7	3.2–3.8	22.1–24.1	11.1–12.0	7.4–8.0	21.4–23.6	10.7–11.8	7.1–7.9
0.65	8.3–9.6	4.2–4.8	2.8–3.2	11.3–13.0	5.7–6.5	3.8–4.3	24.1–26.0	12.0–13.0	8.0–8.7	23.6–25.7	11.8–12.9	7.9–8.6
0.55	9.6–10.8	4.8–5.4	3.2–3.6	13.0–14.8	6.5–7.4	4.3–4.9	26.0–27.8	13.0–13.9	8.7–9.3	25.7–27.8	12.9–13.9	8.6–9.3
0.45	10.8–12.2	5.4–6.1	3.6–4.1	14.8–16.7	7.4–8.4	4.9–5.6	27.8–29.7	13.9–14.8	9.3–9.9	27.8–30.2	13.9–15.1	9.3–10.1
0.35	12.2–13.8	6.1–6.9	4.1–4.6	16.7–19.0	8.4–9.5	5.6–6.3	29.7–32.1	14.8–16.1	9.9–10.7	30.2–33.2	15.1–16.6	10.1–11.1
0.25	13.8–15.8	6.9–7.9	4.6–5.3	19.0–21.9	9.5–11.0	6.3–7.3	32.1–35.2	16.1–17.6	10.7–11.7	33.2–37.3	16.6–18.7	11.1–12.4
0.15	15.8–18.9	7.9–9.5	5.3–6.3	21.9–26.3	11.0–13.2	7.3–8.8	35.2–40.4	17.6–20.2	11.7–13.5	37.3–45.0	18.7–22.5	12.4–15.0
0.08	18.9–21.8	9.5–10.9	6.3–7.3	26.3–30.4	13.2–15.2	8.8–5.1	40.4–45.9	20.2–23.0	13.5–15.3	45.0–53.5	22.5–26.7	15.0–17.8
0.04	21.8–24.5	10.9–12.3	7.3–8.2	30.4–34.3	15.2–17.2	5.1–5.7	45.9–51.8	23.0–25.9	15.3–17.3	53.5–63.0	26.7–31.5	17.8–21.0
0	>24.5	>12.3	>8.2	>34.3	>17.2	>5.7	>51.8	>25.9	>17.3	>63.0	>31.5	>21.0

[a] Probability that the requirement for iron is greater than the usual intake. For the purpose of assessing populations, a probability of 1 has been assigned to usual intakes that are below the 2.5th percentile of requirements, and a probability of 0 has been assigned to usual intakes that fall above the 97.5th percentile of requirements. Usual intakes should be adjusted for intra-individual variance as described in section 7.3.2 (step 1).

Source: adapted from reference (91).

TABLE 7.6

Prevalence of inadequate iron intakes for menstruating women consuming a diet from which the average iron bioavailability is 5%: an example calculation

Probability of inadequacy[a]	Intake range with this probability of inadequacy (mg/day)	Proportion of menstruating women with intakes in this range (%)	Prevalence of inadequacy[b] (%)
1.00	<15.0	2	2
0.96	15.0–16.7	10	9.6
0.93	16.7–18.7	10	9.3
0.85	18.7–21.4	10	8.5
0.75	21.4–23.6	15	11.3
0.65	23.6–25.7	20	13
0.55	25.7–27.8	10	5.5
0.45	27.8–30.2	8	3.6
0.35	30.2–33.2	5	1.8
0.25	33.2–37.3	5	1.3
0.15	37.3–45.0	3	0.5
0.08	45.0–53.5	2	0.2
0.04	53.5–63.0	0	0
0.00	>63.0	0	0
Probability of inadequate intakes for all menstruating women			66.6%

[a] Probability that the requirement for iron is greater than the usual intake. For the purpose of assessing populations, a probability of 1 has been assigned to usual intakes that are below the 2.5th percentile of requirements, and a probability of 0 has been assigned to usual intakes that fall above the 97.5th percentile of requirements. Usual intakes should be adjusted for intra-individual variance as described in section 7.3.2 (step 1).
[b] The prevalence of inadequacy = probability of inadequacy for a given intake range × the percentage of women with intakes in that range.

Having established the prevalence of inadequate intakes, the next step is to simulate how the distribution of intakes would shift upwards as a result of the consumption of iron fortified food(s) (in much the same way as was done in steps 3 and 4 for vitamin A above; see Table 7.4) with a view to finding that level of fortification that would bring the estimated prevalence of inadequacy down to an acceptable level, say 2–3%.

7.3.3.2 Iodine

Based on field experience, WHO has recommended fortification levels for iodine in salt (283). The current recommendation, designed to provide the adult RNI (i.e. 150 µg/day), is to add 20–40 mg iodine/kg salt. This level of fortification assumes no iodine in the usual diet pre-fortification, and that the usual amount of salt consumed is 10 g per day.

7.3.3.3 Folate/folic acid

Numerous studies have demonstrated that a higher intake of folate by some women can reduce their risk of delivering an infant with a neural tube defect (see section 4.2.3). It is generally accepted that women should consume an additional 400 µg/day as folic acid in fortified foods or supplements periconceptionally (*128*). Currently, it is unknown whether the reduction in risk results from the correction of a folate deficiency or through some other as yet unidentified mechanism. However, increasing intake by just 200 µg/day through fortification has been shown to be effective in improving folate status and in lowering the prevalence of neural tube defects in both Canada (*51*) and the United States (*48,49*). Based on this evidence, the Pan American Health Organization has recommended that throughout Latin America food fortification interventions should provide an additional 200 µg folic acid per day (*339*). It is anticipated that at these levels of additional intake, the usual daily intake of folic acid plus food folate will exceed the EAR and approach the RNI for the majority of the target population. In any case, it would be appropriate to start with the estimation of the nutritional gap for folate, which may be around that value, and hence the decision will have a nutritional justification.

It should be noted that folate intakes are conventionally expressed in units of Dietary Folate Equivalents (DFE), where 1 µg folate in food is equivalent to 1 DFE. Because of its higher bioavailability, 1 µg of folic acid actually supplies 1.7 DFE and so less folic acid (the synthetic form of folate that is used as a fortificant and in supplements) is required to meet a given requirement for folate (*128*).

7.3.3.4 Vitamin D

Vitamin D is produced in the skin on exposure to ultraviolet light. At latitudes between 42°N and 42°S, 30 minutes of skin exposure per day (arms and face) is usually sufficient to provide the body with all the vitamin D it needs. However, as discussed in section 4.6, several factors inhibit the ability of the body to synthesize vitamin D and thus increase the risk of vitamin D deficiency. These factors may include living at a more northerly or more southerly latitude (where the days are shorter during the winter season), leaving little skin exposed to ultraviolet light, and having dark skin.

Any decisions about appropriate levels of vitamin D fortification would need to take exposure to sunlight into account. For instance, in situations where exposure to sunlight is adequate but dietary intake of vitamin D is low, it is quite likely that the risk of vitamin D deficiency in a population will be overestimated if based on intake data alone. For this reason, information on the prevalence of rickets in infants and children, low serum 25-hydroxy vitamin D concentrations in the general population, and osteomalacia and/or osteoporosis in women, should be evaluated when predicting the level of vitamin D fortification required.

7.3.3.5 Niacin

Niacin (vitamin B_3) is unique in that it can be synthesized from the amino acid, tryptophan (1 mg niacin can be generated from approximately 60 mg tryptophan). Thus, similar to the situation with vitamin D, there will appear to be a high prevalence of inadequate intakes of the vitamin using only the dietary intake, both before and after fortification, if non-dietary sources of niacin (i.e. synthesis from tryptophan) are not considered. However, because the rate of niacin synthesis from tryptophan is not known with certainty, and probably varies with life stage and physiological status (e.g. in pregnancy and for young infants), the most practical approach may be to ignore the contribution of tryptophan when setting fortification levels. Moreover, the risk of niacin toxicity is low, especially if niacinamide is used as the fortificant (see **Table 7.3**).

As maize contains niacin in a bound form and is low in tryptophan, populations whose staple food is maize (especially maize that is untreated with alkali) are most likely to benefit from niacin fortification (see section 4.4.3).

7.3.4 Bioavailability considerations

The methods used to set EARs already include an adjustment for the bioavailability (i.e. % absorption) of a nutrient from foods, and so when formulating fortification levels using the EAR cut-point method there is usually no need to make any further allowance for this factor. If, however, the bioavailability of the fortificant nutrient is likely to be substantially different from that naturally present in the diet, some further adjustment will need to be made. The efficiency of utilization of the form of the fortificant nutrient may also need to be considered. For example, the conversion rate of synthetic β-carotene to retinol in oil is 2:1, but in the absence of oil, the rate is significantly lower (i.e. 6:1) and the utilization much less efficient.

Micronutrients for which differences in bioavailability may be a factor are listed in **Table 7.7**. Electrolytic iron, for instance, is poorly absorbed, and it is recommended that this particular form of iron fortificant be added at twice the quantity of ferrous sulfate iron, which has a similar bioavailability to non-haem iron in the diet (**Table 5.2**). In contrast, the absorption of some fortificants, such as folic acid and vitamin B_{12}, may be substantially higher than their equivalent (i.e. naturally-occurring) forms in foods (see *section 7.3.3.3*).

Ideally, the absorption of the fortificant nutrient should be confirmed in efficacy trials involving the target population, especially in situations where there is uncertainty about its bioavailability. If this is not possible, then as a minimum, absorption data should be obtained from human studies by other

TABLE 7.7
Examples of micronutrients for which the bioavailability of the form used for fortification differs substantially from their bioavailability in the usual diet

Nutrient/fortificant compound	Proportion absorbed relative to usual diet
Iron	
■ Electrolytic iron	0.5 (compared with non-haem iron in foods)
■ NaFeEDTA[a]	3.0 at high phytate, 1.0 at low phytate (compared with non-haem iron in foods)
■ Ferrous bisglycinate	2.0–3.0 (compared with non-haem iron in foods)
Vitamin A	
■ β-carotene[b]	0.15 from fortified foods in the absence of oil, but 0.5 in oil (compared with retinol)
Folate	
■ Folic acid	1.7 (compared with Dietary Folate Equivalents of natural food folates)
Vitamin B_{12}	2.0 (compared with cobalamin in foods)

[a] NaFeEDTA, sodium iron ethylenediaminetetraacetic acid.
[b] When β-carotene is added as a food fortificant, its bioavailability is higher (the conversion factor β-carotene:retinol is 6:1 in non-oily foods) than that of naturally-occurring β-carotene (in fruits and vegetables), for which the corresponding conversion factor is 12:1.

investigators, and its bioavailability evaluated once the fortification programme is in place.

7.4 Other factors to consider when deciding fortification levels

Experience has shown that in practice, and especially in the case of mass fortification, the amount of micronutrient that can be added to foods is often limited by various safety, technological and/or economic constraints. Of these three limiting factors, cost constraints tend to be the more flexible, whereas safety and technological constraints are more likely to be fixed. However, for some micronutrients there may be ways of overcoming some of the technological constraints. For instance, in the case of iron, undesirable sensory changes in the food vehicle caused by the presence of the fortificant compound might be reduced by using a microencapsulated form of iron instead (see *section 5.1.3.3*). Nor are safety constraints necessarily always cast in stone; with new knowledge and improvements in the precision of ULs, safety constraints may well change over time.

Table 7.8 assesses the strength of each of the three main types of constraint for the range of micronutrients covered by these Guidelines. The assessment of the magnitude of the safety risk is based on the closeness of the EAR to the UL; the closer these two values, the greater the risk. The magnitudes indicated in this table are subjective and are intended only to highlight those areas that may be of concern for a given micronutrient.

TABLE 7.8
Factors that may limit the amount of fortificants that can be added to a single food vehicle

Nutrient	Technological/sensory	Safety	Cost
Vitamin A	X	XXX	XXX[a]
Vitamin D	–	X	X
Vitamin E	–	X	XXX
Vitamin C	XX	X	XXX[b]
Thiamine (vitamin B_1)	–	–	–
Riboflavin (vitamin B_2)	XX	–	–
Niacin (vitamin B_3)	–	XXX[c]	X
Vitamin B_6	–	X	–
Folic acid	–	XXX[d]	–
Vitamin B_{12}	–	–	X
Iron[e]	XXX	XX	X
Zinc	XX	XXX	X
Calcium	X	XX	XXX[f]
Selenium	–	X	X
Iodine	X	XXX	–

–, no constraint; X, a minor constraint; XX, moderate constraint; XXX, major constraint.
[a] If an oil-based form is used to fortify oils or fats, costs can be reduced.
[b] Cost constraints are mainly a consequence of losses during manufacturing, storage, distribution and cooking which mean that a considerable overage is required.
[c] Much less of a concern if niacinamide, as opposed to nicotinic acid, is used as the fortificant.
[d] The risk of adverse effects is minimized by the co-addition of vitamin B_{12}.
[e] Refers to the more bioavailable forms.
[f] Cost constraints are mainly a consequence of the need to add such large amounts.

7.4.1 Safety limits

The safety of fortification can be assessed by comparing predicted micronutrient intakes (in particular the intakes that will occur at higher levels of fortification and at higher intakes of fortified foods, calculated as described in *section 7.3.2*) with the UL (**Table 7.3**). Even if a micronutrient has no recommended UL, high levels of micronutrient additions should be avoided, especially if there is no evidence of derived benefit from levels of intake in excess of the RNI.

7.4.2 Technological limits

The technological limit is defined as the highest possible level of micronutrient addition that does not cause adverse organoleptic changes in the food vehicle. The effects of added micronutrients on the organoleptic properties of the chosen food vehicle must be tested at an early stage, and alternative forms of the fortificant used if necessary (see Part III). Technological incompatibility is usually less of a constraint in the case of food products fortified through targeted or market-driven interventions; such products tend to be distributed to consumers in specialized individual packages, and as final products (see section 7.5.2).

7.4.3 Cost limits

The cost limit is defined as the highest increase in the cost of the food due to fortification that is acceptable to producers and consumers. Indeed, one of the most important criteria for a successful and sustainable food fortification programme in free trade economies is a low proportional increase in product price as a result of fortification. This is especially true of mass fortified products. The issue of cost is usually less of a constraint in the case of targeted and market-driven processed foods, as the price of the product tends to be sufficiently high to absorb the costs associated with fortification.

Table 7.9 shows the annual investment required to provide an adult male with 100% of his EAR of 14 essential micronutrients, taking into account micronutrient losses during production, distribution and storage as well as during cooking, and also any variability in the fortification process which might lead to a lowering of the amount of fortificant delivered (e.g. uneven mixing). The total cost for a dry non-oily food, such as wheat flour, is approximately US$ 4.00 per year, or US$ 0.01 per day. According to these calculations, the most expensive fortificants are calcium (because larger amounts are needed), vitamin A, vitamin E and vitamin C (because of overage needed to compensate for losses). The cheapest – each costing less than US$ 0.02 per year – are thiamine (vitamin B_1), vitamin B_6, folic acid, zinc and iodine.

The above cost estimates apply to the large-scale centralized fortification of a staple, i.e. fortification that is carried out in just a few large industrial units. Under such circumstances, the purchase price of the micronutrients accounts for by far the greatest proportion (at least 80–90%) of the total fortification cost. When fortification is carried out by multiple, smaller-scale enterprises, both the initial investment costs (e.g. of equipment) and the running costs (e.g. of quality control procedures) are proportionally higher, a factor which might hinder the feasibility and sustainability of the programme. Such considerations notwithstanding, in many settings food fortification can be a very affordable way of correcting inadequate micronutrient intakes, and more often than not, the main challenge is finding a suitable industrially-manufactured food vehicle that is consumed in sufficient amounts by the population at risk.

7.5 Adapting the EAR cut-point methodology to mass, targeted and market-driven fortification interventions

The EAR cut-point method can be used to select appropriate fortification levels and to estimate their impact on the prevalence of inadequate intakes for all three

TABLE 7.9
Estimated costs of selected fortificants[a]

	Adult EAR	Nutrient content of fortificant (%)	Cost of fortificant (US$/kg)	Overage[b] (%)	Annual cost of fortificant (US$)[c]
Vitamin A					
■ Vitamin A (SD-250)	429 µg	7.5	42	50	0.136
■ Vitamin A palmitate, 1 million IU	429 µg	30	52	30	0.042
Vitamin D					
■ Watersoluble	5 µg	0.25	33	20	0.035
■ In oil, 1 million IU/g	5 µg	2.5	80	20	0.008
Vitamin E	8 mg	67	26	20	0.163
Vitamin C	37 mg	100	10	250[d]	0.567
Thiamine (vitamin B_1)	1.0 mg	81	24	40	0.018
Riboflavin (vitamin B_2)	1.1 mg	100	38	30	0.024
Niacin (vitamin B_3)	12 mg	99	9	10	0.053
Vitamin B_6	1.1 mg	82	28	20	0.020
Folic acid	188 µg[e]	100	90	50	0.011
Vitamin B_{12}, 0.1% watersoluble	2.0 µg	0.1	38	30	0.043
Iron[f]					
■ NaFeEDTA	7.0 mg	13	15.45	5	0.383
■ Ferrous bisglycinate	7.0 mg	20	25	5	0.402
■ Ferrous fumarate	10.5 mg	33	5.12	5	0.075
■ $FeSO_4$, dried	10.5 mg	33	2.35	5	0.034
■ $FeSO_4$, encapsulated	10.5 mg	16	12.28	5	0.371
■ Electrolytic iron	21.1 mg	97	5.76	5	0.058
Zinc (as oxide)	6 mg[g]	80	3.35	5	0.012
Calcium (as phosphate)	833 mg	39	2.7	5	2.652
Iodine (as potassium iodate)	107 µg	59	20	25	0.002

NaFeEDTA, sodium iron ethylenediaminetetraaectic acid; $FeSO_4$, ferrous.
[a] The cost of supplying enough micronutrient to meet 100% of the EAR of an adult male, daily for one year (via dry food).
[b] The overage is an additional amount that must be added to compensate for losses during production, storage, food production and distribution.
[c] Includes an overage of +20% to cover variability in the fortification process.
[d] Vitamin C is one of the least stable fortificants and a high overage is normally required. If, however, the fortified food is not subject to heat or oxidation, the overage can be much lower.
[e] As folic acid is 1.7 times more bioavailable than naturally-occurring food folates, the EAR for folate has been divided by 1.7.
[f] The EAR for iron depends on its bioavailability from the diet as well as the identity of the iron compound used as the fortificant. The values given here refer to white wheat flour (low extraction), and apply to diets with similar bioavailabilities. If the diet contains large amounts of iron absorption inhibitors, the EAR should be multiplied by a factor of around 2. Reduced iron is not included; its absorption would be at most about half that of electrolytic iron.
[g] Assuming a moderate bioavailability of zinc.

types of intervention – mass, targeted and market-driven. However, in each case, there are some unique issues that need to be addressed; these are outlined below.

7.5.1 Mass fortification
7.5.1.1 Setting levels of micronutrient additions
Many industrialized and some developing countries have a long history of experience with mass fortification. In many cases, fortification levels were selected empirically, that is to say, were based on a combination of experience elsewhere and technological and cost constraints, rather than on any attempt to derive, in a systematic fashion, fortification levels likely to provide the most benefit. This was especially true of situations and settings where food intake data were not available, yet there was a strong desire to move ahead with fortification. However, unless food and nutrient intake data are used as the basis of programme design and evaluation – as described earlier in this chapter – it cannot be known whether those at greatest risk of deficiency in a specific nutrient (and who have the lowest pre-fortification intakes) will consume enough of the fortified food to improve their nutrient intake significantly, and whether those who have the highest pre-fortification intakes will be at risk of excessive intakes after fortification.

Having emphasized the importance of a more rigorous approach to setting fortification levels, it is nevertheless useful to know what fortification levels are already in use for specific foods in other locations. At the very least, knowledge of what levels are used elsewhere will provide some guidance as to what levels of fortification are technologically and economically feasible in which foods. Interestingly, as can be seen from **Table 7.10**, the band of currently used fortification levels for each type of food is relatively narrow. It must be stressed that the impact of fortification at these levels on nutrient intake and nutritional status has only been adequately evaluated in a handful of settings and that these levels cannot be recommended universally. Furthermore, fortification levels in use in one location may be inappropriate in another, and should not be used without confirming their suitability by using the EAR and UL cut-point method, as described in these Guidelines.

7.5.1.2 Constraints
In the case of mass fortification programmes, which tend to rely on staples and condiments as the food vehicle, cost is often the most significant limiting factor. Staples and condiments are consumed frequently and in large amounts, not only by the population directly but also by food industries. Even small variations in price can thus have profound consequences; opposition to fortified products on the grounds of cost, can, for example, lead to an increase in deceptive practices, even smuggling.

TABLE 7.10
Examples of levels of micronutrients currently added to staples and condiments worldwide (mg/kg)

Nutrient	Milk	Evaporated milk	Powdered milk	Margarine	Vegetable oil	Sugar	Wheat flour	Pasta	Corn masa flour	Pre-cooked maize flour	Maize flour	Maize meal	Soy/fish Sauce	Salt
Vitamin A	0.7–1.0	2–3	4.5–7.5	5–15	5–15	5–15	1–5	—	—	2.8	—	1–2	—	—
Vitamin D	0.01	0.01	0.05–0.06	0.02–0.15	—	—	0.014	—	—	—	—	—	—	—
Vitamin E	—	—	—	—	—	—	—	—	—	—	—	—	—	—
Vitamin C	—	—	—	—	—	—	—	—	—	—	—	—	—	—
Thiamine (vitamin B_1)	—	—	—	—	—	—	1.5–7.0	8–10	1–6	3.1	2.4	2–3	—	—
Riboflavin (vitamin B_2)	—	—	—	16	—	—	1–5	3–5	1–5	2.5	—	1.7–2.5	—	—
Niacin (vitamin B_3)	—	—	—	180	—	—	15–55	35–57	25–50	51	1.6	19–30	—	—
Vitamin B_6	—	—	—	20	—	—	2.5	—	—	—	—	2–3	—	—
Folic acid	—	—	—	2	—	—	0.5–3.0	—	0.5–3.0	—	—	0.4–0.5	—	—
Vitamin B_{12}	—	—	—	—	—	—	0.01^a	—	—	—	—	—	—	—
Iron[b]														
— NaFeEDTA	—	—	—	—	—	—	—	—	—	—	—	—	—	—
— Ferrous bisglycinate	—	—	—	—	—	—	—	—	22	—	—	—	250	500^c
— Ferrous sulfate or fumarate	—	—	—	—	—	—	30–45	30	30	30+	—	—	—	—
— Electrolytic iron	—	—	—	—	—	—	45–60	25–35	30–60	20+	—	9–14	—	—
Zinc (oxide)	—	—	—	—	—	—	15–30	—	15–30	—	—	—	—	—
Calcium	—	—	—	—	—	—	2100–3900	—	—	—	—	—	—	—
Iodine	—	—	—	—	—	—	—	—	—	—	—	—	—	15–60

NaFeEDTA, sodium iron ethylenediaminetetraacetic acid.
[a] As recommended at a recent PAHO/WHO meeting (339).
[b] Usually foods are fortified with only one iron compound, but in the case of pre-cooked maize flour trials are currently underway to assess the viability of using more than one iron fortificant.
[c] As encapsulated ferrous sulfate, but to date this has only been used only in experimental trials.

The cost of fortifying one tonne of wheat flour with ferrous fumarate (45 mg Fe/kg), zinc oxide (30 mg/kg), thiamine (6.5 mg/kg), riboflavin (4 mg/kg), niacin (50 mg/kg), folic acid (2.0 mg/kg), vitamin B_{12} (0.010 mg/kg) and vitamin A (2.0 mg/kg) has been estimated to be US$ 5. At a per capita consumption of 100 g of wheat flour a day, this is equivalent to only US$ 0.182 per year or US$ 0.0005 per day per person. Nevertheless, in a country with 10 million consumers, the fortification costs amount to some US$ 5000 per day (US$ 1.825 million per year). At this cost level, some manufacturers might well be tempted to take that as additional profit rather than add the micronutrients.

The cost of fortifying wheat flour with the same micronutrients listed above might increase the price of the flour by US$ 0.30–0.50 per kg, or by 1.0–1.7% relative to that of the unfortified product. Although such increments can be incorporated into the product price, in a free-market economy even small price differentials might be too much to preserve the market share of the fortified product against a non-fortified alternative, especially if the competitive rules are not equal for all. For example, fortification of salt with 20–40 mg iodine/kg using potassium iodate costs US$ 1.25 per tonne, or US$ 0.0000125 per day per person (US$ 0.005 per year per person) assuming a daily consumption of 10 g of salt. This equates to around US$ 45 625 per year for a country of 10 million persons. Thus, although the absolute annual investment is relatively low, this represents an increment in price of 2% over raw salt (assuming the price of salt is US$ 0.06 per kg). Even this modest price increment is disliked by many small producers who fear loss of their market share to the extent that they would avoid adding iodine if not for strict governmental enforcement. Herein lies the reason why salt is currently not more widely used as a vehicle for other micronutrients, even if their addition were technically feasible and biologically efficacious. If, however, mechanisms to overcome impediments of this nature, such as subsidies or effective and reliable enforcement mechanisms, were to be devised, salt may yet become a more attractive option as a vehicle for mass fortification. Salt could also be used in targeted programmes, where price increases due to the cost of fortification tend to be less limiting.

In summary, experience dictates that a mass fortification in an open market economy works best when the increase in the price of the fortified product, relative to the unfortified version, does not exceed 1–2%. However, this is by no means a universal prescription and any decisions relating to cost limits can only be taken by government and industry depending on the situation in any given country.

Annex D describes a procedure that can be used for setting Feasible Fortification Levels for mass fortification programmes based on consideration of safety, technological and cost constraints. If the combined effect of these constraints is to reduce the amount of nutrient that can be added to below that which is required to achieve a given intake goal, then more than one food may need to be fortified or some nutrients may have to be supplied through other strategies, such as supplementation.

7.5.2 Targeted fortification

With targeted fortification, the various constraints on micronutrient additions are generally less restrictive than those that operate in the case of food products subject to mass fortification. Not only is the target group more clearly defined (refugees, displaced persons and young children are usually the main beneficiaries), but the fortified foods are usually in their final form or are offered in defined serving sizes, so that the risk of exceeding ULs is reduced. In addition, the presentation and sensory properties of foods selected for targeted fortification are such that any changes introduced by the addition of micronutrients are more easily hidden, and the cost of fortification is usually compatible with the price of the product or partly borne by the financial supporters of the programme. Nevertheless, it is always instructive to assess technological compatibility and overall cost of targeted fortified foods at the programme planning stage.

7.5.2.1 Blended foods

Guidelines covering the fortification of blended foods for refugees and displaced persons are available elsewhere (*62*) and thus are not discussed in detail here.

7.5.2.2 Complementary foods

That the micronutrient content of breast milk may be considerably lower in undernourished women is a concern in several parts of the world. Nutrients most likely to be reduced in the breast milk of undernourished mothers include vitamin A, all B vitamins except folate, iodine and selenium. The fortification of complementary foods thus provides a means of supplying additional nutrients to infants and children who are still receiving breast milk. However, because infants and young children also require their diets to have a high nutrient density (i.e. a high concentration of nutrient per kcal), in some settings it may be difficult to achieve a low risk of inadequate nutrient intakes even when complementary foods are fortified.

The process of setting the level of fortification for complementary foods is similar to that described earlier in this chapter (see section 7.3.2). The starting point is again the distribution of usual intakes, although in this case is it necessary to consider the intakes from both breast milk and complementary foods for each nutrient being studied. Breast-milk intakes can be estimated from published information on the composition of breast milk (such as that published by WHO, which includes data from both industrialized and developing countries (*340*), and intakes from other sources can be collected using 24-hour recall methods for a representative sample of the group of interest.

Having obtained the relevant intake data, the procedure for setting fortification levels is then much the same as previously, the steps being as follows:

Step 1. Determine the prevalence of intakes that are below the EAR

First, review the intake distributions and determine the prevalence of intakes that are below the EAR; decide if this level of inadequate intakes is acceptable. If it is not, then fortification of complementary foods could be considered.

Step 2. Decide what level of prevalence of inadequate intakes is acceptable

Next, decide on an acceptable prevalence of inadequacy (i.e. the percentage of the children with intakes below the EAR). Often 2–3% is taken to be the maximum desirable prevalence of inadequate intakes. Then determine the level of fortification that will move the prevalence of inadequacy down to this acceptable level.

Step 3. Select a food vehicle

Choose the most appropriate vehicle for fortification, i.e. the one that will reach most of the children, or will reach those with the greatest need.

Step 4. Simulate the impact of fortification

Finally, calculate through simulation the likely impact of fortification of the chosen food vehicle on the prevalence of inadequate intakes and proportion of intakes that are in excess of the UL.

With the exception of iron and zinc, EARs are not defined for infants aged 0–12 months. For this age group, recommended intakes are expressed in terms of Adequate Intakes (AIs), in which case the nutritional goal of a fortification programme would be the raising of the mean intake of the target group to the AI.

Simpler alternative approaches to setting fortification levels for complementary foods do, however, exist. One option is to estimate the size of the gap between the usual median intake and the recommended intake (either the EAR or the AI, depending on the nutrient of interest); this then equates to the amount of micronutrient that needs to be added in order to achieve the desired nutritional goal. Dividing the nutritional gap by the daily amount of food consumed gives the amount of micronutrient that needs to be supplied per gram of the fortified food[1].

---

[1] The fortification level is more conventionally expressed as an amount per 100 g or per serving size (i.e. the amount per gram multiplied by the average serving size, usually 40 g).

7. DEFINING AND SETTING PROGRAMME GOAL

The other option, which is the easier of the two because there is no need for intake data, is to simply add a specific proportion of the EAR (or AI) of the target group in the hope that by so doing the nutritional needs of the majority of the children will be met. Again it is necessary to know how much of a given complementary food is consumed per day, and also what the usual serving sizes are in order to derive a fortification level per 100g of product or per serving size.

The Codex Alimentarius Commission provides recommendations for the composition of certain foods designated for infants and young children. These are subject to a process of continual review and are regularly revised. In the case of supplementary foods for older infants and young children, when the food is supplemented with specific nutrients, the Codex recommendation is to add at least two thirds of the reference daily requirement per 100g of food (*341*). In practice, this means that if an average serving size for this age group is around 40g, each serving should provide between 30% and 50% of the EAR in order to satisfy the daily nutrient needs in 2 to 3 servings a day. Obviously, if detailed dietary information is available, the micronutrient content of complementary foods might be adjusted to the exact characteristics and needs of the target group.

7.5.3 Market-driven fortification

Food manufacturers add micronutrients to their products not just to increase their nutritional value but also to increase their appeal to the health conscious consumer. This business-oriented initiative can play a positive role in public health by improving the supply of essential nutrients that are sometimes difficult to provide in sufficient amounts via mass fortification. So far, the public health impact of fortification of market-driven processed foods has been very modest in developing countries but its importance is expected to be greater in the future, largely as a natural consequence of increasing urbanization and availability of such foods.

The main aim of regulating the level of fortificants in processed foods is preserving the nutritional balance and safety of the diet for the population at large. To this end, minimum levels need to be set to ensure that reasonable amounts of micronutrients are added to food products; these must be stated on the product label, and may be referred to when advertising the product. It is important to also fix maximum levels so as to reduce the risk of an excessive nutrient intake through the consumption of fortified foods, especially for those micronutrients with well-established UL values (see Chapter 11). It may also be desirable to regulate which foods can be fortified (see section 7.5.3.3).

7.5.3.1 Nutritional Reference Values (NRVs)

Guidelines on nutrition labelling that are applicable to all foods including fortified foods have been produced by the Codex Alimentarius Commission (*342*). In an attempt to harmonize the labelling of foods with respect to their nutrient contents, the Codex guidelines define a set of Nutrient Reference Values (NRVs), which are based on the FAO/WHO RNI values for adult males, as a reference for the general populaition. Unlike RNIs, NRVs are not given for specific age or physiological groups but are designed to apply to all family members aged over 3 years. The current NRVs (see **Table 7.11**) are based on the 1996 FAO/WHO RNI values (*210*), and will be adjusted in accordance with the more recent RNI values published by the FAO/WHO (*93*).

TABLE 7.11
Codex Nutrient Reference Values (NRVs) for selected micronutrients

Nutrient	Codex NRV[a]	FAO/WHO RNI for adult males[b]
Calcium (mg)	800	1000
Iodine (µg)	150	150
Iron (mg)	14	13.7
Magnesium (mg)	300	260
Selenium (µg)	–	34
Zinc (mg)	15	7
Biotin (µg)	–	30
Vitamin B_6 (mg)	2	1.3
Folate[b] (µg DFE)	200	400
Vitamin B_{12} (µg)	1	2.4
Niacin (vitamin B_3) (mg)	18	16
Riboflavin (vitamin B_2) (mg)	1.6	1.3
Thiamine (vitamin B_1) (mg)	1.4	1.2
Vitamin C (mg)	60	45
Vitamin A[d] (µg RE)	800	600
Vitamin D[e] (µg)	5	5
Vitamin E (α-tocopherol) (mg)	–	10.0

[a] The Nutrient Reference Value (NRV) is a dietary reference value defined by the Codex Alimentarius Commission for the purposes of harmonizing the nutrition labeling of processed foods and used as a reference for the general population (*342*).
[b] The FAO/WHO RNIs listed here are those published in 1996 (*210*), some of which have since been revised.
[c] 1 DFE = Dietary folate equivalent = 1 µg food folate = 0.6 µg folic acid from fortified foods, which means that 1 µg folic acid = 1.7 DFE.
[d] RE = retinol equivalents (1 µg RE = 3.33 IU vitamin A).
[e] As calciferol (1 µg calciferol = 40 IU vitamin D).

Sources: adapted from references (*210,342*).

7.5.3.2 Setting safe maximum limits for market-driven fortification of processed foods

The fact that market-driven fortified processed foods are usually marketed to all family members, rather than to specific age or physiological groups, presents a number of difficulties in terms of setting maximum limits on the permitted levels of fortificants in such foods. The difficulties are compounded by the fact that the same serving size of the fortified food (breakfast cereals, beverages and nutritional bars, for example) is common to all members of the family. The problem therefore arises that by using maximum limits that are based on the NRVs (i.e. RNIs of adult males; see section 7.5.3.1), unnecessarily large amounts of micronutrients may be delivered to children by fortified foods. In this context, it is worth noting that, for some micronutrients (vitamin A, niacin as nicotinic acid, folate, zinc, calcium and iodine), the UL for children below 8 years of age is very close to the EAR for adult males (see **Tables 7.2 and 7.3**).

Establishing maximum levels for nutrient additions that take into account the above safety concerns thus requires adopting some form of risk assessment appraisal. Such approaches base the calculation of a safe maximum limit on accepted values of the UL for the most vulnerable groups, which in this case are children in the age group 4–8 years. Then, assuming that the amounts of micronutrients provided by the diet and via ongoing mass fortification programmes are known, the maximum micronutrient content per serving size of a market-driven fortified processed food is given by the following equation (a):

$$\text{Maximum micronutrient content per serving size} = \frac{[\text{UL} - (\text{amount of micronutrient provided by the diet} + \text{amount of micronutrient provided by fortified foods in the context of an ongoing mass fortification programme})]}{\text{Number of servings}}$$

In order to apply this equation, it is necessary to estimate the number of servings of processed foods that are consumed. This can done as follows:

The usual serving size for solid foods is generally assumed to be 50 g and that for beverages, 250 ml after reconstitution to liquid. However, for the purposes of this derivation it is better to define the serving size in terms of energy (i.e. in kcal) in order to preserve the nutritional balance of the diet. **Table 7.12** summarizes the usual energy densities of a variety of commercially-available foods, from which it can be seen that the smallest dietary serving size is 40 kcal. Thus, a serving of solid foods (50 g) contains 5 dietary servings, a serving of milk or cereal-based beverages, 6 dietary servings, and sugar-based beverages, 1 dietary serving.

TABLE 7.12
Energy densities of common food presentations

Food presentation	Usual serving size	Energy density per serving	Energy density per 100 g or 100 ml
Solid	50 g	160 kcal	320 kcal
Milk or cereal-based beverages	250 ml	200 kcal	80 kcal
Sugar-based beverages	250 ml	100 kcal	40 kcal

If it is assumed that 30% of an individual's daily energy intake (2000 kcal) is derived from fortified processed foods, the amount of energy provided by these foods would be:

$$2000 \text{ kcal} \times 0.3 = 600 \text{ kcal}.$$

In terms of the number of the smallest dietary serving size, expressed as an energy density (i.e. 40 kcal), this amount of energy equates to:

$$600 \text{ kcal}/40 \text{ kcal} = 15 \text{ servings}.$$

Thus, the previous equation can be transformed as follows:

$$\text{Maximum micronutrient content per 40 kcal serving size} = \frac{[\text{UL} - (\text{amount of micronutrient provided by the diet} + \text{amount of micronutrient provided by fortified foods in the context of an ongoing mass fortification programme})]}{15}$$

Box 7.3 illustrates the use of this procedure for milk and sugar-based beverages.

Under normal circumstances, and after considering nutrient amounts supplied by the diet, it is unlikely that the maximum safe limits per usual serving size for the nutrients mentioned in **Table 7.13** (with the exception of calcium) will be in excess of 30% of the RNI in the case of solid foods and milk- or cereal-based beverages and in excess of 15% of the RNI in the case of sugar-based beverages.

7.5.3.3 Keeping the nutritional balance

Some micronutrients were intentionally omitted from the discussion in the preceding section, because either they do not have a recognized UL (health risks

> **BOX 7.3**
>
> **Example: setting maximum safe levels for the fortification of milk and sugar-based beverages with vitamin A**
>
> **1. Milk**
>
> A milk beverage is to be fortified with vitamin A. The fortified product is aimed at a population in which the daily intake of retinol (preformed vitamin A) through the diet and from ongoing mass fortification programmes by children is approximately 300 µg.
>
> Given that the UL for vitamin A in children aged 4–8 years is 900 µg (Table 7.3), the maximum content of vitamin A per 40 kcal serving size will be:
>
> (900 − 300 µg vitamin A)/15 servings = 40 µg vitamin A/serving.
>
> By using the relevant conversion factor (Table 7.14), we can calculate the maximum safe vitamin A content for a 250 ml serving of milk, as follows:
>
> 40 µg vitamin A × 5.0 = 200 µg vitamin A.
>
> Expressed as a percentage of the adult male RNI (see Table 7.1), the maximum vitamin A content of a 250 ml serving of the fortified milk is:
>
> 200/600 × 100 = 33%,
>
> and expressed as a percentage of the current NRV (see Table 7.11), the maximum vitamin A content of a the same sized serving of milk is:
>
> 200/800 × 100 = 25%.
>
> **2. Sugar-based beverages**
>
> A similar calculation for a sugar-based beverage yields a maximum vitamin A content of 100 µg (i.e. 40 µg × 2.5) per 250 ml of beverage (or reconstituted powder), which represents 17% of the adult male RNI and 12.5% of the current NRV for this vitamin.

have not, as yet, been identified), or their UL is high enough to not to raise serious concerns about the safety of high intakes from fortified foods. However, in the interests of maintaining an adequate balance in the diet, it is recommended that these other nutrients be added to processed fortified foods in roughly the same proportion as those micronutrients for which large intakes are undesirable. In practice this means limiting micronutrient additions to between 15% and 30% of the adult RNI in the case of solid foods and milk- or cereal-based beverages, and to half of these values (i.e. 7.5–15%) in the case of sugar-based beverages.

TABLE 7.13
Calculated maximum micronutrient content[a] per 40 kcal-sized serving, assuming no other sources of micronutrient in the diet

Nutrient[b]	UL (children aged 4–8 years)	Maximum amount Per 40 kcal serving	Maximum amount As a % of the RNI[c]
Vitamin A (as retinol) (μg RE)	900 μg	60 μg	10
Niacin (as nicotinic acid[d]) (mg)	15 mg	1.0 mg	6
Folic acid (mg)	400 μg	27 μg	7
Iron (mg)	40 mg	3 mg	22
Zinc (mg)	12 mg	0.6 mg	4
Calcium (mg)	2500 mg	167 mg	17
Iodine (μg)	300 μg	20 μg	13

UL, Tolerable Upper Intake Limit; RNI, Recommended Nutrient Intake.
[a] Maximum levels listed here should be reduced by an amount proportional to the amount of nutrient supplied by the diet (including though mandatory mass fortification programmes).
[b] There are other micronutrients with UL values, but they are not included here because it would be very difficult to approach the UL through the consumption of fortified foods.
[c] As a percentage of the RNI for adult males.
[d] Niacinamide can be used without this restriction.

TABLE 7.14
Factors for converting maximum micronutrient amounts per 40 kcal-sized servings to maximum amounts for different food presentations and serving sizes

Food presentation	Usual serving size	Conversion factor Per usual serving size	Conversion factor Per 100 g or 100 ml
Solid	50 g	4.0	8.0
Milk or cereal-based beverages	250 ml	5.0	2.0
Sugar-based beverages	250 ml	2.5	1.0

These recommendations are in line with Codex guidelines on nutrition claims and their use, which are only expressed in terms of percentage of the NRV serving for minerals and vitamins (see *section 7.5.3.1*). The Codex Guidelines for Use of Nutrition Claims (*343*) stipulate that a food can only be described as a "source" of a specific nutrient if it supplies 15% of the NRV per usual serving, (or 15% of the NRV per 100 g (solid food), or 5% of the NRV per 100 ml (liquid food), or 5% of the NRV per 100 kcal). In order to qualify as being "high" in a specific nutrient, a food product must contain twice as much of the nutrient as a "source" does. It means that many foods could be classified as a "source", but very few products – mostly those naturally rich in micronutrients – could be classified as "high" in specific micronutrients.

It is generally recommended that nutrient content claims be restricted in accordance with these rules, even if the food product contains – for technological purposes or naturally – more than 30% of the NRV. Claims based on percentages in excess of 30% of the NRV in a given fortified food should be discouraged, on the grounds that such claims might mislead consumers as to what constitutes a properly balanced diet.

Summary

- Authorities taking the decision to launch a micronutrient fortification programme should not do so without collecting food and nutrient intake data, supported by various ancillary information, especially, biochemical data on nutritional status. Such data are necessary to make an informed judgment about the types and amounts of specific nutrients to add to which foods. Given the long-term effort and investment that is needed to implement and sustain fortification programmes, and the need to protect individuals in populations consuming the fortified foods, both for deficiencies as well as for excesses, an initial investment in collecting adequate food intake data is highly recommended.

    — Biochemical and clinical data can reveal which micronutrients are insufficient in the usual diet and indicate the prevalence and severity of specific micronutrient deficiencies in different population groups.

    — Information on the distribution of usual dietary intakes of nutrients within population groups provides the most useful basis on which to justify and design a micronutrient fortification programme to correct micronutrient deficiencies.

    — Knowledge of dietary patterns, although useful, is not sufficient information for making final decisions about which nutrients to add to which foods, and how much of each nutrient to add.

- The amount of micronutrient added to the diet through food fortification should be designed such that the predicted probability of inadequate intakes of that specific nutrient is ≤2.5% for population subgroups of concern, while avoiding risk of excessive intakes in other subgroups of the population.

- Due to technological, safety and cost constraints, it may not be possible to add the amount of nutrient(s) needed to ensure adequate intakes in almost all members of a population by mass fortification. In that case, fortification of several food vehicles, other types of fortification, or supplementation, should be considered.

- While these Guidelines provide information on the rationale for fortification and the implementation of fortification programmes, the final decisions concerning which micronutrients to prioritize in a specific location should be made on the basis of local information and public health priorities.

CHAPTER 8
Monitoring and evaluation

Monitoring and evaluation are essential components of any food fortification programme, systems for which should be developed at the outset of a programme, ideally during the design and planning stages. Monitoring and evaluation provide an opportunity not only to assess the quality of the implementation and delivery of a programme, but also the degree to which it reaches its targeted households and individuals, and achieves its nutritional goals. More importantly, the results of monitoring and evaluation exercises provide programme planners and policy-makers with the necessary information to make decisions about whether to continue, expand, replicate or end a programme.

8.1 Basic concepts and definitions

For a fortification programme to be effective, the chosen food vehicles have to be available nationwide or, at least, in the specific geographical areas targeted by the programme. In practice, this means that the product must be available to purchase from local retail stores or outlets that are accessible to the targeted segments of the population. Furthermore, the fortified products have to be purchased by the target families, and consumed with sufficient frequency and in appropriate amounts by the targeted individuals. Throughout this process, that is to say, from the factory to the retail stores, and right up until the time of consumption by targeted individuals, it is vital that the product maintains its expected quality. Thus to ensure that the planned impact is achieved, a programme's *operational performance* (or *implementation efficiency*) must be monitored; this is best accomplished through a system of continuous data collection at key delivery points. When bottlenecks or operational inefficiencies are identified, information must be directed to the programme entity responsible for implementing remedial actions and for re-directing the programme as needed. This set of actions constitutes programme *monitoring*.

In the context of food fortification, the term "monitoring" thus refers to the continuous collection, review and use of information on programme implementation activities, for the purpose of identifying problems, such as non-compliance, and informing corrective actions so as to fulfil stated objectives (6). The ultimate purpose of monitoring a fortification programme is to ensure that the fortified product, of the desired quality, is made available and is accessible to consumers in sufficient amounts.

The term "evaluation" on the other hand is used to refer to the assessment of the effectiveness and the impact of a programme on the target population. In the case of food fortification, evaluations are undertaken with the aim of providing evidence that the programme is indeed reaching its nutritional goals, be this an increase in the intake of a fortified food or of specific nutrients, or an improvement in the nutritional status, health or functional outcomes of the target population. Programme evaluation should not be undertaken until a programme has been shown – through appropriate monitoring – that it has been implemented as planned, and is operating efficiently. A poorly implemented programme is unlikely to achieve its desired impact, and thus, resources should not be wasted in undertaking evaluations until programme operational inefficiencies have been corrected.

A schematic representation of a model monitoring and evaluation system for fortification programmes is shown in **Figure 8.1**; this model provides a framework for the various monitoring and evaluation activities that are described in this chapter.

The framework model distinguishes two main categories of monitoring, *regulatory monitoring* and *household/individual monitoring*. The former, regulatory monitoring, encompasses all monitoring activities conducted at the production level (i.e. at factories, packers), as well as monitoring at customs warehouses and

FIGURE 8.1

A monitoring and evaluation system for food fortification programmes

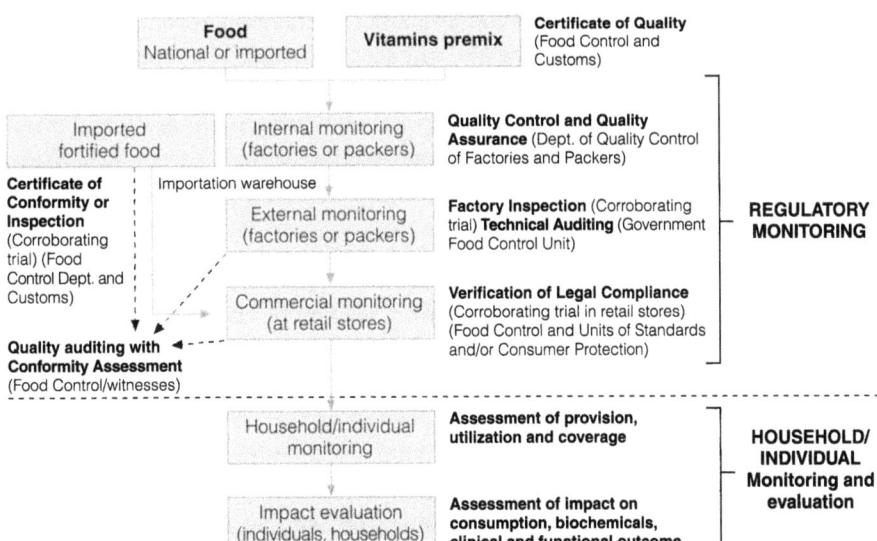

at retail stores, by concerned regulatory authorities as well as by producers themselves as part of self-regulation programmes. Production level regulatory monitoring comprises both *internal* and *external monitoring;* regulatory monitoring at the retail level is referred to here as *commercial monitoring*. The primary aim of regulatory monitoring is to ensure that the fortified foods meet the nutrient, quality and safety standards set prior to programme implementation.

The other category, household/individual monitoring, as its name implies, involves households and their members and has the following objectives (adapted from Habicht et al. (*344*):

— to ensure that targeted individuals and households have access to the fortified food and that the fortified food is of the expected quality (i.e. to measure service *provision*);

— to ensure that targeted individuals and households purchase and consume the fortified food (i.e. to monitor service *utilization*);

— to ensure that targeted individuals and households consume the fortified food in appropriate amounts and frequency (i.e. to measure *coverage*).

Once regulatory and household monitoring have demonstrated that the programme is operating in a satisfactory manner, evaluation of the programme at the household and at the individual level can be undertaken to assess its impact. This is generally referred to as *impact evaluation* (**Figure 8.1**) Some of the data obtained through household monitoring, for example, data on consumption of fortified foods and/or micronutrient intakes, can also be used in programme evaluation (see section 8.4).

Table 8.1 summarizes the key features of each of the three principal framework components of monitoring and evaluation identified above, i.e. regulatory monitoring, household monitoring and impact evaluation. The remainder of this chapter is devoted to discussing each of these components in more detail and concludes by outlining the minimum requirements for a monitoring and evaluation system for a fortification programme (section 8.5).

8.2 Regulatory monitoring

As shown in **Figure 8.1**, regulatory monitoring comprises three parts – internal monitoring, external monitoring and commercial monitoring:

- *Internal monitoring* refers to the quality control and quality assurance (QC/QA) practices conducted by producers, importers and packers.

- *External monitoring* refers to the inspection and auditing activities carried out at production centres (factories and packers) and importation custom sites. Governmental authorities are responsible for external monitoring, which is

TABLE 8.1
Purpose and function of the various components of monitoring and evaluation systems for fortification programmes

Component	Purpose	Specific function
Regulatory monitoring	To ensure that fortified foods meet nutrient quality and safety standards throughout their shelf-life (i.e. from factory to retail store); comprises: — internal monitoring; — external monitoring; — commercial monitoring.	Regulatory monitoring can address questions such as: — Is GMP applied? — Is HACCP in place (when applicable)? — Is QA/QC correctly done? — Are inspection and technical auditing functions at the factory and at packing facilities implemented satisfactorily? — Is verification of legal compliance at retail stores carried out as planned?
Household/ individual monitoring and evaluation	To assess: — provision; — utilization; — coverage.	Household monitoring can address questions such as: — Is the fortified food accessible to the target population? — Is the fortified food of acceptable quality? — Does the targeted population purchase the fortified food? — Is the fortified food being stored, handled/prepares as intended? — Does the targeted population consume the fortified food in appropriate amounts/frequency?
Impact evaluation	To assess impact on outcomes of interest, such as: — consumption of fortified food; — intake of specific nutrient(s); — nutritional status (i.e. biochemical indicators); — health; — other functional outcomes (e.g. growth, cognition).	Impact evaluations can address questions such as: — Has the targeted population reached a pre-established acceptable level of a given outcome of interest (e.g. is prevalence of iron deficiency <20% among pregnant women; is 70% of the target population consuming fortified product; or does 80% of the target population have an adequate intake of a particular micronutrient? (These are examples of *adequacy*[a] evaluations.) — Does the targeted population have improved outcome(s) since the intervention was implemented (before-and-after); or does the targeted population have better outcome(s) after the intervention compared with a control group; or did targeted population have a greater improvement in outcome(s) following the intervention compared with a control group? (These are examples of *plausibility*[a] evaluations.) — Has the group randomly assigned to receive fortified food achieved a greater improvement (before-and-after) in outcome(s) compared with a randomized control group? (This is an example of a *probability*[a] evaluation.)

GMP, good manufacturing practice; HACCP, hazard analysis critical control points; QA/QC, quality assurance/quality control.
[a] The different types of impact evaluation are described in greater detail in section 8.4 of these Guidelines.

implemented as a mechanism to assure compliance with standards and regulations.

- *Commercial monitoring* is similar to external monitoring in that it is generally the responsibility of the government and its purpose is to verify that the fortified products comply with standards, but is conducted at the level of retail stores.

For each stage of the monitoring process, it is helpful to establish indicators that can be used to measure success. In the case of fortification programmes, success criteria can be expressed in terms of the proportion of samples containing a specified minimum amount of a given nutrient at various stages in the lifecycle of the product, i.e. at the time of production (the Production Minimum), at the point of sale (the Retail or Legal Minimum) and at the point of consumption (the Household Minimum). A sample set of success criteria for monitoring purposes are presented in **Table 8.2**.

To be effective, a monitoring system requires a set of established procedures, methodologies and reporting requirements, all of which make a contribution to ensuring the continuous assessment of a programme. A clear delineation of responsibilities and an efficient feedback mechanism, which facilitate the establishment and implementation of corrective measures when operational problems arise, are also essential. **Table 8.3** (*345*) outlines how some of these facets of

TABLE 8.2

Suggested criteria for measuring success at various monitoring stages for food fortification programmes (expressed as a percentage of samples that must comply with minimum levels and Maximum Tolerable Levels)

Monitoring stage	Minimum levels			Maximum Tolerable Level[d]
	Household[a]	Retail[b]	Production[c]	
Internal	100	100	≥80	<20
External (inspection)	100	≥80	–	<20
Household	≥90	–	–	<10

[a] The Household Minimum Level is the amount of nutrient that must be present in the food at the household level before being used in meal preparation. This value is estimated to reach a nutritional goal after considering losses during food preparation (specific additional intake of certain nutrients).
[b] The Retail Minimum Level (or the Legal Minimum Level) is the nutrient content of the fortified food at retail locations at the moment of sale. Usually it is 20–30% larger for vitamins and iodine, and 3–5% larger for minerals, than the Household Minimum Level.
[c] The Production Minimum Level is the nutrient content of the fortified food in the factory, which considers an overage for losses occurring during production, distribution and storage. It is the decision of the manufacturer/importer which overage to use to ensure that the product retains the Retail Minimum Level during the duration of its commercial life.
[d] The Maximum Tolerable Level (MTL) is the maximum allowed content of a specific micronutrient in a fortified food to assure that none of the consumers receives an amount near to the Tolerable Upper Intake Level (UL).

8. MONITORING AND EVALUATION

TABLE 8.3
Suggested regulatory monitoring activities for a food fortification programme

Monitoring stage	Action/indicator (success criteria)	Frequency/timing	Methodology and entity responsible for action
Internal monitoring (quality control and assurance)	GMP applied	Daily.	*Method:* Follow a GMP manual approved by company directors. *Responsible:* Factory manager.
	HACCP system in place, where applicable	Daily.	*Method:* Follow a HACCP manual approved by company directors. *Responsible:* Factory manager.
	Premixes and preblends available in sufficient amounts for at least 15 days of production	Daily.	*Method:* Continuous inventory of micronutrient premixes and preblends in existence and use. Confirm that batches of premix are used in the same order in which they were produced. *Responsible:* Factory manager.
	Dosage is in the correct proportion	At least once per shift.	*Method:* Ensure premix flows according to the production rate so that the theoretical average is as expected and the Production Minimum Level is always attained. *Responsible:* Factory quality control department.
	Corroborating tests (at least 80% of samples fulfil the Production Minimum Level and less than 20% reach the Maximum Tolerable Level)	At least every 8 hours; if success criteria are not fulfilled, frequency of sampling should be increased to every 2–4 hours.	*Method:* Take a random sample(s) from packaging line. A fast semi-quantitative assay can be used at shorter intervals, but at least one daily-composite sample should be analysed using a quantitative assay. *Responsible:* Factory quality control department.

183

TABLE 8.3
Suggested regulatory monitoring activities for a food fortification programme *(Continued)*

Monitoring stage	Action/indicator (success criteria)	Frequency/timing	Methodology and entity responsible for action
External			
Factory (inspection and technical auditing)	Fortification centre carries out QC/QA procedures and maintains up-to-date registers	At least once every 3–6 months; frequency of visits should be increased to 1–4 times/month if problems are detected.	*Method:* Conduct auditing to verify performance of the QC/QA procedures and registry, and that fortification centres adopt GMP. *Responsible:* Food control authorities.
	Corroborating tests (at least 80% of individual samples fulfill the Legal Minimum Level and less than 20% reach the Maximum Tolerable Level)	Combine testing with visits to examine QC/QA and GMP procedures; if intentional or serious mistakes are suspected, plan a Quality Audit for Evaluation of Conformity.	*Method:* Collect 5 individual samples of packaged product and take 5 samples from the production line, and test for compliance. *Responsible:* Food control authorities.
At importation sites (applies to imported/donated products)	Obtain Certificate of Conformity[a] of sale from country of origin	Each time a product lot enters the country.	*Method:* Examine documentation, quality and labelling of products in the customs warehouses. *Responsible:* Importation officials in collaboration with food control authorities.
	Corroborating tests (at least 80% of individual samples fulfill the Legal Minimum Level and less than 20% reach the Maximum Tolerable Level)	Combine with examination of importation papers. If intentional or serious mistakes are suspected, plan a Quality Audit for Evaluation of Conformity.	*Method:* Randomly select 5 individual samples from the lot and test for compliance with the Legal Minimum Level and the MTL. *Responsible:* Importation officials in collaboration with food control authorities.

Commercial (inspection at retail stores)	Corroborating tests (at least 80% of samples of each brand fulfill the Legal Minimum Level and less than 20% reach the Maximum Tolerable Level)	Systematic and continuous examination of the product distributed to all regions of the country; each region should be visited at least once a year.	*Method*: Visit stores to collect samples; send samples to official laboratories for quantitative assays. At the local level, semi-quantitative assays may also be used to confirm presence of fortificant if fraud is suspected. *Responsible*: Local personnel from public institutions (e.g. representatives of ministries of health, industry, consumer protection organizations).
Quality Audit for Evaluation of Conformity	Verify production or stored batch complies with standards when analysed using statistical sampling criteria	Whenever it is necessary to take legal actions; can also be requested and financed by producers to certify production lot for exportation.	*Method*: Visit fortification centres suspected of non-compliance with regulations and standards, or when required by exporting industry. Follow technical recommendations of the Codex Alimentarius Commission (*345*) or any equivalent guidelines suitable for this activity. *Responsible*: Personnel of the public agency for food control: as visits to fortification centres are performed under suspicions of non-compliance of regulations and standards, these activities should be carried out in the presence of independent witnesses.

GMP, good manufacturing practice; HACCP, hazard analysis and critical control point; MTL, Maximum Tolerable Level; QC/QA, quality control/quality assurance.

[a] The Certificate of Conformity is a statement that the imported product complies with a set of specific standards.

monitoring might be implemented in practice for each of the three stages of regulatory monitoring, internal, external and commercial.

Table 8.3 lists an additional monitoring stage, namely quality audits for evaluation of conformity. This is the formal examination and testing of a batch of a fortified food product for compliance with standards. It should be reserved for special circumstances, which can either be when intentional non-conformity is suspected (and legal action is required) or when certification of a production lot prior to exportation is necessary.

8.2.1 Internal monitoring (quality control/quality assurance)

Broadly speaking, *quality assurance* (QA) refers to the implementation of planned and systematic activities necessary to ensure that products or services meet quality standards. The performance of quality assurance can be expressed numerically in terms of the results of quality control procedures. *Quality control* (QC) is defined as the techniques and assessments used to document compliance with established technical standards, through the use of objective and measurable indicators that are applicable to the products or services.

Detailed information about QC/QA can be found in any one of the many technical manuals that are devoted to this subject and in publications on good manufacturing practice (GMP) (*346*). In these Guidelines the topic of QA/QC is viewed from a purely public health perspective and focuses on indicators and criteria that are relevant to the process of food fortification. Thus in the context of food fortification, **quality assurance** consists of establishing the following procedures:

— obtain from the providers a certificate of quality[1] for any micronutrient mixes used;

— request, receive and store in a systematic, programmed and timely manner the ingredients and supplies for the preparation of a preblend[2];

— produce the preblend according to a schedule that is adjusted to the rate of food manufacturing and fortification;

— control the adequate performance of the preblend equipment;

— appropriately label and deliver the preblend;

---

[1] The micronutrient mixes must be accompanied by a document that certifies their nutrient content. This is usually the case for products shipped by international companies dedicated to this task.
[2] A **preblend** is the combination of the micronutrient mix with another ingredient, often the same food that is to be fortified, with the purpose of reducing the dilution proportion and improving the distribution of the micronutrient mix in the food and guaranteeing that there will be not be separation (segregation) between the food and micronutrient particles.

— use the preblend in the same order of production (i.e. first in, first out);

— verify appropriate functioning of the feeder machines and the mixers in a continuous and systematic manner;

— ensure that the product is adequately packaged, labelled, stored and shipped.

It is possible that other process variables, such as pH and temperature/time exposure, could affect the stability of added micronutrients and should also be considered in the design of quality assurance programmes.

The **quality control** procedures will typically consist of taking samples of the fortified food, either by batch or in a continuous manner depending on the system of production, and determining their micronutrient content. Irrespective of the sampling method, the number of samples required will be governed by the consistency and reliability of the fortification process. A highly homogeneous and consistent operation, regardless of the size of the batch or the rate of production, will need less sampling than one with variable results. Nevertheless, even in the most reproducible conditions it is important to take and analyse samples routinely in order to verify and keep track of whether the technical standards are being met.

Figure 8.2 illustrates the features of a dynamic sampling system suitable for a continuous production process. Under optimal operation, one sample of a product per 8-hour shift might be sufficient; this would be categorized as a *relaxed* intensity of sampling. If the technical specifications of the product are not attained (i.e. the micronutrient content is lower than the factory minimum or higher than the Maximum Tolerable Level), then sampling frequency should

FIGURE 8.2

Suggested frequency and intensity of sampling for monitoring compliance with standards

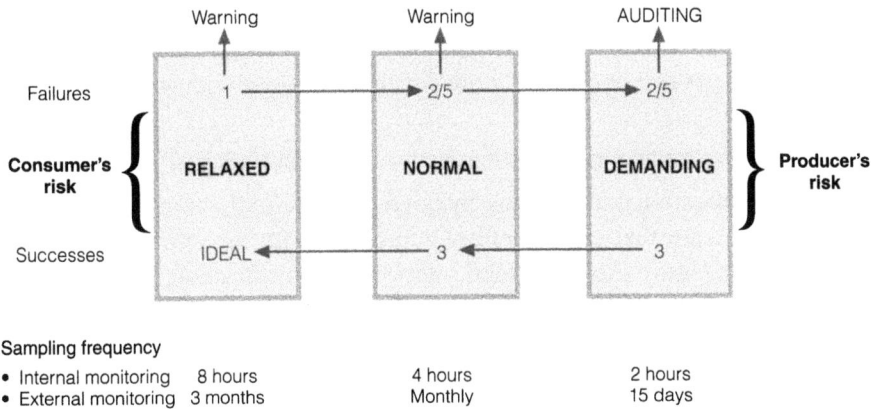

be increased from the relaxed intensity to a *normal* intensity and corrective actions taken. In a "normal" situation, if 2 out of 5 consecutive samples of the product fail to meet the technical requirements, then the intensity of sampling should be changed to a *demanding* intensity, and corrective actions implemented. Again, if 2 out of 5 consecutive samples do not achieve the technical requirements, then the production should be stopped until the source of error is found and the necessary corrective measures introduced.

When production is reinitiated, sampling should start at the demanding intensity, be switched to a normal and then back down to a relaxed intensity if, each time, three consecutive samples satisfy technical requirements. The relaxed situation implies a degree of consumer risk; if sampling is infrequent, there is a greater chance of some non-compliant batches reaching the market. When sampling is frequent (i.e. as in the demanding situation), the likelihood of detecting even a minor deviation from the standard is increased, and prompts producers to expend time and resources in the resolution of the problem (the producer's risk). Neither the relaxed nor the normal sampling intensity should be viewed as positive or negative; they simply reflect the performance of the fortification process at the moment of the assessment. Results of QC must be carefully recorded and kept, because they document the history of the efficiency and also the producer's supervision of the fortification process.

Because results are needed quickly (so that corrective actions can be implemented promptly), QC procedures demand fast and simple analytical assays. These assays do not necessarily need to have high analytical resolution (i.e. be able to discriminate between small concentration ranges), but it is essential that they are able to determine whether fortification standards are being met (i.e. micronutrient content not less than the production minimum nor more than the Maximum Tolerable Level). In this regard, semi-quantitative assays are potentially very useful and attempts have been made in recent years to develop test kits based on semi-quantitative assays. Test kits for the measurement of iodine in salt, for example, have been developed but, to date, have met with limited success; those currently on the market, have been found to be of questionable reliability (*347*). Clearly, further research is needed in this area before semi-quantitative tests can be applied more widely in the food industry.

8.2.2 External monitoring (inspection and technical auditing)

Some form of external monitoring by governmental food control authorities is essential to assure that producers are complying with the approved technical standards that ensure the quality and safety of food fortification. Awareness that their product might be checked at any time usually provides producers with a strong motivational force to carry out an acceptable production process with the appropriate QA/QC procedures. In industrialized countries, it is usually sufficient to confirm once a year (or even less frequently) the nutrient content indicated on the food labels from samples taken in the market (see Commercial monitoring, section 8.2.3). However, in much of the developing world, where it is very difficult to trace and to retrieve a defective batch once a food product reaches retail stores, it is advisable to also conduct external monitoring at the factory level.

External monitoring combines two types of actions:

- checking the performance and the records of the producers' quality assurance procedures (*technical auditing*);
- confirming that the technical specifications for the product are being met at factories, packaging sites and points of entry into the country (*inspection*).

Ideally, inspection and verification of legal compliance should be based on the analytical assessment of the micronutrient content of a food product by means of a quantitative assay. All samples should contain the fortificant; at least 80% of samples from factories, importation sites and warehouses should present the Legal Minimum amount, and less than 20% of samples should have a micronutrient content that is above but always near the Maximum Tolerable Level (**Table 8.2**). If this is found not to be the case, then more frequent visits to the factory to carry out technical auditing and inspection activities are justified (see **Figure 8.2**).

Imported products should be treated in a similar manner to locally produced foods, only instead of checking the producers' documented AQ/QC procedures, the certificate of conformity provided by the country of origin should be examined. However, food control authorities can corroborate compliance of the technical standards in samples of the imported shipments.

The intensity of sampling and factory inspection frequency depends on the reproducibility of the fortification process and should be determined for each type of industry under the specific conditions of each country. For example, for salt fortification by small industries this might be every 15 days, for sugar industries every month, and for wheat flour industries every 6 months. In theory, sampling should follow a statistically based approach, such as that recommended by the Codex Alimentarius Commission (*345*). In practice, however, the number of samples and the analytical work required can overwhelm the available human, financial and material resources of the food control entities in many developing countries. For day-to-day monitoring and routine inspection visits, the Codex sampling procedures are often impractical and unrealistic and are thus best reserved for situations that require a quality audit for evaluation of conformity (e.g. for cases when the product requires a certificate of conformity for exportation, or if there is a legal controversy that might lead to serious penalties) (See **Table 8.3**).

A simpler, low-cost monitoring system, based on the concept of *corroborating tests*, has been successfully adopted by some countries in Central America. These tests consist of checking compliance with fortification standards in a small number of samples (e.g. 5–10 product samples from factories) during the moment of the technical auditing visit; samples are taken from the production line and also from storage areas. At least 80% of the samples should contain the Legal Minimum of the micronutrient, and less than 20% should be above, but never too far from the Maximum Tolerable Level. If these criteria are not fulfilled, then a warning statement must be provided and more frequent visits for technical auditing and inspection should be planned to the factories responsible for the product. In extreme cases, a quality audit for evaluation of conformity might be necessary (**Table 8.3**). The concept of corroborating tests is based on the principle that quality is the main responsibility of producers; governmental authorities only act to represent the public, and to guarantee that monitoring is indeed carried out.

8.2.3 Commercial monitoring

As is the case for any other industrially produced food, fortified foods, irrespective of whether fortification is voluntary or in response to public health interest, must be correctly identified with a label. A label should include at least the brand of the product, the address of the responsible entity, and the Legal Minimum Level of the nutrient and, if industry development allows, also the date of minimum durability, the batch number and the production date.

As mentioned in the previous section, in industrialized countries external regulatory monitoring is generally limited to a confirmation of micronutrient content and label claims in samples obtained from retail stores. In the event of a breach of standards, mechanisms exist for the recall of defective products and retraction of misleading claims. Strict governmental enforcement of regulations and stiff penalties for non-compliance, means that it is very rare for a producer to take the risk of not complying with regulations and on the whole, the procedure works well. In the developing world, as indicated previously, it is not always possible to trace and retrieve a defective batch once a food product reaches the market place, and so it is necessary to monitor for compliance with quality standards and label claims at the both the factory and retail levels (see also section 8.2.2).

In many settings, especially in the developing world, commercial monitoring can be particularly useful for identifying brands and factories that deserve closer auditing. A system based on the use of corroborating tests, as suggested for factories above, can equally well be applied to the commercial setting; one or two samples of each brand from each store might be used to check for standard compliance. If anomalies are found, then a technical comprehensive auditing of the responsible factory or importation firm would be warranted. Semi-quantitative assays to detect the presence of micronutrients might be useful for monitoring at retail stores, and as an enforcement tool at the local level. However, any legal action must be based on results obtained from quantitative assays carried out as part of a quality auditing visit to the responsible factory.

A nation-wide programme to fortify vegetable oils with vitamins A and D_3 was established in Morocco in 2002. The system devised for monitoring the quality of the fortified product is described in detail in **Annex E**, and serves to illustrate the practical application of the principles of regulatory monitoring introduced here.

8.3 Household monitoring

It is generally assumed that having established through regulatory monitoring that a fortified product is of the required quality at the retail store level, the same product will be of a similar quality once it reaches households and individuals. Because the product may have deteriorated during storage, confirmation of this assumption is always recommended. Nor can it be assumed that just because fortified foods are available to buy from shops, they will necessarily be consumed by the target population; consumers may well purchase non-fortified foods in preference to fortified products (if both fortified and non-fortified foods are available locally). Even if officially only fortified products are available at retail stores, consumers may be able to acquire non-fortified (probably cheaper) foods via non-official means, such as smuggling and from door-to-door sellers.

8.3.1 Aims and objectives

In short, the aim of household monitoring is to assess whether or not a programme is providing appropriately fortified products in sufficient amounts and at affordable prices to the targeted population. More specifically, household monitoring can answer questions such as:

- Are the fortified products accessible (i.e. available and affordable) to the targeted households and individuals? Are they of expected quality and are they available from retail stores in targeted regions/communities?

- Are the fortified products being purchased by the targeted households, taking into account tastes and preferences, and patterns of consumption? If not, why are the fortified products not being purchased? Is it because they are unaffordable (cost), because their taste and appearance is altered by the fortification process, or is it because they are not part of the usual consumption pattern of the targeted population?

- Are the fortified products being purchased and consumed in sufficient amounts by specific household members to meet programme nutritional goals (i.e. to increase their micronutrient intake and/or to meet a predefined level of micronutrient requirements)? If not, is it because of cultural practices concerning the appropriateness of feeding these products to specific household members (based on age, physiological status, etc.), or is it because of tastes and preferences of specific household members, or because of inequitable food distribution within the household?

- Which individuals/population groups are not being reached by the fortification programme and why?

- Are individual family members consuming sufficient amounts of fortified products to increase their intake of specific micronutrients (and/or to meet programme nutritional goals for specific age/physiological groups)?

In effect, monitoring at the household level addresses three key aspects of programme performance, that is to say, provision, utilization and coverage (see section 8.1). Household monitoring activities designed to assess each of these aspects of food fortification programme performance are outlined in **Table 8.4**; in each case, suitable indicators and data collection methodologies are proposed.

8.3.2 Methodological considerations

As **Table 8.4** indicates, there are a variety of approaches that can be used to gather data for the purposes of assessing programme performance in terms of provision, utilization and coverage. Primary data collection as part of the programme's overall monitoring and evaluation system is one option. Alternatively, and this is often a more practical solution, it may be possible to join with – or "piggy-back" on to – other programmes that have ongoing or regular data collection components. For example, some countries in Central America carry out school censuses at regular intervals; it is then a relatively simple matter to collect samples of fortified products, such as vitamin A-fortified sugar or iodized salt, by asking pupils to bring a small sample from home to school. Other routine data collection systems which might provide opportunities for "piggy-backing" include 30-cluster surveys, sentinel sites monitoring, and lot quality assurance sampling (LQAS) monitoring systems (*6,348–350*). These types of simple monitoring systems are widely used to monitor immunization coverage, universal salt iodization and other primary health care interventions. If such systems are not already in place, they can be established specifically for the fortification programme. Guidance on how to implement relatively simple data collection systems, and examples of their successful application in health care settings, is available elsewhere (*6,351–353*).

8. MONITORING AND EVALUATION

TABLE 8.4
Suggested household monitoring activities for a food fortification programme

Aspect of programme performance	Indicator (success criteria)	Frequency/timing	Methodology and entity responsible for action
Provision	Volume of product sold at an affordable price in retail stores in target regions (specific criteria to be determined)	At least annually.	*Method*: Either through new data collection or by adding appropriate questions (i.e. "piggy-backing") onto existing data collection vehicles, such as: — cross-sectional community surveys; — cross-sectional household surveys; — school surveys or censuses; — 30-cluster surveys; — sentinel site monitoring; — lot quality assurance sampling (LQAS); — market surveys. *Responsible*: Programme monitoring and evaluation unit (if applicable), individuals responsible for the existing data collection programme that is being added to, or researchers.
Utilization	Number or proportion of households purchasing fortified product regularly Number or proportion of targeted households in which fortified product is present Number or proportion of household members consuming fortified product regularly	At least annually.	*Method*: As for Provision, excluding market surveys which do not apply here. *Responsible*: As for Provision.

GUIDELINES ON FOOD FORTIFICATION WITH MICRONUTRIENTS

TABLE 8.4
Suggested household monitoring activities for a food fortification programme (*Continued*)

Aspect of programme performance	Indicator (success criteria)	Frequency/timing	Methodology and entity responsible for action
Coverage	Proportion of households or household members consuming product with expected frequency and in adequate amounts to meet programme nutritional goals (acceptable level to be determined) Observed changes in nutritional status since implementation of fortification programme through intake of fortified products and regular diet (acceptable changes to be determined)	Once a year until acceptable coverage levels are achieved; thereafter every 3–5 years.	*Method*: Household surveys, either specific to the programme or as an add-on to existing or planned surveys, depending on availability of resources locally. In order to derive an appropriate denominator for coverage estimates, a representative sample of the target population is, however, required. *Responsible*: Programme monitoring and evaluation unit (if applicable) or researchers.

Market surveys are one way of collecting data on the price and availability of fortified products in retail stores; such data are useful for monitoring service provision. Many countries already operate routine systems for collecting price data for a number of food commodities, in which case fortified foods can simply be added to the list of products being monitored. The monitoring of programme utilization and coverage, however, necessitates data collection at the household or individual level. Any of the simple data collection systems mentioned above can be used to collect information relating to utilization. Conducting representative household and community surveys is another option, but these tend to be more costly. Again, it is possible to take advantage of, or piggy-back on, existing data collection vehicles or surveys that are being conducted at the household level. In addition, qualitative approaches, which include observations, informant interviews and focus group discussions, may be useful for gathering information about programme implementation and service delivery, use of the fortified products and users' perceptions about the fortified versus the non-fortified foods.

Coverage of a fortification programme is usually assessed by determining what proportion of at-risk individuals consume the fortified products in sufficient amounts and with sufficient frequency. Thus, to evaluate coverage, information on the number of at-risk individuals is necessary. This can be obtained from either a census or by surveying a representative sample of the population. Estimates of the intake of the fortified product(s) and/or of the micronutrient(s) of interest are also required.

Two approaches are available for evaluating programme coverage. The first involves assessing the total dietary intake of the micronutrient of interest, with and without considering the consumption of the fortified food. This allows the percentage of the population, analysing each of the target groups independently (e.g. preschool-aged children, adolescents, women), that moves from having intakes that are below the relevant EAR to having intakes that are above the EAR to be estimated. The proportion of the population that moves from below to above the EAR provides a measure of the success of the programme. The second approach is to estimate the additional intake that would be supplied through consumption of the fortified food. In this case, the measure of the programme's success is given by the proportion of the population fulfilling that additional intake. Success criteria will inevitably vary according to the specific objectives of the programme and should be set accordingly. However, it can be helpful to set stricter criteria for measuring coverage of targeted fortification programmes, in terms of the proportion of the population that will benefit, to ensure that those most in need of fortified foods actually receive them.

8.4 Impact evaluation

The main purpose of evaluating any intervention is to determine whether or not it is reaching its overall goals. In the case of food fortification programmes, the primary objective is to improve the nutritional status of the target population. Impact evaluations of most health and nutrition programmes, including food fortification interventions, are however rarely performed, in part because they are perceived as being complex, costly and sometimes threatening. The results of impact evaluations are nevertheless important decision-making tools, providing answers to important questions such as:

- Has the intake of a specific fortified food increased to expected levels following a food fortification programme?

- Has the intake of specific nutrients of interest increased to expected levels following a food fortification programme?

- Has the nutritional status of specific groups (for selected nutrients) improved, as a result of the fortification programme?

- Has the fortification programme reduced the prevalence of specific micronutrient deficiencies?

- Has the fortification programme reduced the prevalence of poor functional outcomes, such as growth faltering, morbidity from infectious diseases, child mortality, and poor cognitive and motor development?

- Has the fortification programme been more effective in improving status of certain micronutrients and/or among certain age/physiological groups than others?

The following subsections review a range of methodologies that can be used for food fortification programme evaluation, highlighting in each case the purposes and settings for which they are most appropriate. Although not all fortification programme evaluations will necessarily require the more sophisticated and therefore the more costly methodologies, impartiality is always vital. In order to ensure that impact evaluations are impartial, it is recommended that they are carried out under the auspices of independent research groups or international agencies. Ideally, funds for monitoring and evaluation, should be allocated at the time of programme design and budget allocation, but this is not to say that funds cannot be complemented by donor agencies at a later date.

8.4.1 Impact evaluation design

There are a number of different ways in which the evaluation of the impact of a food fortification programme can be tackled. However, the choice of methodology should be dictated by the specific purpose of the evaluation, and by the availability of resources. The level of precision required to satisfy the needs of decision-makers regarding the effectiveness of their programme is another important factor to bear in mind when selecting an evaluation design.

Habicht et al. (*344*) have devised a useful way of classifying the various approaches to evaluating public health interventions. The classification is based on the premise that the choice of the evaluation method depends on the precision of data required by decision-makers to be able to say that the programme being evaluated has been effective. Three levels of inference are identified: *adequacy*, *plausibility* and *probability*. Application of this classification to fortification programme evaluation is presented in **Table 8.5**.

8.4.1.1 Adequacy evaluation

An *adequacy* evaluation is the appropriate choice if the objective is to assess whether the prevalence of a particular micronutrient deficiency is at or below a pre-determined level. For example, the goal of a fortification programme may be to reduce the prevalence of iron deficiency among children to 10% or less (or any other cut-off point used to define a public health problem). In this case, adequacy would be achieved if the evaluation showed that the prevalence of iron deficiency at the time of the evaluation was lower than the 10% pre-established cut-off point. Similarly, if a programme sought to raise the level of intake of fortified wheat flour by a target population group to a certain pre-determined level, an adequacy evaluation would simply have to demonstrate that this level (or a higher level) of intake has been reached by the targeted population.

Adequacy evaluations are the simplest (and least costly) type of evaluation to carry out, primarily because they do not require randomization or the use of a control group (**Table 8.5**). Nevertheless, adequacy evaluations demand the same level of scientific rigour as any other type of evaluation. Appropriate study designs for this type of evaluation include one-time cross-sectional surveys that focus on the outcome of interest.

8.4.1.2 Plausibility evaluation

A *plausibility* evaluation seeks to demonstrate, with a given level of certainty, that the reduction in say, the prevalence of iron deficiency, is related to the fortification programme being evaluated. Many factors unrelated to food fortification can reduce the prevalence of iron deficiency, and thus the reduction can be wrongly attributed to the fortification programme unless the evaluation takes these factors into consideration. For example, if public health measures to control parasites and infections have been implemented, or if development programmes to raise incomes have resulted in an increased intake of animal products in the targeted population, a failure to control for these external effects could

TABLE 8.5
Evaluating the impact of fortification programmes on nutritional status: a range of approaches

Evaluation type	Aim of the evaluation	Evaluation design requirements
Adequacy	To assess whether the prevalence of specific micronutrient deficiencies (or the intake of specific micronutrients) is acceptable or such that there is a public health problem.	Adequacy evaluations require a cross-sectional survey of nutrient intakes, or of clinical, functional or biochemical indicators of deficiency, at a certain point in time. Prevalence data must be evaluated against established criteria of adequacy, or of a public health problem. Assessment should focus on deficiencies in those micronutrients that are of primary interest, and which can be supplied in fortified foods.
Plausibility	To be able to state that it is plausible that food fortification was the cause of changes in nutritional status.	Plausibility evaluations require a quasi-experimental design such as: — a cross-sectional study which compares households (or individuals) that consumed fortified foods with a comparable group that did not; — a longitudinal study in which measures are recorded in the same individuals before and after a period of fortification; — a longitudinal study in which measures are recorded before and after a period of fortification in a group that received fortified foods, and also in a control group that did not; this allows changes due to other factors (e.g. food prices, national economy) to be accounted for; — a case-control study which compares cases who consumed fortified foods with controls who did not but who are similar in many relevant characteristics, such as socioeconomic status, place of residence (i.e. geographic location, urban vs. rural, household composition), gender, age (i.e. matched controls).
Probability	To determine, with a level of probability that was established before the evaluation, that observed changes in nutritional status are due to fortification.	Probability evaluations require a double-blind, randomized, experimental design that compares responses to fortified foods with non-fortified foods. This requires: — randomization of participants in the "fortified" and "non-fortified" groups; — before-and-after measurements in the same subjects; — that neither the participants nor the evaluators know which treatments are being consumed by whom, during the intervention or during the data analysis (i.e. a double-blind study).

wrongly attribute the reduction in iron deficiency to food fortification. It is therefore important for plausibility evaluations to control for these potential confounding factors and biases through the careful selection of an appropriate study design and through the use of multivariate data analysis techniques. Plausibility evaluations use quasi-experimental or case–control designs (**Table 8.5**): they require either the comparison between an intervention and a control group (who did not receive the intervention), or before-and-after information on a group who received the intervention (a pre–post design), or both (i.e. before-and-after information on both an intervention and a control group).

8.4.1.3 Probability evaluation

Probability evaluations provide the highest level of confidence that the food fortification programme is responsible for the observed reduction in the prevalence of deficiency. Only probability methods can establish causality; these necessitate the use of randomized, controlled experiments, carried out in a double-blind manner whenever possible (**Table 8.5**). The probability evaluation is based on the premise that there is only a small known probability (usually $P < 0.05$, i.e. a less than 5% chance) that the observed differences in iron deficiency (for example) between the group that was randomly assigned to receive fortified foods and the non-fortified food control group are due to chance.

Probability evaluations are complex and expensive to perform because they need a randomized sample and a control group. They may not be feasible in usual field conditions, either for practical reasons or for ethical reasons. For example, if the fortified product is different in appearance and/or taste, it will be impossible to carry out the intervention in a double-blind manner. Similarly, it may not be practical to randomize the population into a food-fortified and a control group. Moreover, using a control group often raises ethical concerns. For these reasons, probability methods are more commonly used for small, pilot efficacy trials (i.e. interventions carried out under controlled conditions to determine efficacy), than for effectiveness trials (large-scale interventions carried out under real-life field conditions, and facing usual implementation constraints). Probability evaluations are the reference standard of efficacy research.

Note that the questions listed above (page 14) assume either a plausibility or a probability evaluation design, rather than an adequacy design. This is because the formulation of these questions implies a change or an improvement that is attributable to the fortification programme. Adequacy evaluation designs can address similar questions, but they would have to be phrased with reference to pre-established criteria of adequacy, rather than with respect to a change attributable to the programme. For example, the first question:

> Has the intake of a specific fortified food increased to expected levels following a food fortification programme?

would become:

> Is the intake of a specific fortified food at the expected level (say, is 90% of the population consuming salt fortified at the mimimum household level)?

Adequacy criteria could also be expressed in terms of biochemical indicators; for instance:

> Is the prevalence of vitamin A deficiency among preschool-aged children lower than say 20% (or any other pre-established criteria) following the food fortification programme?

8.4.2 Methodological considerations

8.4.2.1 Selection of outcome indicators

Outcome indicators that can be used to assess the impact of fortification programmes include measures of intake (which can also be used as indicators of utilization – see section 8.3; Table 8.4); clinical and biochemical indicators of nutritional status (see **Tables 3.1, 3.4, 3.6, 4.1, 4.3–4.5, 4.7, 4.8, 4.10, 4.11, 4.13–4.16**); and functional indicators such as growth, morbidity, mortality or development. Examples of each type of outcome indicator are given in **Table 8.6**, along with suitable methods for their measurement.

Given that the goal of food fortification is to improve the nutritional status of a population, biochemical markers would normally be the indicators of choice for evaluating the impact of fortification programmes. However, the measurement of biochemical status indicators requires considerable resources and technical expertise, for example, for collecting blood samples in the field and for conducting high-quality laboratory analyses, which means that this is not always a practical, or indeed a feasible, option. Fortunately, there are cheaper and less complex alternatives to measuring biochemical status indicators for assessing the impact of a programme, such as measuring the consumption of a fortified product or the intake of a particular micronutrient of interest. These measures are suitable alternatives to biochemical indicators in cases where strong evidence of their validity has been obtained from either rigorous efficacy trials[1] or from effectiveness trials conducted in similar conditions as the programme being evaluated. For example, if it has been established in efficacy trials that consumption of a certain minimum amount of a given fortified product results in a desirable change in one or more biochemical indicators (and prevents micronutrient deficiency), other fortification programmes using the same food vehicle can rely on

---

[1] An efficacy trial is one that applies an intervention under controlled conditions to determine the magnitude of effect that can be achieved under the best possible circumstances (*344*). Effectiveness trials, on the other hand, test the impact of an intervention under real life conditions, and given usual operational inefficiencies that occur under normal field conditions.

TABLE 8.6
Impact evaluation of a food fortification programme: suggested outcome measures

Outcome measure	Methodology and responsible entity
Intake indicators methods:	*Method:* Any of the following dietary assessment
Adequate or increased intake of fortified food(s)[a]	— weighed intake; — 24-hour recall;
	— food frequency questionnaire;
Adequate or increased intake of specific micronutrient(s) of interest	— assessment of usual intake. *Responsible:* Independent researchers.
Nutritional status indicators	*Method:* Recommended biochemical and clinical
Adequate or improved biochemical and clinical status indicators for micronutrient(s) of interest	indicators for selected micronutrients are listed in Tables 3.1, 3.4, 3.6, 4.1, 4.3–4.5, 4.7, 4.8, 4.10, 4.11, 4.3–4.16. *Responsible:* Independent researchers.
Functional outcomes	*Method:* Standard approaches to the measurement of
Adequate outcomes or improvements in functional outcomes such as growth, morbidity, mortality and motor and cognitive development	these functional outcomes should be used, for example: — for growth, anthropometry; — for morbidity, 2-week recall or surveillance data; — for mortality, recall data; — for child cognitive and motor development, the appropriate battery of tests and scales. *Responsible:* Independent researchers.

[a] Monitoring of the intake of fortified products can also be done as part of household monitoring (see **Table 8.4**).
[b] An impact evaluation should only be performed once programme monitoring has indicated that programme is operating in a satisfactory manner and therefore, is in theory capable of achieving its nutritional goals. Full impact evaluation need only be done once, as long as regular monitoring ensures appropriate fortification levels at all stages (i.e. in factories, retail stores and households), adequate utilization of the product and adequate coverage of the targeted population.

consumption data to measure their impact. This technique is commonly employed in evaluations of salt iodization and immunization programmes. In the case of the former, coverage information is used to measure success, an approach that is valid because there is strong evidence that iodized salt, consumed regularly and in sufficient amounts, is effective in preventing iodine deficiency. The selection of outcome indicators is discussed further in section 8.5 in the context of the minimum requirements for monitoring and evaluation systems for fortification interventions.

8.4.2.2 Data requirements

In order to be able to conduct an impact evaluation using any of the indicators and methodologies listed in **Table 8.6**, it is necessary to first calculate the number of subjects that will need to be surveyed (i.e. the sample size) so as to ensure a result of adequate precision and sensitivity (i.e. be able to detect differences of a particular size when they exist). Ideally, a random procedure should be used to select subjects for study.

Specific data needs for each category of impact evaluation are as follows:

- *Adequacy evaluations* require data on the chosen outcomes, and also a minimum amount of information about the study subjects (such as age, sex and physiological status) to facilitate interpretation of the results.

- *Plausibility evaluations* demand more detailed information about the study subjects in order to account for confounding factors. However, the more information that is collected on possibly confounding or other explanatory factors, the more rigorous the evaluation design will need to be if it is to demonstrate that the outcome achieved is related to the intervention. It is therefore prudent to collect information on factors unrelated to the fortification programme, but which may have contributed to the changes observed in the outcome of interest. Data from other programmes implemented in the area, on say community improvements, and on household and individual sociodemographic characteristics can all help strengthen the analysis and interpret the findings. This type of information can also be used to understand pathways and mechanisms, and to help interpret lack of impact.

- For *probability evaluations*, if a double-blind experimental study design is used, control for confounding influences is not required. However, it is always useful to have information on intermediary outcomes to help describe mechanisms and dose–response relationships, and to identify subgroups of the population that may have benefited more (or less) than others from the intervention.

8.4.2.3 Timing of an impact evaluation

As noted at the start of this chapter, an evaluation of the impact of a fortification programme should not be undertaken until a certain level of operational performance has been achieved. Say, for example, commercial monitoring establishes that levels of a micronutrient in a product available from retail stores are only 20% of what they should be, conducting an impact evaluation of such a poorly functioning programme would only be a waste of time, effort and money. It is therefore important that fortification programmes establish a priori the minimum criteria for the quality of service delivery that it must achieve before any efforts to evaluate its impact are undertaken.

The timing of programme evaluation is will also depend on how quickly an impact on the biochemical indicators of interest can be expected. In other words, how soon after a programme has been implemented and has been found to be operating satisfactorily should an impact evaluation be undertaken? Both the type of intervention (fortification versus supplementation, for example) and the nutrient(s) of interest are key factors to consider. In relation to the former, the amount of nutrient(s) delivered daily in fortified foods is usually much less than that which can be administered in a supplement; moreover, the fortified foods may not be consumed every day, or in the expected amounts. The combined effect of these factors is that it will take longer for the biological impact of a micronutrient fortification programme to become detectable than it will for a supplementation programme, probably by as much as several months (especially in the case of effectiveness trials). For instance, it takes about 6–9 months before the effect of iron fortification on iron status is seen.

The rate of change in nutritional status indicators varies substantially by nutrient, and also according to the sensitivity of the indicator. It takes about 1–2 years from the start of a salt iodization programme to see a significant reduction in goitre. Some individuals may take even longer than this to recover, especially if they are also iron deficient (*86*). On the other hand, urinary iodine is a fairly responsive indicator of iodine intake, and should increase significantly within a few weeks of the commencement of an increased iodine consumption. On the whole, changes in biochemical indicators of vitamin status tend to be more rapid than those in indicators of mineral status. For instance, population serum folate and plasma homocysteine concentrations respond within 6 months of the introduction into the diet of flour fortified with folic acid (*49,52*). Similarly, consumption of sugar fortified with vitamin A produces measurable impacts after only 6 months (*46*).

8.4.2.4 Counfounding factors

Finally, when planning an impact evaluation it is important to recognize that a number of factors can affect the ability of individuals to respond to fortification. Particularly significant in this regard is the prevalence of parasitic infestations and infections in a population. Some parasites cause large, continuing micronutrient losses; hookworm, for example, causes intestinal loss of blood and therefore increased losses of iron, vitamin A, vitamin B_{12} and several other nutrients. Parasite control programmes are obviously an effective strategy in these situations and should be instigated in conjunction with food fortification.

The presence of parasites and infections can also affect the sensitivity of indicators of nutritional status, which can make the impact of a fortification programme more difficult to detect. For example, haemoglobin and serum ferritin are responsive to changes in iron status but are also affected by inflammation and infectious disorders. If these conditions are widespread, iron status can only really be assessed using a combination of indicators, that is serum ferritin in combination with serum transferrin receptors or erythrocyte zinc protoporphyrine, and an indicator of inflammation, such as C-reative protein (*75*) (see also **Table 3.1**). This approach has been adopted with good effect in both Viet Nam (*28*) and in Morocco (*44*) to demonstrate the efficacy of iron fortification of fish sauce and salt, respectively. The presence of malaria presents particular challenges: malaria not only leads to a substantial reduction in haemoglobin concentrations, but also affects many other nutritional status indicators, including serum ferritin, serum transferrin and transferrin receptors, plasma retinol and erythrocyte riboflavin (*152*). Simultaneous assessment of malaria parasites (by blood smears) or more accurately, of malaria antigens using test strips (*152*), and of indicators of inflammation (such as alpha-1 glycoprotein, and C-reactive protein), will assist in the detection of individuals whose test results may be affected by malaria.

8.5 What is the minimum every fortification programme should have in terms of a monitoring and evaluation system?

This chapter has highlighted the importance for food fortification programmes of having a well-planned monitoring and evaluation system. These systems should be designed in such a way that the information provided by monitoring and evaluation is used effectively for decision-making and for overall programme management. In order for this to happen, responsibilities for data collection at the different levels must be clearly established and the system must include feedback loops, which allow the information to flow (in a timely manner) to the entities responsible for taking action at the different levels.

Regulatory monitoring is an essential part of any monitoring and evaluation system and should always be implemented, at least to some degree. Information from internal, external and commercial monitoring activities should be shared regularly with all sectors engaged in the food fortification programme. Feedback activities should include the sharing of information about successes and any follow up on corrective measures required when problems were detected.

Of equal importance is household monitoring. Its value lies in its ability to provide a general appraisal of the impact of the programme, and in the absence of an effective system of nutritional surveillance, it also provides information about the importance of food fortification in the diet of target populations. The annual cost of household monitoring has been estimated at less than US$ 10 000 per fortified food (O. Dary, personal communication, 2004). Despite its relatively low cost, household monitoring is often neglected in many programmes. In many settings, household monitoring is dependent on external donors for financial support, a factor which limits its permanence and sustainability.

The chapter has also stressed the urgent need to measure the impact of food fortification programmes, again to support decision-making, and, in particular, to assist programme planners and policy-makers in making decisions about programme continuation, modification, expansion or termination. Different types of impact evaluations can be employed; these vary in their level of sophistication and in the intensity of resources required. Decisions about which specific type of evaluation and which outcome indicators to use should be driven primarily by programme objectives and the level of precision required to be able to attribute impact to the programme itself (i.e. this will determine whether an adequacy or a more complex plausibility design is needed, for example).

The choice of outcome indicator(s) for impact evaluations is a pivotal one. Questions that can help guide the selection of an appropriate of outcome indicator are:

- Can intake measures be used instead of more invasive (and often more costly) biochemical indicators?
- How often do impact evaluations have to be carried out?

The answer to these questions largely depends on the availability and strength of evidence from efficacy trials and previous effectiveness evaluations of comparable programmes conducted in similar environments and population groups. The results of only one or just a few efficacy trials are usually sufficient to prove that a fortified food can change the nutritional status (and its associated biological indicators) in a human population, in which case it might not be necessary to repeat such experiments in each community (see also section 8.4.2.1). It thus follows that the first step in planning an impact evaluation is usually to determine whether or not there is strong evidence from existing efficacy trials that the planned intervention causes a given impact when conducted under controlled conditions.

If strong evidence from efficacy trials can be established, effectiveness trials can then be implemented to test whether the same impact can also be achieved when the intervention is delivered under normal field conditions and programme constraints. In the case of fortification programmes, if other effectiveness trials indicate that an impact can be obtained over a given period of time with an intake of a specific amount of micronutrients through the consumption of fortified products, there is no need to invest in the more resource intensive and complex demonstrations of impact on biochemical indicators. It may be sufficient to ensure that the targeted population consumes the fortified food of expected quality in sufficient amounts and with adequate frequency. However, before conclusions obtained from one community can be extrapolated to another, it is important to assure that the conditions are similar. It may be necessary to conduct efficacy trials to corroborate findings once every 5–10 years, especially if environmental, dietary and health conditions of the targeted population change rapidly. This objective might be combined with the function of general nutrition surveys to monitor the evolution of the nutritional status of the population.

Obviously, in the absence of strong evidence from efficacy trials, there are no short-cuts and a detailed impact evaluation (efficacy trial or probability evaluation), involving appropriate biochemical indicators, will need to be carried out. The comments made previously about the timing of evaluations (section 8.4.2.3) and the need to consider potential confounding factors (section 8.4.2.4) become especially pertinent in these circumstances.

Summary

- A well-designed, well-managed monitoring and evaluation system is essential for ensuring the success and sustainability of any food fortification programme. As integral components of the programme, monitoring and evaluations activities should be formulated and budgeted for during the very early planning stages.

- Some degree of regulatory monitoring is critical. Of the three main categories of regulatory monitoring – internal monitoring (conducted at factories and packers), external monitoring (conducted at factories and packers) and commercial monitoring (conducted at retail stores) – internal monitoring is a must. In settings where effective enforcement mechanisms exist, it is usually sufficient to confirm compliance with regulations in samples taken from retail stores (commercial monitoring). Elsewhere it is prudent to conduct external monitoring at both the factory level and at retail stores.

- Impact evaluations should only be carried once it has been established, through regulatory and household monitoring, that the programme has achieved a predetermined level of operational efficiency.

- Although rigorous impact evaluations of food fortification programmes are urgently needed, not all programmes will require the most costly and sophisticated designs. Judicious choices will have to be made in selecting the most appropriate evaluation for each particular situation.

CHAPTER 9
Estimating the cost-effectiveness and cost–benefit of fortification

Notwithstanding the limitations mentioned in section 1.4, food fortification may often be the least expensive way of achieving a particular nutritional goal, such as a specified reduction in the prevalence of anaemia, iodine deficiency or subclinical vitamin A deficiency. Put another way, fortification is frequently more *cost-effective* than other public health interventions that have the potential to achieve the same health or nutritional outcome, such as supplementation. Indeed, several studies have demonstrated that fortification is not only cost-effective (i.e. is a cheaper way to increase micronutrient intake compared with other interventions that have the same aim), but also has a high *cost–benefit* ratio (i.e. is a good investment).

In this chapter the concepts of cost-effectiveness and cost–benefit are formally defined. Techniques for estimating the cost-effectiveness of an intervention and for performing a cost–benefit analysis are also outlined, and illustrated in the latter half of the chapter by a series of example calculations for a hypothetical low-income country. The methods employed can be readily modified and applied to other countries. Although both cost-effectiveness and cost–benefit analyses are widely used as decision-making tools by policy-makers working in the public health arena, their application to food fortification is a relatively new development. To date, only interventions involving iron, iodine and vitamin A have been evaluated in these terms, and consequently form the focus of the material presented here.

9.1 Basic concepts and definitions

9.1.1 Cost-effectiveness

Cost-effectiveness is defined as the cost of achieving a specified outcome. In the case of food fortification, examples of the desired outcome might include: averting one case of subclinical vitamin A deficiency, averting one case of anaemia, or averting one case of goitre or of iodine deficiency.

Two outcome measures that are frequently employed in cost-effectiveness assessments of health interventions are the "cost per death averted" and the "cost per disability-adjusted life-year saved" (or cost per DALY saved). The former, the cost per death averted, has been successfully used to assess the cost-effectiveness of various fortification and supplementation interventions, but in this context its application requires making various critical assumptions (see section 9.2.1). For example, costs per death averted have been estimated for vitamin A supplementation for children and for iron supplementation for pregnant women (groups that are particularly susceptible to deficiencies and therefore frequently targeted in intervention programmes). However, it is a less useful calculation in the case of iodine fortification, principally because mortality outcomes are relatively rare, the main benefit being increased productivity (see section 9.3.2).

The advantage of the other widely used effectiveness measure, the cost per DALY saved, lies in the fact that it combines mortality and morbidity outcomes into a single indicator (*354,355*). This measure has been employed to good effect to assess the effectiveness of various health interventions, including fortification and supplementation, as part of WHO's CHOICE project (see **Box 9.1**). However, relative to the alternative measure, the cost per death averted, its calculation is more demanding in terms of data requirements and the assumptions that must be made (see section 9.2.1)

Cost-effectiveness analysis is a particularly useful exercise for comparing different interventions that share the same outcome, for example, for comparing supplementation with vitamin A with fortification with vitamin A, or for comparing vitamin A supplementation with immunization. In both cases the shared outcome is the number of deaths averted. The two pieces of information required for the calculation of the cost-effectiveness of an intervention are: the unit cost of the intervention (i.e. the cost per person assisted per year), and some measure of the effect of the intervention (i.e. the proportion of the target population that achieves some specified outcome). The cost estimates, being less resource intensive, tend to be easier to obtain than the estimates of the effect, which require (at a minimum) a baseline and a follow-up assessment, and (ideally) a control group.

BOX 9.1

Choosing interventions that are cost-effective: WHO's CHOICE Project

CHOICE stands for "CHOosing Interventions that are Cost-Effective", and is a tool developed by WHO to help decision-makers select those interventions and programmes that provide the maximize benefits for the available resources. By generalizing the cost-effectiveness analysis, the application of the CHOICE model indicates which interventions provide the best value for money.

Application of the CHOICE model to data from WHO's Africa D region (mainly West Africa) has demonstrated that micronutrient interventions are potentially highly cost-effective[1]. In **Figure 9.1** the average cost per DALY saved by hypothetical programmes for zinc supplementation in the under-fives (coverage, 80% of the target population), iron supplementation in pregnant women (coverage, 50% of pregnant women), vitamin A/zinc fortification (coverage, 80% of the general population), and iron fortification (coverage, 80% of the general population) are compared. Both the fortification programmes achieve relatively low costs per DALY saved. The same iron and vitamin A/zinc fortification programmes are compared in **Figure 9.2**, but this time with the following interventions: oral rehydration (coverage, 80% of the target population), case management of pneumonia (coverage, 80% of the target population), and disinfection of water supply at point of use combined with water use education (coverage, 100% target population). Whereas all of these programmes were found to be highly cost-effective, the fortification programmes were particularly so.

FIGURE 9.1

Cost-effectiveness of micronutrient supplementation and fortification

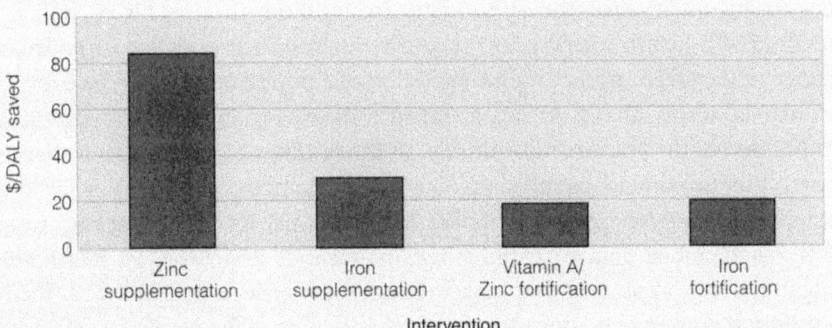

FIGURE 9.2

Cost-effectiveness of selected interventions affecting children

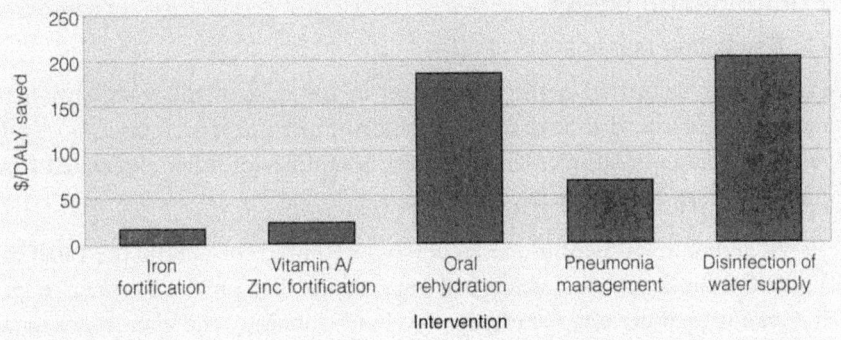

---

[1] Further information about the CHOICE project, including a description of the methodology employed, can be found on the WHO web site at: http://www.who.int/choice/en/.

9.1.2 Cost–benefit analysis

Cost-effectiveness analyses are valuable tools for comparing interventions that share the same outcome; if however, the objective is to compare interventions with different outcomes, or to compare interventions whose potential benefits or outcomes extend beyond health, then a cost–benefit analysis is needed. In its simplest form, a cost–benefit analysis compares the monetary cost of an intervention with the monetary value of the outcome (i.e. the benefit). The outcomes or benefits may be increased productivity (e.g. iron fortification makes adults less anaemic and hence more productive) or possibly lower health care system costs (e.g. mothers who are less anaemic will incur fewer complications during childbirth). Since cost–benefit analyses can be used to compare the relative merits of health interventions with other kinds of government spending, they are especially helpful for advocating for increased resources for nutrition and health.

A cost–benefit ratio calculation requires much the same unit cost and effect data as a cost-effectiveness analysis. Again, the cost data are typically easier and cheaper to obtain than the effect data. In addition, the benefit or rather the outcome of a health intervention (e.g. a reduction in prevalence of goitre or a change in the mean urinary iodine excretion of a population) has to be expressed in financial terms, that is to say, assigned a monetary value. Most cost–benefit studies do not do this directly, but rely on the findings of other studies that have linked the proximate health outcome to a financial benefit. For example, cost–benefit analyses involving iodine interventions, which are seeking to estimate the financial gain of eliminating one case of goitre (as an intermediate outcome), turn to studies that have estimated the costs associated with the loss of productivity per child born to a mother with goitre. The worked example presented in section 9.3.2 adopts this approach.

9.2 Information needs

9.2.1 Estimating unit costs

Unit cost calculations (i.e. the calculation of the cost of the intervention per person per year) need to take into account not just the recurrent costs of supplying fortificants or supplements, but also a number of other associated costs. For fortification, these typically include:

— the initial investment in the technology required for adding the fortificant to the food vehicle (which will vary depending on the number of processing facilities and the existing level of technology, the micronutrient and the nature of the packaging, storage and/or handling of the final product that is required);

— the cost of "social marketing" to attain public acceptance of (or preference for) the fortified food;

— the cost of quality control and quality assurance by producers and of government monitoring and evaluation activities.

In the case of supplementation, the additional costs may include the time and logistics costs of the distribution of the supplement (which are not always reported), and again, the costs associated with monitoring and evaluation. Typical costs incurred by a wheat flour fortification programme (with iron and zinc) are set out in **Table 9.1**; these include the initial investment costs (amortized over expected lifetime of the equipment), recurrent costs, and the cost of monitoring and evaluation.

The estimated unit costs of various past supplementation and fortification programmes, compiled by Levin et al. (*357*), are listed in **Table 9.2**. According to these data, unit costs for supplementation are consistently higher than those for fortification. Supplementation costs are 10–30 times higher than fortification costs in the case of iodine, 3–30 times higher for iron, and 1.5–3 times higher for vitamin A. The cost differential is largely dependent on what proportion the target population is of the whole population; fortification becomes increasingly cost-effective the higher the proportion of the population in need of the intervention.

Although now rather out of date, the unit cost data reported by Levin et al. (*357*) do provide some useful insight into the relative cost-effectiveness of supplementation and fortification as strategies for correcting micronutrient deficiencies. For instance, in the case of vitamin A, if supplementation costs 2–2.5 times as much as fortification per person, supplementation is potentially the more attractive option when the target group comprises less than 40–50% of the population (e.g. children aged less than 2 years). However, for iron the situation is reversed: per person iron supplementation is at least 10 times more costly than fortification but the prevalence of anaemia is well over 10% in most developing country populations. In this case then, mass fortification would most likely be the more cost-effective strategy. It should be stressed that these conclusions are based on average data and cannot be applied to all settings; the relative cost-effectiveness of supplementation and fortification will vary markedly across countries according to both the unit cost of the intervention and the fraction of population targeted.

Another factor to consider in the supplementation versus fortification debate is the effectiveness of the intervention itself; this can be highly variable. In the case of vitamin A deficiencies, both supplementation and fortification have been shown to be effective in impact evaluations (*33,46*). In areas of endemic iodine deficiency, salt iodization programmes have also been shown to be highly effective (*25,359*). However, the evidence for the effectiveness of iron interventions is less clear cut (see section 1.3.1.1). Recently completed studies from China and Viet Nam, involving soy and fish sauces, respectively, suggest that

TABLE 9.1
Hypothetical annual costs of wheat flour fortification with iron and zinc (assumes an annual flour production of 100 000 tonnes at 1 mill using a continuous fortification system)

	Cost of iron fortification (US$)	Additional cost of including zinc (US$)	Total costs (US$)
Industry costs			
Capital investment	820	0	820
Recurrent costs			
Equipment (maintenance, depreciation)	600	0	600
Ferrous sulfate fortificant[a]	57 090	NA	57 090
Zinc sulfate fortificant[b]	NA	102 600	102 600
Quality control	7 920	2 880[c]	10 800
Total industry costs	66 430	105 480	171 910
Industry costs per tonne fortified wheat flour	0.66	1.05	1.72
State costs			
Capital investment and maintenance	2 625	0	2 625
Mill inspection and monitoring			
Salaries and transportation	3 500	0	3 500
Laboratory analysis and reports (including technician salaries)	1 500	96[d]	1 596
Quality assurance and monitoring training	1 000	500[e]	1 500
Programme monitoring (i.e. dietary intake, travel, per diems, analysis, reports)	1 400	0	1 400
Evaluation			
Travel, per diems, collection of biological samples	3 000	0	3 000
Laboratory analysis and reports (including technician salaries)	5 000	3 600[f]	8 600
Total state costs	18 025	4 196	22 221
Total programme costs	84 455	109 676	194 131
Total cost per tonne fortified wheat flour	0.84	1.10	1.94
Total cost per capita (assuming an intake of 150 g per person per day)	0.05	0.06	0.11

[a] Cost of the ferrous sulfate (US$ 8.65/kg (pure iron)), plus an additional 33% to allow for shipping costs, added to 100 000 tonnes wheat flour at 66 ppm.
[b] Cost of the zinc sulfate (US$ 34.20/kg (pure zinc)), plus an additional 33% to allow for shipping costs, added to 100 000 tonnes wheat flour at 30 ppm.
[c] Assuming 2 samples are analysed per day, for 360 days per year at a cost of US$ 4 per sample.
[d] Assuming 1 sample per month is collected from the marketplace and analysed in duplicate, for 12 months of the year at a cost of US$ 4 per sample.
[e] An additional 50% of the cost of quality assurance and monitoring training was included to cover the zinc assessment.
[f] Programme evaluation based on serum zinc analysis in a sample of 1 500 preschool-aged children: assuming a cost of US$ 4 per sample, and a total of three assessments conducted in a 5 year period (i.e. baseline, after 12–15 months, and 5 years post-programme initiation), the cost is US$ 18 000 over the 5-year period or US$ 3 600 per annum.

Source: adapted from reference (*356*).

TABLE 9.2
Estimated unit costs of selected micronutrient interventions

Intervention	Country, year of programme	Cost per person (US$)	Cost per person (1987 US$)	Cost per person per year of protection (1987 US$)[a]
Iodine				
Oil injection	Zaire, 1977	0.35	0.67	0.14
Oil injection	Peru, 1978	1.30	2.30	0.46
Oil injection	Bangladesh, 1983	0.70	0.76	0.25
Oil injection	Indonesia, 1986	1.00	1.05	0.21
Salt fortification	India, 1987	0.02–0.04	0.02–0.04	0.02–0.04
Water fortification	Italy, 1986	0.04	0.04	0.04
Vitamin A				
Sugar fortification	Guatemala, 1976	0.07	0.14	0.14
Capsule	Indonesia/Philippines, 1975	0.10	0.21	0.42
Capsule	Haiti, 1978	0.13–0.19	0.23–0.34	0.46–0.68
Capsule	Bangladesh, 1983	0.05	0.05	0.10
Iron				
Salt fortification	India, 1980	0.07	0.10	0.10
Sugar fortification	Guatemala, 1980	0.07	0.10	0.10
Sugar fortification	Indonesia, 1980	0.60	0.84	0.84
Tablets	Kenya/Mexico, 1980	1.89–3.17	2.65–4.44	2.65–4.44

[a] Different interventions supply vitamin and mineral requirements for different lengths of time. The cost per year has therefore been adjusted to take account of these differences in the duration of protection provided by the intervention.

Sources: references (*357,358*).

fortification with NaFeEDTA has been instrumental in reducing iron deficiency anaemia among women (*28*). On the other hand, despite the fact that iron supplementation has proved to be efficacious in controlled trials (*360*), many iron supplementation programmes have been relatively ineffective in improving anaemia status, even in targeted subgroups. One possible explanation for this is apparent discrepancy is that in many cases iron deficiency is not the main cause of the observed anaemia, but rather it is some other factor.

9.2.2 Cost-effectiveness analyses

Most cost-effectiveness analyses rely on a single indicator or outcome measure to reflect the change brought about by the intervention, usually a measure of nutritional status. However, in terms of the magnitude of the calculated cost-effectiveness, different outcome measures do not always yield the same result. Possible outcome indicators for iron, for example, include the change in mean haemoglobin level, the change in mean haemoglobin level of the initially deficient population, and the proportion of the population removed from anaemia. The first measure gives equal weight to improvements in haemoglobin status irrespective of the initial level of deficiency, the second gives equal weight to all those initially deficient (again, irrespective whether the deficiency was severe or mild), and the third will give a higher weight to improvements in the mildly deficient, but will ignore improvements that don't "bump" people over the threshold, even if their haemoglobin status improves. (As explained in Chapter 3, anaemia is an imperfect indicator of iron status due to the fact that in many populations anaemia has multiple causes).

The most useful outcome or effect measures for cost-effectiveness analyses tend to be those which also provide information on the causes of the change in nutritional status. This is particularly helpful when making comparisons with other studies, which may have employed a different outcome measure. If restricted to using only a single outcome measure, then it is desirable to select the one that can be linked to other outcomes of interest. In the iron example above, the proportion of the population removed from anaemia is the most useful effect indicator, because it is possible to link anaemia status (i.e. anaemic/not anaemic) to productivity outcomes or to pregnancy complication outcomes.

The cost-effectiveness of fortification interventions is likely to vary considerably according to the prevailing conditions, since it is heavily dependent on the following factors:

- the food vehicle used, the storage conditions and the stability of the fortificant during storage;

- the initial level of deficiency in the population (e.g. improvements in iron status may be easier to obtain in initially more deficient populations, because their iron absorption is more efficient and because the cost per case of anaemia averted is lower if more of the population is anaemic);

- dietary patterns, especially with respect to the consumption of foods which inhibit or enhance absorption of the micronutrient of interest in the same meal;

- marketing and processing patterns, and whether the chosen vehicle is consumed by all households in the groups likely to be deficient, including the poor and those living in remote areas.

Despite the inherent variability in the cost-effectiveness of food fortification interventions, it is not necessary to perform analyses for all programmes and for all conditions. Nevertheless, information should be obtained for a selection of programmes operating under a range of conditions.

9.2.3 Cost–benefit analysis

Undertaking a cost–benefit analysis of a fortification programme is generally more involved and certainly more demanding of data (and assumptions) than is a cost-effectiveness analysis. However, only cost–benefit analyses permit comparisons across a broad range of benefits, including non-health outcomes. Issues to bear in mind when undertaking cost–benefit analysis include the following:

- What benefits should be included? Some benefits (e.g. lower health care costs because of improved iron status, and thus reduced numbers of maternal deaths) may be important, but hard to calculate in the developing country context. Omitting important benefits will make the results more conservative.

- Should non-market benefits be taken into account? The effects of food fortification, for example, improved productivity in women, will only partially show up as market benefits. Fortification may well result in important non-market benefits, such as better child-care, which will affect the market productivity of the next generation. Ideally then, non-market benefits should be valued, by using shadow prices or contingent valuation methods.

- How can future benefits be incorporated? Ideally, the present value of the future benefits stream should be included, appropriately discounted, say by 3% (the social rate of discount typically employed in cost–benefit-type analyses). Nevertheless, even this low rate of discount still favours interventions with immediate benefits (e.g. those targeted at adults) relative to those with future benefits (e.g. those targeted at children).

- Cost–benefit analysis (unless equity weights are used) tends to favour interventions that benefit the rich more than the poor (the rich have higher wages, and consequently higher productivity losses when they die or fall ill), and similarly those benefiting men rather than women (as men are the more economically productive, at least in terms of market benefits).

- Because of the assumptions required, it is sometimes desirable to present the results of a cost–benefit analysis in natural units (e.g. in terms of productivity (for iron-deficiency anaemia) or morbidity rates (for vitamin A deficiency) as well as in monetary values.

It is possible to undertake cost–benefit analyses prospectively (i.e. incidence studies), but this necessitates making assumptions about how a new fortification programme will affect the future time path of outcomes, discounting all costs and benefits to the present *(361)*. The alternative is a prevalence study, in which costs of fortification are compared with the existing costs attributable to deficiency. The latter requires fewer assumptions, is simpler to undertake, and may be quite useful for advocacy purposes (see Chapter 10). In the series of worked examples presented in these Guidelines, a prevalence method has been used to estimate the cost–benefit ratio of interventions to correct deficiencies of iodine and iron (see sections 9.3.2 and 9.3.3).

9.3 Estimating the cost-effectiveness and cost–benefit of vitamin A, iodine and iron interventions: worked examples

For the purposes of illustrating of application of cost-effectiveness and cost–benefit analysis methodologies to food fortification, example calculations are set out below for three micronutrients, namely, vitamin A, iodine and iron. Country-specific data required to perform these calculations is given in **Table 9.3** for a hypothetical large, low-income developing country P. These data would be needed to replicate the cost–benefit and cost-effectiveness calculations for another country. Use of generally accepted fortification costs (i.e. those set out in Table 9.3 and which are derived from historical programme data) is recommended, unless country-specific data are available.

The sample calculations require several key assumptions to be made concerning the economic consequences of deficiency (**Table 9.4**). Assumptions must also be made about the effectiveness of a given fortification programme. Although it is clear that effectiveness of fortification depends on the chosen food

TABLE 9.3

Country-specific data required for cost-effectiveness and cost–benefit calculations, country P

Annual per capita GDP	US$ 430
Child death rate	117.4 per 1 000
Proportion of children ≤5 years in population	25.6%
Share of labour force in agriculture	25%
Prevalence of subclinical vitamin A deficiency, children ≤5 years	30%
Cost per person per year of vitamin A fortification	US$ 0.10
Prevalence of goitre, women of childbearing age	15%
Cost per person per year of iodine fortification	US$ 0.10
Prevalence of anaemia (population average)	37.25%
Cost per person per year of iron fortification	US$ 0.12
Infant mortality rate	80 per 1 000
Maternal mortality rate	200 per 100 000
Cost per pregnancy of iron supplementation	US$ 1.70

For the purposes of illustrating of application of cost-effectiveness and cost–benefit analysis methodologies to food fortification, example calculations are set out below for three micronutrients, namely, vitamin A, iodine and iron. Country-specific data required to perform these calculations is given in **Table 9.3** for a hypothetical large, low-income developing country P. These data would be needed to replicate the cost–benefit and cost-effectiveness calculations for another country. Use of generally accepted fortification costs (i.e. those set out in Table 9.3 and which are derived from historical programme data) is recommended, unless country-specific data are available.

TABLE 9.4
Key assumptions in estimating cost-effectiveness and cost–benefit of selected micronutrient fortification

Micronutrient	Assumptions	Reference(s)
Vitamin A	The relative risk of mortality for children with subclinical vitamin A deficiency (compared with those that are non-deficient) is on average 1.75:1.	(362)
Iodine	Of all births to women with goitre, 3.4% are cretins (productivity loss 100%), 10.2% are severely mentally impaired (productivity loss 25%), and the rest suffer minor IQ loss (productivity loss 5%).	(103, 104, 355, 363)
Iron	Productivity loss associated with anaemia is 5% (light manual work), 17% (heavy manual work) and 4% in all other kinds of work.	(361)
	The odds ratio associated with 10 g/l increase in haemoglobin is 0.80 for maternal mortality, and 0.72 for perinatal mortality in Africa (0.84 in other regions); prenatal supplementation with iron is associated with 11.7 g/l improvement in haemoglobin.	(364)

vehicle, the composition of the usual diet, and the pre-existing level of deficiency in the population, it is rarely possible to accurately account for such variations, due to a lack of field data. Under such circumstances, it is instructive to conduct a sensitivity analysis, according to the key assumptions made. This involves repeating the calculations several times, varying each of the key parameters in turn. If the cost-effectiveness ratio does not change dramatically, or the cost–benefit ratio remains robust (i.e. benefits remain large relative to costs), as the parameters are changed, then greater confidence can be placed in the conclusions.

9.3.1 Vitamin A supplementation: a cost-effectiveness calculation

Cost–benefit calculations cannot readily be undertaken for interventions involving vitamin A. Although there are subsequent productivity effects, the more immediate benefit of vitamin A supplementation in children is a reduction in child morbidity and mortality. For this reason, it is rather more helpful to estimate the cost-effectiveness of vitamin A fortification or supplementation (expressed as the cost per death averted or the cost per DALY saved), which can then be compared with other public health interventions that have the potential to achieve the same outcome.

The calculation of the cost-effectiveness of vitamin A fortification, using the cost per death averted as the outcome measure, hinges on the assumption that all child deaths due to vitamin A deficiency (VAD) can be averted by vitamin A fortification. If this assumption is made, the calculation is simply a matter of estimating the proportion of all child deaths that are due to VAD, this being equivalent to the number of deaths that can be averted by fortification.

The population attributable risk due to vitamin A deficiency (PAR_{VAD})[1] is calculated from the prevalence of VAD in children and probability or risk of dying from VAD, according to the following formula:

$$PAR_{VAD} = [Pre_{VAD} \times (RR_{VAD} - 1)]/[1 + Pre_{VAD} \times (RR_{VAD} - 1)]$$

where:

Pre_{VAD} = the prevalence of vitamin A among children in the under-6 years age group; and

RR_{VAD} = the relative risk[2] of mortality for children with subclinical VAD.

Then, based on the values given in **Tables 9.3** and **9.4**, in country P,

$$PAR_{VAD} = (0.3 \times 0.75)/(1 + 0.3 \times 0.75) = 0.183.$$

In country P, the child death rate (i.e. in the under-fives) is 117.4 per 1000. Hence the number of child deaths per year that theoretically could be prevented by eliminating VAD in this population group is:

$$0.183 \times 117.4 = 21.48 \text{ per } 1000.$$

Suppose that the unit cost of vitamin A fortification per year is US$ 0.10. This represents the cost of providing 100% of the daily requirements of vitamin A for the population in wheat flour, or 75% of the daily requirements of preschool-aged children via margarine (O. Dary, personal communication, 2004). If, in country P, children under 5 years of age account for 25.6% of the population (Table 9.3), then the cost of fortification per child aged under 5 years is:

$$0.10/0.256 = 0.39, \text{ or US\$ 0.39 per year.}$$

The cost per death averted is therefore:

---

[1] The population attributable risk (PAR) is defined as the proportion of cases in the total population that are attributable to the risk factor.
[2] The relative risk (RR) is defined as the ratio of the probability of disease development among exposed individuals to the probability of disease development in non-exposed individuals.

0.39/0.02148 = 18.16, or US$ 18.16 per year.

This cost can then be compared with that of alternative interventions which save children's lives, such as immunization and treatment of infectious disease. The costs per death averted for the latter are typically significantly higher, which suggests that vitamin A fortification would be a very cost-effective intervention for reducing childhood mortality in country P.

9.3.2 Iodine: a cost–benefit analysis

In the cost–benefit calculation for iodine described here, goitre prevalence is used to indicate iodine deficiency and the main economic consequence of iodine deficiency is assumed to be productivity losses in those children born to mothers with goitre (see **Table 9.4**). Although in many respects urinary iodine excretion is a better indicator of iodine deficiency (it tracks improvements in iodine intake more rapidly (6), at present, such data are not widely available for many countries. Nor is the relationship between urinary iodine excretion and birth outcomes well documented, although it is anticipated that this will become clearer in the future.

Based on the assumptions given in **Table 9.4**, the average percentage productivity loss per birth to a mother with goitre is:

$$(100\% \times 0.034) + (25\% \times 0.102) + (5\% \times 0.864) = 10.27\%.$$

The per capita productivity loss in country P, where the prevalence of goitre in women is 15%, is given by the formula:

Productivity loss per capita = Prevalence of goitre × Average productivity loss × Wage share in GDP × Per capita GDP.

Note that instead of multiplying an average productivity loss by an average wage expressed in units of currency, and applying a factor which equates to the proportion of the population that works in the market labour force, we use here a simplification, as follows:

We assume that the average wage in the population is given by:

Average wage = (Per capita GDP × Wage share in GDP)/ Employment proportion,

where the employment proportion is the market labour force as a share of the total population.

If the wage share in GDP in country P is 40%, then application of the above formula gives a per capita productivity loss of:

$$0.15 \times 0.1027 \times 0.40 \times 430 = 2.65, \text{ or US\$ 2.65}.$$

If the unit cost of iodine fortification is US$ 0.10 per person per year (*359*), then the cost–benefit ratio of iodine fortification is 0.10:2.65 or 1:26.5. If the costs of fortification are as low as US$ 0.01, as has been suggested by Dary (personal communication, 2004) for parts of central America, then the cost–benefit ratio will be even greater. This is a very favourable cost–benefit ratio. These calculations make the critical assumption that iodine fortification programmes are 100% effective, i.e. that they completely remove the possibility of goitre in the population in the long term.

9.3.3 Iron fortification: a cost–benefit analysis

The cost–benefit analysis for iron outlined below uses the prevalence of anaemia as a proxy indicator of iron deficiency. However, it is generally accepted that only about half of the cases of anaemia are in fact iron-deficiency anaemia; conversely, there are a considerable number of iron deficiency cases that are not associated with anaemia (see section 3.1.1). Despite its being an imperfect indicator of iron deficiency, anaemia is nevertheless used in this analysis in the absence of alternative inexpensive and easy-to-apply tests of iron deficiency (see discussion in Ross & Horton (*365*). The present cost–benefit calculation further assumes that the main economic effect of iron deficiency is a loss of manual work, i.e. productivity. Based on the assumptions given in **Table 9.4**, the productivity loss for a known prevalence of anaemia ($Pre_{anaemia}$) is given by the formula:

Productivity loss associated with anaemia over all market work + Additional productivity loss associated with anaemia in light manual labour + Further additional productivity loss associated with anaemia in heavy manual labour,

that is,

4% × Wage share in GDP × Per capita GDP × $Pre_{anaemia}$ + 1% × Wage share in GDP × Per capita GDP × $Pre_{anaemia}$ × Light manual share + 12% × Wage share in GDP × Per capita GDP × $Pre_{anaemia}$ × Heavy manual share.

Although the prevalence of anaemia (Pre_{anemia}) is not necessarily congruent with presence of iron deficiency, it is nevertheless an appropriate indicator to use here since the estimates of productivity losses employed (see **Table 9.4**) are derived from studies involving iron interventions in anaemic populations, not specifically iron-deficient populations.

According to statistics produced by the International Labour Organization (ILO), in low-income countries light manual labour represents about 70% of all market work, 60% in lower-middle income countries, and 50% in upper-middle income countries (*366*). For the purposes of this calculation, it can be assumed that 57.5% of the work in agriculture is heavy manual labour (based on the assumption that half of work in agriculture and construction is heavy manual work, and that construction represents 15% of work in agriculture (*366*).

If in country P, the proportion of employment in agriculture is 25%, the overall prevalence of anaemia in the population is 37.25%, and light manual labour represents 60% of all market work (the country being in the lower-middle income category), then the per capita productivity losses associated with iron deficiency are as follows:

$$(4\% \times 0.4 \times 430 \times 0.3725) +$$
$$(1\% \times 0.4 \times 0.6 \times 430 \times 0.3725) +$$
$$(12\% \times 0.4 \times 0.144 \times 430 \times 0.3725)$$
$$= 4.04 \text{ US\$}.$$

For a unit fortification cost per person of US$ 0.12 (based on data from Venezuela (*39*), this produces a cost–benefit ratio of 0.12:4.04. However, as mentioned above, iron fortification cannot correct all anaemia (i.e. it is not 100% effective), and a further adjustment to account for this fact needs to be made.

According to the Venezuelan study conducted by Layrisse et al. (*39*), iron fortification led to a 9% reduction in the prevalence of anaemia. However, the study was limited to children aged 7, 11 and 15 years, and was based on a before-and-after comparison, rather than on an intervention/control design. Layrisse's conclusions are, however, supported by the results of a well-controlled study from Morocco involving double-fortified salt (with iron and iodine). In this case, fortification, albeit at a higher concentration, achieved a 15% decline in the prevalence of iron-deficiency anaemia in children aged 6–14 years, for an estimated annual cost of US$ 0.22 (*44*).

If it is assumed that in country P the same absolute decrease in anaemia prevalence can be obtained as was achieved in Venezuela (for the whole population, not only children), then the proportional reduction in anaemia due to the fortification programme would be:

$$0.09/0.3725, \text{ or } 24\%.$$

So, if the economic benefit of averting iron deficiency in the population is US$ 4.04 per person, and the cost of fortification is US$ 0.12 per person and the effectiveness is 24% (i.e. a fortification programme reduces the prevalence by 24%), then the cost–benefit ratio becomes:

$$0.12 : 4.04 \times 0.24 \text{ or } 1 : 8.$$

This is a fairly high cost–benefit ratio, and suggests that iron fortification would be a prudent investment in country P. The cost–benefit ratio for iron fortification is lower than that calculated for iodine (see previous section). However, if benefits are assessed in terms of reduced mortality (as opposed to productivity losses), iron fortification produces the better cost–benefit ratio. Additional benefits for both iodine and iron, not taken into account here, include improvements in cognitive development and in school performance in children.

9.3.4 Iron supplementation: a cost-effectiveness calculation

Studies have established that iron supplementation during pregnancy is associated with a 11.7 g/l improvement in haemoglobin levels. In turn, a 10 g/l improvement in haemoglobin levels is associated with an odds ratio of 0.80 for maternal mortality rates (MMR), and an odds ratio of 0.84 for perinatal mortality rates (taken as 40% of the infant mortality rate (IMR)). Based on these data (see **Table 9.4**), it can be assumed that iron supplementation in pregnancy produces a reduction in the MMR from 200/100 000 to 137/100 000 **live births** (or from 2 to 1.37 per 1000 **live births**), and a reduction of the perinatal mortality rate from 32 per 1000 to 23 per 1000 **live births**.

Hence, for an investment of US$ 1700 per 1000 pregnancies, 9.63 deaths are averted (9 perinatal deaths and 0.63 maternal mortalities). This equates to a cost per death averted of US$ 176.5.

While on the surface it appears that iron supplementation during pregnancy is a less cost-effective strategy than vitamin A fortification in children (the cost per death averted is about 10 times higher – see section 9.3.1), it should be remembered that iron supplementation also has immediate productivity benefits that would not be conferred by vitamin A.

Summary

The *cost-effectiveness* of an intervention is expressed in terms of the cost of achieving a specified outcome. Analyses of cost-effectiveness are particularly useful for comparing different interventions that share the same outcome. In assessments of health interventions, the two most widely used effectiveness measures are "cost per death averted" and the "cost per disability adjusted life-year saved" (cost per DALY saved). Both measures can be applied to micronutrient interventions. Although the latter measure combines mortality and morbidity outcomes into a single indicator, its calculation is generally more demanding in terms of data needs and assumptions.

A *cost–benefit* analysis compares the monetary cost of an intervention with the monetary value of a specified outcome (i.e. the benefit). Because cost–benefit analyses are able to compare interventions whose potential benefits or outcomes extend beyond health, they can be used to evaluate the relative merits of health interventions and other kinds of government spending. Cost–benefit analyses are thus especially helpful for advocating for increased resources for nutrition and health.

Cost-effectiveness and cost-benefit analyses have shown that:

- Both iodine and iron fortification have the potential to achieve high cost–benefit ratios, given the prevailing levels of micronutrient deficiency and the economic situation of many low-income countries.
- Food fortification with vitamin A is highly cost-effective in reducing mortality in children, as is supplementation with iron in pregnant women.
- Fortification becomes increasingly cost-effective the higher the proportion of the population in need of the intervention.

CHAPTER 10
Communication, social marketing, & advocacy in support of food fortification programmes

In common with other health promotion programmes, all food fortification programmes share two objectives:

(i) to create an enabling environment – in this case, one that makes adequately fortified foods widely available and provides the means for individuals to acquire them;

(ii) to help individuals adopt healthful behaviours – in this case, behaviours that enhance the contribution of fortified foods to their micronutrient status.

Fulfilment of these objectives not only requires political commitment and corporate support, but also that national laws and regulations, manufacturing and marketing practices, and community norms, policies and structures be strengthened or modified in some way so as to bring adequately fortified foods to those who need them most. Furthermore, individuals are likely to need guidance and encouragement before they willingly incorporate fortified products into their diets, modify their dietary practices that affect the absorption of nutrients in foods, and adopt household storage and cooking techniques that maximize the nutrient value of the foods they eat. Throughout the entirety of this individual behaviour–environment change continuum, communication plays a critical role.

To increase its chances of success, a fortification programme needs to be supported by a range of well-coordinated communication activities that promote individual, community, corporate and political change. In this respect it is important to be aware that messages about the benefits of fortification can be communicated in a number of different ways, using a variety of techniques, to very different effect depending on the intended audience. By outlining some of the options available, the main purpose of this chapter is, therefore, to help micronutrient programme managers understand the different communication needs of various sectors and so direct their communication activities more efficiently.

10.1 Communication strategies: the options

There are a number of recognized methodologies that are available to programme managers for communicating messages about the benefits of micronutrient fortification; these include nutrition education, social marketing and advocacy (see **Table 10.1**). Experience has shown some approaches to be particularly useful for encouraging individuals to adopt healthier behaviours (e.g. health communication, nutrition education, social marketing); others have helped foster community support, led to the introduction of laws or regulations or mobilized entire countries for periodic health actions (e.g. advocacy, social mobilization). In practice, however, it is not simply a question of choosing one approach over another, but finding the right blend of strategies and tactics that together achieve programme objectives (*367*).

A useful framework for analysing communication needs, in which education, marketing and legislation are viewed as interconnected approaches to managing social and health issues, has been suggested by Rothschild (*373*). By describing the relationship between various activities in terms of individual decision-making and perceived costs and benefits (**Figure 10.1**), Rothschild's framework can assist in identifying which approaches are best suited to which tasks.

TABLE 10.1
Nutrition promotion methods defined

Concept	Definition
Nutrition education	Any set of learning experiences designed to facilitate the voluntary adoption of eating and other nutrition-related behaviours conducive to health and well-being (*368*).
Health communication	The crafting and delivery of messages and strategies, based on consumer research, to promote the health of individuals and communities (V. Freimuth in (*369*).
Social marketing	"The design, implementation, and control of programmes aimed at increasing the acceptability of a social idea, practice [or product] in one or more groups of target adopters. The process actively involves the target population, who voluntarily exchange their time and attention for help in meeting their health needs as they perceive them" (*370*).
Advocacy	Persuading others to support an issue of concern to an individual, group or community. May involve, "the strategic use of the mass media as a resource to advance a social or public policy initiative" (*371*).
Social mobilization	A broad scale movement to engage large numbers of people in action for achieving a specific development goal through self-reliant effort. Social mobilization is most effective when it is composed of a mix of advocacy, community participation, partnerships and capacity-building activities that together create an enabling environment for sustained action and behaviour change (*372*).

FIGURE 10.1
Relationship between individual decision-making and the perceived costs and benefits of any new behaviour, idea or product

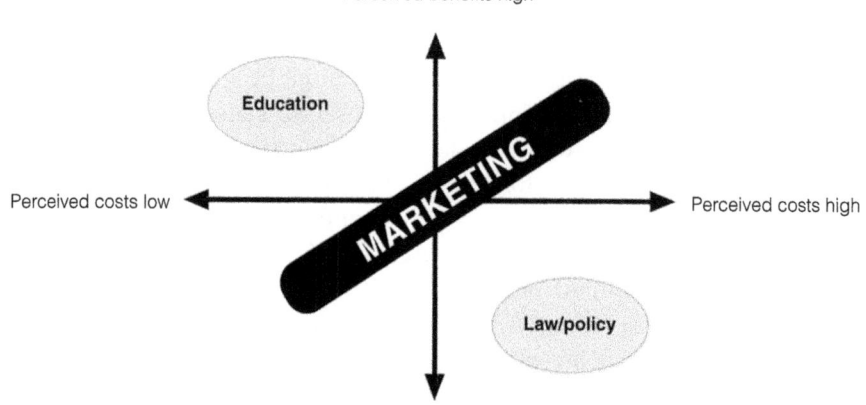

Source: reproduced from reference *(374)*, with the permission of the publishers.

10.1.1 Education

The upper left-hand quadrant of Figure 10.1 is occupied by education or "providing knowledge". This approach is most effective when the benefits of a change are obvious, and the change does not appear costly to the person or group being asked to make the change. It had been assumed in the past that only a minimal amount of communication was needed to "educate" the public, opinion leaders in the scientific community and industry about the benefits of adding nutrients to foods. However, experience with salt iodization has demonstrated that in reality a far more negotiated approach is required.

Fortified products are developed to address a biological need for micronutrients. However, at the individual level this need is largely unrecognized because people neither crave micronutrients nor realize that they are deficient. Instead, a population's need for micronutrients is defined by the health community, usually in terms of a biochemical, clinical or some other marker of deficiency. Since raw data on the prevalence of deficiency are often difficult for the general public to understand, by themselves they do not suffice for providing individuals with a believable rationale for changing their shopping, food preparation or dietary habits. What is needed instead is a more user-friendly message, preferably one that is tailored to suit the information needs and cognitive ability of the recipients (see **Box 10.1**).

Lack of ambiguity in educational messages is vital. Whenever technical experts disagree, the public tends to ignore all scientific evidence until such time

> **BOX 10.1**
>
> **Education as a communication strategy: keys to success**
>
> Educational approaches work best when the recipient of the information has already expressed a desire or commitment to perform the desired behaviour and is now seeking information on what to do and how to do it.
>
> Information for the purpose of providing knowledge must be simple, clear and unambiguous. It should be:
>
> — adjusted to the cognitive abilities of the learner (i.e. according to age, educational level, literacy and language of maximum understanding);
>
> — adjusted to the communication medium be it oral, visual, or tactile (e.g. mixing instructions);
>
> — answer factual questions such as What? Whom? Where? How?

a unified message has emerged. For fortification programme managers it can sometimes be difficult to achieve a consensus between competing claims of effectiveness, safety, quality and cost of a given intervention. For instance, whereas public health professionals tend to advocate the most appropriate fortificant levels for maximum impact, or recommend use of those fortificant compounds that offer the highest bioavailability, producers will try to minimize changes in product quality and cost. A process which successfully negotiates these varying perspectives among public and private sectors is critical to developing a product profile that has the support of both government and industry – and that ultimately will be accepted by the consumer. Hence, at the outset of food fortification programmes, it is important to attempt to integrate and translate the technical language and jargon of the public health, food science and business sectors into a common vocabulary that all the various professionals involved can understand. Technical language and jargon should be reserved for professional communications; the public will require a more carefully crafted approach altogether, and one that is based on the appearance of scientific consensus in order to achieve maximum penetration.

10.1.2 Laws, policy and advocacy: communicating with policy-makers

In direct contrast to education, and occupying the diagonally opposite quadrant in Figure 10.1, laws (or regulations) are used to prompt societal change when a change appears to be costly and to compromise individual benefits. In the context of health, most laws and regulations are aimed at achieving the collective good over individual desires or profit. Rothschild defines law as "the use of coercion to achieve behaviour in a non-voluntary manner" (*373*), but in

> **BOX 10.2**
>
> **Advocacy as a tool for communicating with policy-makers: keys to success**
>
> Advocacy frames issues for public attention, the media and policy-makers. For maximum impact, advocacy should be:
>
> — focused on one or a very limited number of issues;
>
> — get to the point quickly and end quickly;
>
> — add emotional content and localization;
>
> — answer the question: Why should we care?

practice laws can really only persuade, as individuals or entities can always choose whether or not to obey a law or regulation according to their own cost–benefit calculation.

When any concerned group organizes to change a law or policy, their primary tool is *advocacy*. Thus the recipient of advocacy is an individual or group with the power to change the law or regulation, i.e. policy-makers. The primary message that needs to be communicated is why this individual or group should care (**Box 10.2**). "Ideally, policy-makers should incorporate scientific information when . . . making decisions. In reality, many decisions are based on short-term demands rather than long-term study, and policies and programmes are frequently developed around anecdotal evidence. Existing health data are often under-utilized and sometimes ignored" (*375*).

Some advocacy groups (and indeed governments and corporations) actively court the mass media to draw attention to a particular issue and to present their standpoint. Micronutrient programme managers wishing to use the media in this way are advised to develop good working relationships with key journalists and thus earn a reputation for being a reliable source of information. It is helpful to develop fact sheets, press briefings and other background materials that can be used by the news media, but in order to maximize their impact, these usually need to be combined with a "newsworthy" event, such as the release of new data, a public meeting or a decision taken by the government. Although media success can be measured by the volume of exposure or "airtime", ensuring that a story is presented the way it was intended is equally, if not more, important. This can be extremely difficult as the news media is increasingly an "entertainment industry," and what drives story placement is often linked to what brings high levels of audience attention. Strategies for increasing media coverage are presented in **Box 10.3**.

BOX 10.3

Using the media: keys to success

Chances of obtaining media coverage are enhanced by:

— conflict, controversy or injustice;

— community involvement;

— irony;

— a hard news "link" (timeliness);

— images, i.e. pictures, video films, photographs, graphs, and expert interviews.

10.1.3 Social marketing

The central part of Figure 10.1 is occupied by marketing, or, more specifically, by social marketing. Social marketing is the use of marketing techniques developed by the private sector (i.e. commercial marketing) to achieve public sector goals. In the area of public health, this technique has been used successfully to support family planning, HIV prevention, oral rehydration, hand washing, and immunization, as well as various nutrition programmes, such as infant feeding, salt iodization, iron supplementation and dietary diversification programmes (*376,377*)

Commercial and social marketing are alike in that both attempt to influence individuals to make choices concerning their behaviour, and/or the products or services (the "offering") they use by increasing the perceived value of the offering and mitigating the perceived obstacles to its use. In commercial marketing, consumers buy a product or service that they judge to be a fair trade for the sum of money paid. The profits generated through this exchange are distributed back to the company that produced the product or service and its stockholders.

The term "social marketing" is generally used to describe the promotion of those "causes judged by persons in positions of power and authority to be beneficial to both individuals and society" (*378*). The potential consumer in a social marketing programme might be asked to use a product (e.g. a polio vaccine, a vitamin A capsule, soap), a service (e.g. well-baby visit, preventive dental checkup) or adopt or modify a behaviour (e.g. mix an oral rehydration solution, refuse an offer of a cigarette, breastfeed exclusively for 6 months). Usually, the potential consumer or "adopter" initially feels no need or desire for this product, service or modified behaviour, and, in fact, uses or does something else instead.

When the exchange is completed, the consumer or adopter will have given up time, a previously held belief or attitude, money, or even all three to acquire the offering. In a social marketing programme, unlike the commercial marketing scenario, the return to the "stockholders" is better health and welfare for the society. However, when social and private sector entities combine to market socially beneficial products, such as fortified foods, a reasonable monetary profit is usually also generated. This means that the venture can be made self-sustaining, and thus avoid having to rely on constant inputs from governments or donor agencies (*379,380*).

As the objective is largely a voluntary exchange, social marketing works best when it involves potential consumers in every aspect of a programme. Potential consumers need to be consulted about product or service development as well as its cost (or "price"), image ("product positioning"), distribution (or "place") and promotion. These factors are referred to as the four "Ps" of social marketing, and are analysed in the context of food fortification in **Box 10.4**.

Social marketing programmes require considerable investment in order to create awareness of the offerings and to demonstrate their value to potential adopters to the extent that adopters are willing to exchange their time, money or dearly held beliefs or habits for them. Social marketing programmes rely heavily on communication, and need time to develop to their full potential. However, social marketing is not just about communication; no amount of advertising, or advocacy, social mobilization, education, information or health communication can sell an inferior product that is badly packaged and distributed and/or unfavourably priced. For these reasons, social marketing objectives should be defined, alongside other programme objectives, at the planning stage of a fortification programme. Social marketing indicators should also be developed at this time; these can used, in combination with other programme indicators, to evaluate programme implementation and performance (see Chapter 9). Consumer behaviour and its antecedents can be useful complementary measures of programme success.

10.2 Communication to support social marketing programmes

As indicated in the previous section, the right mix of social marketing and other strategies can make all the difference to the success of a public health programme. Food fortification programme managers can make use of any one of a number of published resources to guide the development of the communication component of a social marketing programme to support their own fortification initiative. *CDCynergy. A communications guide for micronutrient interventions* is one such resource that not only provides step-by-step guidance in such matters, but draws on examples of successfully marketed micronutrient

BOX 10.4

Keys to success in social marketing: the four "Ps" for fortified foods

Product positioning

- A high quality fortified product should be produced in accordance with good manufacturing practice, WHO technical guidelines or some other form of guidelines and regulations.
- Product presentation should be attractive, tasty and in all ways appealing to the potential consumer.
- Positioning of the product is derived through research with the potential consumer. It makes a promise that can be kept. Eventually this will become a "brand".

Price

- The fortified product should be packaged in quantities and priced so as to be affordable to the potential consumer.
- Different quantities/price points might be developed to satisfy different groups of consumers.

Place

- The fortified product needs to be widely distributed (including rural areas) using commercial food distribution channels, where appropriate.
- All physical barriers to obtaining the fortified product should be eliminated.

Promotion

- Product promotion should be driven by the product's positioning.
- The benefits of fortified foods and the limitations of non-fortified substitutes need to be presented in terms that are meaningful to the consumer.
- The act of purchasing fortified foods needs to be presented as "new", and then eventually, as "normal".
- The consumer should be persuaded to adopt consumption practices that enhance the absorption of micronutrients.
- The consumer should be educated to store fortified foods in ways that protect the product and prolong its shelf-life.

programmes from around the world[1]. In this particular guide, all promotional materials production and messaging is based on a systematic, data-driven process that is centred on the intended audience or the consumer. This process requires the following activities:

- Qualitative and quantitative research to define participating audiences, consumer attitudes and barriers to change.

- Data analysis to define and segment audiences into like groups for communication.

- Research and pre-testing to determine the most motivating benefits for these target audiences.

- Message creation based on key benefits. For each segment, messages must answer the question, "What is the benefit to me?" Background and qualitative research can define the key messages that answer that question.

- Promotions and other activities that are disseminated via channels appropriate to each audience segment.

This approach can be applied to other communication strategies, including advocacy and nutrition education, to make them more tailored and effective. Social marketing research methods can also be used to interact with all participants in a micronutrient programme, i.e. not just potential consumers, but also industry representatives, and government and nongovernmental organizations (NGOs).

The guidance and suggestions for communicating the benefits of fortification that is provided in this part of the Guidelines is necessarily generic. It is recommended that social marketing research be conducted in each country or region in order to identify the right mix of messages and communications that are going to support fortification programme goals to best effect.

10.2.1 Building collaborative partnerships

In some parts of the world, the formation of alliances or networks has led to a more effective collaboration between the main partners involved in the control of MNM. These partnerships typically include representatives from bilateral and multinational agencies, international and national NGOs, research and academic institutions, foundations and increasingly, industry. The Network for Sustained

---

[1] *CDCynergy. A communications guide for micronutrient interventions* is a comprehensive CD-ROM that helps plan, implement and evaluate communications programmes. The CD-ROM is available, free of charge, from the Centres for Disease Control and Prevention and can be ordered online via: http://www.cdc.gov/nccdphp/dnpa/immpact/tools/order_form.htm.

Elimination of Iodine Deficiency[1] and the Global Alliance for Improved Nutrition (GAIN)[2] and the Flour Fortifcation Initiative[3] are among the better-known examples. The primary role of these alliances has been to mobilize decision-makers with regard to the public health dimension of MNM and to provide support for food fortification programmes.

Within this atmosphere of multisectoral collaboration, the primary role of the food industry is to produce, distribute and market a good quality, competitively-priced fortified product. Ideally, fortification should add no more than a few per cent of product cost to the product price, have no detrimental impact on product quality and not create imbalances in the business or competitive environment. The public sector, on the other hand, is responsible for creating an environment that allows the private sector to invest in fortification. This enabling environment should minimize unfair competition from lower quality or cheaper unfortified foods that make it difficult to pass added costs of fortification on to the consumer.

Inevitably there will be some tension between the public sector emphasis on consumer rights and on equity and health issues, and the private sector focus on consumer demand, commercial viability and revenue generation. Balancing the public and private perspectives requires developing communication channels for negotiating a number of potentially contentious issues, such as:

- Increasing sales is a fundamental goal of private sector marketing. However, this is not necessarily a public or national goal, and for some food vehicles, such as sugar or salt, increased consumption – or sales – is not an explicit goal of the programme. Messages should lead consumers to the fortified product, but not necessarily to increase overall consumption of the commodity (i.e. sugar, oil, salt, flour).

- Whereas private companies strive to maximize revenues, the public sector strives to maximize accessibility and minimize any price rise. A balance thus needs to be struck whereby producers are fairly compensated, while avoiding any sharp price increases for at-risk consumers.

- Logos and endorsements awarded by governments or NGOs can be powerful promotional tools. The difficulty here lies in the fact that, while the private sector promotions are designed to maximize market share, public campaigns cannot be seen to be favouring specific companies. One possible solution is to use public promotions that are generic to fortification, to the micronutrients concerned, to the seal of recognition or to the food vehicle.

---

[1] Further information is available via the Internet at: http://www.sph.emory.edu/iodinenetwork/.
[2] Further information is available via the Internet at: http://www.gainhealth.org.
[3] Further information is available via the Internet at: http://www.sph.emory.edu/wheatflour/.

> **BOX 10.5**
>
> **Engendering Collaborative Partnerships: The role of a multisectoral fortification task force or committee**
>
> Although informal work groups can provide channels for communication, a more formal body, where members officially represent the interests of their organizations, can be more effective in opening communication channels in the right way along the chain – from high-level decision-makers through to consumers. A multisectoral task force or committee is useful for securing commitment, gaining consensus and for coordinating the contributions of various sectors or disciplines (*380*). Participation should include stakeholders involved in the technical implementation of fortification, as well as those offering credible channels to key audiences, institutions and decision-makers. While participants will vary according to national circumstances, the core group might include:
>
> - government health, regulatory and food control agencies involved in regulation, monitoring and surveillance, as well as agencies that deal with special financing needs;
> - companies involved in the production of the choosen food vehicle, value-added processing, and the wholesale and retail distribution of the fortified product;
> - academic and research institutions (which provide technical input as well as credibility);
> - NGOs (which offer support, resources and channels of communication to a range of constituencies).
> - Consumer organizations.

In some settings, the best way to make sure that lines of communication between programme partners are open may be to establish a formal multisectoral task force or committee. The role and membership of such a body are discussed further in **Box 10.5**.

10.2.2 Developing messages for government leaders

For many national governments, fortification is an attractive option because it offers an opportunity to achieve national health and nutrition goals that – by shifting the costs to the market – can be substantially financed by the private sector. Naturally, government departments and agencies vary in their priorities and so some will have a greater interest in certain outcomes than others. For instance, the potential for improved productivity and national economic development will be of particular interest to departments responsible for finance and revenue. Messages framed by national economic circumstances are thus more likely to strike a chord with policy-makers working in these areas[1]. Other examples include:

- Messages defining reduced health care costs will have particular resonance among officials responsible for health budgets[2].

- Outcomes such as improved cognitive ability and improved school performance can be persuasive for agencies investing in educational programmes.

- Agencies dealing with industrial development or public works are most likely to be motivated by estimates of depressed productivity and economic loss.

Depending on national circumstances, some government departments may have very specific concerns about the impact of fortification and thus may be prime targets for advocacy. Having identified, through social marketing research, the specific interests and concerns of each group, advocacy or education sessions can then be tailored to address these. For instance:

- In some countries, government agencies are involved in the production, distribution or subsidy of staple foods. Fortification will impact the budget of ministries or agencies responsible for the financing of these activities.

- Sometimes the selected fortification vehicle (often wheat flour) is imported, in which case, officials may have specific concerns about promoting a product that has a negative impact on the national balance sheet.

- Since fortification is more cost-effective when adopted by larger or more modern industries, agencies responsible for small business development may be concerned about the social and economic impact on small producers, their families and communities.

- Creating an enabling environment for private investment often involves providing exemptions from specific taxes and duties. The ministries responsible for administering these revenue-creating programmes are often deluged with exemption requests.

10.2.3 Developing messages for industry leaders

From the point of view of private producers, fortification cannot be allowed to negatively impact fundamental business goals, i.e. sales and profits. Any new

---

[1] A number of tools are available for estimating the economic impact of micronutrient deficiencies based on national statistics for prevalence, gross domestic product, workforce structure, health care utilization and other country-specific factors. *Profiles*, a computer simulation developed by the Academy for Education Development, Washington, DC, USA is one such tool. More information is available through the internet at http://www.aedprofiles.org/. Another is that developed by the Micronutrient Initiative, Ottawa, Canada, details of which are given in the report titled, *Economic consequences of iron deficiency* (365).

[2] The *Profiles* simulation (see above) includes a methodology for measuring the reduction in health expenditures.

product launch carries with it the risk of consumer resistance and, therefore, a loss of sales and reduced profits. Messages for industry can address this concern by highlighting past successful commercial experiences or ongoing trials that indicate little or no consumer resistance to fortified products.

Although from the consumer perspective, fortification usually entails only a very small annual cost, for a large producer, it can mean a large initial investment. To help overcome any reticence on the part of industry to make the necessary investment, messages directed at the industry sector need to stress public sector commitment to creating an "enabling market environment", that is to say, one that allows business to make a reasonable profit or at the very least recoup their investment. While this involves a number of technical, commercial and regulatory factors, a key element is the creation of consumer awareness and demand. Therefore, messages to industry should also highlight public sector commitment to developing communication channels and to providing support for credible health claims and public endorsements, such as official logos.

Beyond the basic messages about enabling conditions of sales and profits, a number of other messages may be useful for securing industry commitment to fortification programmes. Again, depending on the results of research involving industry and government sector representatives, messages that express the following ideas may be helpful:

- In the eyes of public or government relations departments, the promise of an improved public image and better government relations is often perceived as a benefit to business.

- For technical audiences, fortification could be presented as an opportunity to improve product quality. For example, in the case of flour millers, adding micronutrients can be framed as restoring milled flour to the original nutritional quality of the whole grain.

- For production managers in developing countries, reference to fortification in North America and Europe can suggest industry best practice.

- For some companies, expanded market share and consumer brand loyalty may be perceived as a potential business benefit of fortification. However, although some companies may benefit more than others, there is little evidence that national fortification increases sales overall.

Nor should the power of the argument that fortification is "Doing the right thing" be underestimated. While largely focused on the bottom line, industry does have a social conscience. Moreover, industry is very concerned about consumer awareness and the reaction to a new product. This interest is not confined to the industry sector; policy-makers and business leaders are also sensitive to potential consumer reaction. For government leaders, consumers are also political constituents, and they too need to anticipate potential public reaction to fortification. Therefore, even though they may not be a direct audience for advocacy, understanding the consumer is critical to answering the concerns of leadership audiences and for developing effective messages.

10.2.4 Developing consumer marketing strategies and education

The goal of consumer marketing and education is to create a perception of value in fortification, so that consumers will accept the new product, choose fortified over non-fortified products, and if necessary, pay a slightly higher price. Creating consumer demand for fortified foods, particularly among lower income consumers, can encounter steep barriers, especially in a highly-competitive environment (see **Box 10.6**).

BOX 10.6

Fortified products and consumer barriers

Possible consumer barriers to fortified foods and products include the following:

- Research in many countries indicates that nutritional benefits, while an important feature, is a low purchase priority. Price, taste, packaging, accessibility and convenience are almost invariably of higher priority.

- The need for micronutrients is often unrecognized by the consumer, and must be made visible. This is a difficult task.

- The benefits of fortification are subtle. Because fortified foods offer a preventive rather than a therapeutic benefit, no immediate satisfaction is felt. Moreover, benefits such as improved school performance and greater productivity accrue only years into the future. Promoting prevention and future benefits is often particularly challenging.

- While the incremental price increase associated with fortification is nearly invisible, low-income consumers are keenly sensitive to any price differential. Consumers, particularly the poor who tend to be at the greatest risk of MNM, are also the most likely to purchase cheaper products or to seek alternatives.

- Staple foods are often seen as pure or natural products. Consumer resistance may emerge from misinformation about adding "foreign" substances or "additives." These range from apprehensions about toxicity or changes in the sensory qualities of a food, to fears about the true goal of the fortification programme.

- Staple foods and condiments are part of cultural identity and consumers may simply resist giving up the old for the new.

- In some cases, there is resistance from sometimes more affluent market segments who feel that they do not need additional micronutrients, and believe they are being forced to purchase and consume fortified products.

Consumer marketing strategies can be divided into two categories, "push" and "pull". A push or *supply-driven* strategy pre-empts the choice between a fortified and unfortified product by universal, and usually mandatory, regulation. In theory, while prices may rise as a result of the introduction of mandatory fortification, there will be no price difference between competitive products as a result of fortification. With little consumer choice or price competition, the consumer plays a less active role and thus communication strategies need to focus on ensuring consumer acceptance, awareness and education.

When fortified foods compete with less expensive non-fortified products in the market-place, a *demand-driven* or pull strategy is needed. In this scenario, a perception of value must be created to compensate for the price difference and the fortified product must be positively differentiated from the competition in order to develop an active consumer preference. Communication strategies focused on generic consumer awareness and understanding may not always be sufficient and sometimes more aggressive commercial marketing techniques are required in order to provide a competitive edge for fortified products.

A collaborative alliance of government, industry and NGO representatives, along the lines previously described (see section 10.2.1) offers opportunities to reach consumers through a broad mix of public and private sector communication channels. These range from government broadcast television and radio, through health or outreach centres, to various points of sale. Each of these sectors also brings their own distinct brand of experience and expertise: public sector agencies and many NGOs have long experience in health and nutrition communications, and in public education activities to raise health awareness and promote healthy behaviours. The private food sector provides expertise in consumer marketing, with which to create product demand and consumer purchasing preference. Opening multisectoral channels of communication and cooperation is central to capitalizing on the unique strengths of each sector.

10.3 Sustaining the programme

Even after fortified products have been launched and established in the market place, consumer and professional awareness remains critical to sustaining fortification programmes. Maintaining consumer support ensures that when governments change, fortification-friendly policies are sustained. Likewise, consumer awareness will help to secure stable and continued industry support despite changes in market conditions which may tempt companies to withdraw from the programme or not comply with regulations, despite initially supporting fortification.

Continued collaboration between organizations and agencies involved in communications and quality assurance is also vital to sustaining interest in fortification. For example, when awarding public sector symbols – logos, seals of approval or other forms of endorsement – product quality must be regularly assured. The added value of the public symbol is only as good as the products with which it is associated and ultimately it is the credibility of the organization(s) standing behind the endorsement that is at stake. In countries where government food control and enforcement is not fully functional, consumer organizations offer a means by which to monitor the marketplace. Under such circumstances, empowering consumer organizations to work with government and industry – by collecting samples or publishing results of product analysis – can be an important strategy to ensure quality assurance and evaluation.

Summary

The chances of success of a fortification programme are greatly improved if it is supported by a range of activities that collectively help to create an enabling environment for fortification. In practice this means promoting change at all levels – individual, community, corporate and political.

Various ways of communicating messages about the benefits of fortification exist, including nutrition education, social marketing and advocacy. Education strategies work best when the benefits of change are obvious (the perceived benefits are high) and the change does not appear costly to the individual or group being asked to make the change (i.e. perceived costs are low). Conversely, regulatory approaches may be more appropriate when the perceived benefits of the change are low and the perceived costs are high. All fortification programmes will benefit from some form of social marketing, i.e. the use of commercial marketing techniques to achieve public sector goals. Social marketing is at its most effective when it involves the consumer in every aspect of a programme, from product development to product positioning, placement, pricing and promotion, and is based on qualitative and quantitative research that has defined the key consumer groups, their attitudes and barriers to change.

Messages must be unambiguous and tailored to match the information needs and cognitive abilities of the recipient.

Establishing some form of collaborative network or alliance can be a good way of opening and maintaining communication channels among principal stakeholders. This can also provide a forum for negotiating any conflicts of interest that may arise between the private and public sectors.

CHAPTER 11
National food law

Governments have a key role to play in ensuring that food fortification is effective for the population group(s) most at risk from micronutrient malnutrition, but is safe for the population as a whole. Food laws and related measures, together with a broader food control system, are the primary tools that are available to governments for establishing an appropriate level of control over food fortification practices.

This chapter examines some of the technical and legal issues that are involved in the development of national food fortification law. The discussion focuses on the regulation of the composition of fortified foods and the labelling and advertising of pre-packaged fortified food products. Other elements of national food laws, for example those dealing with industry licensing, support or sanctions are beyond the scope of these Guidelines. When establishing provision for fortification within national food law, regulators will need to take account of existing regulations on international trade and the global agreements that today increasingly govern that trade. For this reason, the chapter commences with a brief overview of the international systems for setting food standards and the current global agreements on international trade.

11.1 The international context

Two global trade agreements are relevant to food, both of which are administered by the World Trade Organization (WTO). These are:

- the Agreement on the Application of Sanitary and Phytosanitary Measures (the SPS Agreement);

- the Agreement on Technical Barriers to Trade (the TBT Agreement) (*381*).

Food fortification measures, whether mandatory or voluntary, are most likely to be covered by the latter, i.e. the TBT Agreement. This agreement recognizes that:

> No country should be prevented from taking measures that are necessary for the protection of human health at the levels it considers appropriate, subject to the requirement that they are not applied in a manner which would con-

stitute a means of arbitrary or unjustifiable discrimination between countries where the same conditions prevail or a disguised restriction on international trade, and are otherwise in accordance with the provisions of this Agreement.

In other words, countries may adopt provisions that restrict trade for legitimate reasons – health being one of them – providing such measures are in accordance with the five governing principles laid down in the TBT Agreement. These five governing principles act to ensure that unnecessary obstacles to international trade are not created. The key elements of the TBT Agreement relating to coverage, definitions, legitimate objectives and governing principles are explained in **Annex F**.

The TBT Agreement encourages the use of international standards, except where they would be ineffective or inappropriate in the national situation (see www.codexalimentarius.net and **Annex F**) *(382)*.

11.2 National food law and fortification

Food law, operating in concert with the broader food control system, is the mechanism commonly used by governments to set technical provisions for fortified foods, the most important of which relate to their composition, labelling and claims. (Claims are statements that manufacturers make in order to inform consumers about their products.) Food law may also be used to impose broader controls on the food industry, and to establish monitoring and public information systems in support of food fortification.

Food law typically has a number of objectives, the most important of which is the protection of public health. Other frequently cited objectives are:

— the provision of adequate information to enable informed choice;

— the prevention of fraud and misleading or deceptive conduct;

— fair trade.

To meet these objectives, fortification provisions in food law should not only ensure that all compositional parameters applicable to both fortificants and food vehicles deliver safe and appropriately efficacious public health outcomes but also that the labelling, claims and advertising of fortified foods is factual and not misleading, and provides sufficient information to enable appropriate consumption.

11.2.1 Forms of food law: legislation, regulation and complementary measures

Food law commonly comprises proclaimed or decreed legislation that establishes the legal framework and the broad principles, accompanied by subordinate technical regulations that give detailed effect under or within such legislation. Thus food fortification requirements may be established either in an act of the governing legislature (such as a food- or health-related act), or in technical food regulations. An example of an act that is solely dedicated to mandatory fortification is the Philippines' Act Promoting Salt Iodization Nationwide (*6*). This law establishes policy, applicability, industry support, public information and sanctions, and is supported by rules and regulations for the implementation of salt iodization and related purposes; these rules include a technical standard for iodized salt. Other countries use technical regulations (also called standards or other such similar terms), to mandate the specific legal requirements for food fortification, but rely on parent legislation to ensure appropriate implementation. One advantage of setting fortification provisions in regulation, rather than in legislation, is that amendments can be made more quickly and easily, providing of course, that the power to administer regulations is delegated from the primary governing legislature to an appropriate subsidiary or statutory body.

Regardless of the way in which national food law is constructed, all those involved in the food production and distribution system (including importers) must understand the applicable laws and, above all, comply with them. To this end, and to ensure that food law achieves its public health objectives, it must be:

— certain in its operation (i.e. clearly and unambiguously expressed for those engaged in the activity to which the regulation is directed);

— supported by an appropriately structured and resourced information dissemination system and enforcement capability.

Under certain circumstances, complementary measures to government legislation or regulation can be used to fulfil regulatory objectives. These measures take the form of industry self-regulation or a co-regulatory mechanism between industry and government in which government decides the appropriate level of involvement. Such measures are respectively administered by industry alone or jointly by industry and the government sector, and are best suited to matters of process or intermediate outcome. A complementary system only works well when the following recognized "success factors" are present:

— the level of risk to public health and safety, or potential harm to consumers, is low;

— the product is relatively homogeneous across the product category and consumers can readily identify it with the industry;

— the industry is competitive, but also cohesive and represented by an active industry association;

— the industry and/or its association is responsive to consumer complaints;

— companies are keen to enhance their future viability and are concerned about their reputations, future customers and the wider community.

11.2.2 Regulating food fortification: general considerations

Before deciding on the format and detail of fortification provisions, it is vital that regulators understand the factors that shape their country's food supply patterns. Important considerations might include the balance between domestically-produced and imported fortified products; the micronutrient composition of the imported product; the capacity of the domestic industry to produce or increase production of the fortified product; and the industry's overall cohesiveness. Having this understanding is especially pertinent if imported fortified products are going to make a significant contribution to the intake of micronutrients. If compositional parameters in national regulation do not accommodate the fortified imports (e.g. if the minimum iron fortification level set by a newly-introduced law was higher than the iron content of the imported product), an unintended diminution of micronutrient supply may occur, unless the domestic industry can quickly fill the gap.

Regulators also need to be aware of the present level of community nutritional knowledge and any planned nutrition education initiatives, so as to be able to determine the appropriate balance between label information and education, and the type and amount of information required or permitted in labelling and advertising. In this regard, and as previously indicated, regulators also need to bear in mind their obligation to international trade agreements and to international standards (see section 11.1).

Finally, any amendment of a food law that requires industry to change its production practices and/or product labelling should incorporate a transition period. It inevitably takes some time before all domestic manufacturers and importers become aware of new regulatory requirements and are able to modify their production and/or labelling operations accordingly. It may also be appropriate for foods produced in accordance with a previous version of the law to continue to be sold for a given period.

11.3 Mandatory fortification

If a food product is subject to mandatory fortification, then the manufacturer is legally obliged to add one or more micronutrients to that food. Mandatory fortification can reach the general population or an identified target group, depending on the consumption pattern of that food. For instance, fortification of a staple food, such as wheat flour, would increase the majority of the population's intake of a fortificant micronutrient, whereas fortification of, say, formula infant milk or complementary foods would increase the micronutrient intake of a specific population group only. The conditions appropriate to the selection of mandatory fortification as either a population wide (mass) or specific population group (target) intervention were discussed in Chapter 2 of these Guidelines.

Mandatory fortification is written into food law, usually in the form of regulation which specifies a legal minimum, and where appropriate, a legal maximum level for each micronutrient in the identified food or category of foods. Providing there are no technological impediments, one food or category of foods could be required to contain several added micronutrients. This tends to apply to foods targeted at specific population groups having multiple nutritional needs and whose food variety may be limited.

11.3.1 Composition

In its simplest form, a regulatory requirement governing the composition of a fortified food might be written as follows:

[*Nominated food*] must [*contain*]:

(i) no less than [*x*] mg/kg of [*micronutrient name*],

and, where appropriate

(ii) no more than [*y*] mg/kg of [*micronutrient name*].

Each of the key terms (i.e. those in italic typeface) are discussed in more detail below, with particular reference to the implications for, and possible approaches to, mandatory regulation.

11.3.1.1 The nominated food

The name of the food or food category selected for fortification must be generally and unambiguously understood, or else explicitly defined or described in the regulation. The identity of the selected food(s) should correspond to the food(s) used to derive the level of fortification required to achieve pre-set programme nutritional goals (see section 7.3). Matching as closely as possible to the identity of the foods used in the calculations enables more accurate predictions of programme impact on micronutrient intake to be made.

Potential areas of ambiguity or difficulty to be aware of include the following:

- The definition of a food or a food category may be as broad or as narrow as required. For example, the nominated food could simply be given as "flour", which might mean all flours derived from all types of grain available in a country. Alternatively, a much narrower description could be employed, for instance, "all flour from one or more [specified] grains", or "flour having [particular compositional characteristics]" (which might be defined by extraction rates); or "flour destined for [a particular use], such as bread making.

- Where necessary, regulations should stipulate whether they apply to foods sold only at the retail level, or only at the wholesale level (for use as ingredients in processed foods), or both. However, more precise descriptions of foods or food categories, in the form of say, "food ingredient destined for [a particular purpose]", for example, bread-making flour or table salt, will automatically determine the market level at which the bulk of the product is sold.

- If necessary, the use of mandatorily fortified wholesale ingredients in certain processed foods could be more precisely controlled by stipulating that such ingredients either should always be or should never used be in particular foods, depending on the level of dietary intake of a given micronutrient that fortification is designed to achieve.

11.3.1.2 "Contain" or similar term

The term "contain", or some such similar term, refers to the *total* amount of micronutrient in the food. In other words, the legal minimum and maximum levels apply to the amount of both naturally-occurring and fortificant micronutrient present in a food, not just to the amount of fortificant that is added. This approach suits those micronutrients whose different chemical forms have similar bioavailabilities; more complex regulation is needed in cases where there are significant differences in bioavailability between naturally-occurring and fortificant forms of the micronutrient in question.

Food manufacturers can adopt slightly different strategies for calculating the amount of micronutrient that needs to be added in order to exceed the minimum requirement depending on whether or not a maximum level is also established by regulation. In cases where only a minimum requirement is set, and providing that the cost of the fortificant is not prohibitive, manufacturers can ignore a food's natural content of a given micronutrient, thus risking exceeding the legal minimum by at least the natural content. However, if a total maximum level of micronutrient is also prescribed, the food's natural content must be taken into account to ensure the total does not exceed the maximum permissible limit. In cases where the natural content is likely to be negligible, the legal minimum (x) and maximum levels (y) approximate to the range of permitted micronutrient addition.

11.3.1.3 Legal minimum and maximum levels

Procedures for determining the legal minimum (x) and maximum (y) total micronutrient content of a fortified food are set out in Chapter 7 of these Guidelines. In conceptual terms, legal minimum levels are established on the basis of efficacy, whereas maximum levels are determined on the basis of safety or other more conservative criteria. Both the legal minimum and the maximum level serve to protect human health, and thus could be used to justify any restrictions on trade under the relevant international trade agreements.

Sometimes manufacturers need to add extra amounts of micronutrient (an overage) to account for any subsequent losses of fortificant during production, storage and distribution, thereby ensuring that the food meets at least the legal minimum at the relevant distribution point. When calculating overages, manufacturers should bear in mind any maximum levels that may also apply to the food at that same distribution point.

The regulatory limits (i.e. the minimum and maximum levels) represent the extremes of the total permitted micronutrient content of the fortified food at the point(s) in the distribution chain to which the regulation applies. Generally this is taken to be at the point of retail sale. Theoretically then, no individual food sample taken for testing from a retail outlet should have a micronutrient content outside of these boundaries. However, as explained elsewhere in these Guidelines, in some countries regulatory monitoring or enforcement policies may allow a small defined deviation or tolerance from the legal requirements as appropriate to the prevailing conditions (see Chapter 8).

11.3.1.4 Name of micronutrient

The term used to identify the added micronutrient can have significant ramifications for both manufacturers and those involved in related monitoring activities. Usually the generic name of the micronutrient, for example, "iodine", is used; this generally corresponds to that which is measured in laboratory analysis for monitoring purposes. However, most analytical methods employed in the food control system do not discriminate between naturally-occurring and fortificant forms of a micronutrient (a notable exception being folic acid).

Many commercial micronutrient fortificants contain other chemical entities that contribute to the molecular weight (MW) of the compound. For example, iodine is commercially available as potassium iodate (KIO_3, MW = 214), of which about 60% is iodine, or as potassium iodide (KI, MW = 166), of which about 76% is iodine. A regulatory requirement expressed as "mg/kg of [micronutrient name]", refers to the amount of micronutrient (i.e. iodine), not to the amount of the chemical compound (e.g. potassium iodate). This form of expression thus ensures that the same amount of the *actual* micronutrient is added, irrespective of the chemical composition of the fortificant compound used. For example, salt fortification with iodine at a level of 20 mg iodine/kg of salt (assuming a negligible natural content) requires the addition of about 34 mg of potassium iodate or about 26 mg of potassium iodide per kg of salt.

TABLE 11.1
Relationship between legal minimum and maximum levels for iron with regard to its relative bioavailability from selected fortificants

Mineral compound	Legal minimum level	Maximum level
Ferrous sulfate	Natural iron content + Minimum amount iron from ferrous sulfate	Natural iron content + Maximum amount iron from ferrous sulfate
Electrolytic iron[a]	Natural iron content + 2 × Minimum amount iron specified for ferrous sulfate	Natural iron content + 2 × Maximum amount iron specified for ferrous sulfate

[a] The bioavailability of iron from electrolytic iron is approximately half that of iron ferrous sulfate, so twice as much needs to added to deliver an equivalent amount of iron.

11.3.1.5 Permitted micronutrient compounds

Because commercially available fortificant compounds vary in their chemical composition and bioavailability, not all compounds are appropriate for use in all foods (see Part III). This gives rise to a number of options for regulators: regulations can either include a list of all the permitted micronutrient fortificant compounds (leaving the food manufacturer free to chose which particular compound to use), or it can permit the use of specific compounds in given categories of foods. Regulations can go further and stipulate the identity and purity requirements of the permitted compounds, or make reference to pharmacopoeias and other technical publications that set out such requirements.

For some micronutrients, most notably iron, significant differences in the bioavailability of the various iron-containing chemical compounds can affect the efficacy of fortification and thus the amount of fortificant that needs to be added (see section 5.1). **Table 11.1** shows how the legal minimum and maximum levels of total iron can be expressed in order to account for significant differences in the relative bioavailability of iron from the added fortificant compounds through the use of multiples of a reference amount. In this example, the minimum and maximum amounts for ferrous sulfate are given by the sum of naturally-occurring iron and iron that is contributed by the added ferrous sulfate. Regulatory amounts applicable to the second compound, electrolytic iron, are calculated assuming the same base amount of naturally-occurring iron but double the amount of iron from ferrous sulfate, iron being the more bioavailable from the latter.

11.3.2 Labelling and advertising

The purpose of a food labelling is to identify the food inside the package and to provide the consumer with information about the food and its appropriate handling and use. Basic information such as product name; "use by" or "best before" date; storage instructions and directions for use; and ingredient list is as for all foods and is not discussed further in these Guidelines. In this context consideration may be given to the Codex General Standard for the Labelling of Pre-packaged Foods (*383*).

In the case of fortified foods, governments may establish regulations on labelling, claims and advertising requiring manufacturers to provide certain nutritional information to consumers. The usefulness and detail of such information will depend on the level of nutritional knowledge of target consumers, the assigned role of the label in fulfilling educational objectives of the fortification programme and the cost-effectiveness of this approach compared with alternative communication strategies.

11.3.2.1 Micronutrient declaration

How much qualitative or quantitative nutritional information, such as a standardized listing of the nutrient content of a fortified food, to include on the label (apart from any reference to the micronutrient in the name of the food such as "iodized" or "iron-enriched/fortified" or its declaration as a fortificant ingredient) is an important decision for regulators. Such decisions should be made in the context of the target population's nutritional knowledge and future nutrition education initiatives. For instance, symbols or pictorial presentations, rather than quantitative information, may be more efficacious among target populations with a high illiteracy rate and/or comparatively little knowledge of nutrition. The cost burden of providing nutritional information, initially borne by the manufacturer but subsequently passed to the consumer, is another factor to consider. Several Codex texts provide general guidance regarding labelling and claims and may be helpful to regulators; these are the Codex Guidelines on Nutrition Labelling (*342*) and the Codex Guidelines for Use of Nutrition Claims (*343*) (see also **Annex F**).

Quantitative micronutrient declaration requirements can pose a particular challenge to manufacturers and regulators because of the labile nature of some micronutrients with time. In many regulatory systems, the veracity of label information applies to the product at the point of sale; external monitoring for compliance also tends to occur at this stage. Specific mention of such matters is made in section 3.5 of the Codex Guidelines on Nutrition Labelling (*342*). Regulators may also wish to consider the need for "best before" dates on long shelf-life fortified foods, especially if the non-fortified versions are exempt from date marking (e.g. solid sugars or food grade salt). Stipulating a best-before date provides a means of linking the nutrient declaration to the shelf-life period.

11.3.2.2 Nutrition and health-related claims

Claims are statements that manufacturers voluntarily make to inform consumers about their products. Nutrition and health-related claims focus on the nutritional properties of the food, or its nutritional and, where permitted, health benefits for consumers. Nutrition and health claims are especially relevant to voluntarily fortified foods, and are discussed in more detail in the section on voluntary fortification (see section 11.4.2). Two issues are, however, specific to mandatory fortification. Although there is little incentive for manufacturers to voluntarily make nutrition and health-related claims about their products when all the foods in one category are fortified, if the mandatorily fortified food constitutes only a portion of the entire food category (e.g. table salt *vis a vis* all salt), then manufacturers may choose to make lawful claims about the nutritional properties and potential benefits of consumption of their fortified products. Under these circumstances, the issues for regulators are the same as for voluntary fortification (see section 11.4.2).

Secondly, some mandatorily fortified raw ingredients are used in the manufacture of highly-processed energy-rich foods. The processed foods themselves thus become fortified, albeit indirectly and to a lesser extent. Regulators might wish to consider whether any restrictions should be placed on the ability of indirectly fortified processed foods to bear nutrition and health-related claims that refer to, or are based on, the fortified nature of the product.

11.3.3 Trade considerations

Prescribing mandatory fortification requirements in regulation may impose trade restrictions on imported products, either because they are unfortified or they have been fortified differently. These trade restrictions may cause difficulties for a country's trading partners. Nevertheless, it is clear from WTO jurisprudence that not only do countries have the right to determine the level of health protection they deem to be appropriate – providing such measures do not *unnecessarily* restrict trade – but also the protection of human health is one of several legitimate objectives that countries can cite in justification of a trade restriction (see section 11.1) (*384*).

Such considerations aside, different fortification requirements between nations may well create some practical difficulties for intercountry trade. Nations in the same region, with similar public health nutrition problems and food cultures, may benefit from finding a common position on fortification policy and regulation that could be uniformly adopted. This would not only provide for intraregional trade and potential economies of scale, but also increase the leverage of the region, where necessary, to source an imported fortified product according to the region's particular specifications. Although, mandatorily fortified food moving in international trade can be imported not only by countries with compatible mandatory fortification regulations but also by those countries whose voluntary fortification regulations accommodate the composition of the imported food, the product labelling may need to be modified so that it is nationally compliant. The need for labelling modification will depend on the flexibility of the labelling requirements of the importing country.

11.4 Voluntary fortification

Voluntary fortification occurs when a manufacturer freely chooses to fortify foods. It is practised widely in most industrialized countries and increasingly in developing countries. The extent to which a manufacturer's decision to fortify a food is voluntary and independent does, however, vary depending on the micronutrient and the prevailing sociopolitical and legal environment. In some cases, the impetus for voluntary fortification flows from government – in the form of incentives, collaborative arrangements or an expectation of cooperation with specific voluntary fortification permissions – often as a milder alternative to mandatory fortification. In several industrialized countries, the regulations governing the fortification of some basic commodities, such as salt and margarine, represent examples of this particular brand of voluntary fortification.

More commonly, voluntary fortification is driven by a desire on the part of industry and the consumer to increase micronutrient intake as a means of obtaining possible health benefits. Perhaps not surprisingly, commercial considerations are frequently decisive factors in the development of voluntarily fortified food products. Such products are promoted, through labelling and advertising, on the basis of their health and nutritional features.

The proliferation of fortified products that has occurred in recent years could have important implications for future micronutrient intakes and dietary habits. Most significantly, increased consumption of fortified products may result in intakes of certain micronutrients that pose potential risks to public health. Therefore, governments are advised to exercise an appropriate degree of control over voluntary fortification, either in the form of food regulation or through cooperative arrangements (e.g. a code of practice). The regulation of voluntary fortification should not only be consistent with overall regulatory objectives, but should also take account of the Codex General Principles for the Addition of Essential Nutrients to Foods (*385*) (see **Annex F**).

As in the case of mandatory fortification, there are several key issues that need addressing when developing regulations for voluntary fortification, in particular, issues which relate to the composition, labelling and advertising, and the trade of fortified products. These are discussed in greater detail below, but in essence are as follows:

- the range of foods suitable for fortification;
- the range and concentrations of micronutrients appropriate for different categories of foods;
- the mode of regulatory expression (i.e. whether there is a need for absolute limits or whether more flexible mechanisms for establishing compositional parameters would be more workable);
- the identity of, and purity specifications for, the listed fortificant compounds;
- controls on nutritional and health claims as well as advertising, and the appropriate level of detail of nutrition label information.

11.4.1 Composition

11.4.1.1 Range of foods

There is considerable debate and certainly no international consensus regarding the extent to which regulators should seek to minimize public health risks due to MNM, particularly in relation to the range of foods that are eligible for voluntary fortification. To date, the debate has centred on whether the choice of foods or food categories for voluntary fortification should be decided by governments, or left entirely to manufacturers, in which case the prevailing technological and/or commercial constraints – such as whether the fortificant adversely affects product characteristics or the cost is dissuasive or prohibitive – will largely determine which products are fortified and which are not.

One view is that, without some regulatory constraint, the proliferation and promotion of fortified foods has the potential to modify food choices and dietary behaviour in ways that are not commensurate with the maintenance of health and well-being. These concerns anticipate that the commercial promotion of voluntarily fortified foods would enhance their appeal to consumers who would expect to gain a health benefit from the consumption of such foods. Furthermore, if consumers responded regularly to such promotional activities, this could lead to dietary distortions in which fortified foods are favoured over naturally nutritious foods. It might also confound consumers' perception and understanding of the nutritional contribution of various foods to a healthful diet, and thus undermine efforts to educate them about the nutritional value of different foods and the importance of a varied diet for ensuring adequate intakes of essential nutrients. Collectively, these influences may have a detrimental effect on the quantity, quality and ratio of intakes of certain macronutrients, and thus constitute a long-term health risk for the population.

Of greater concern is the possibility that some promoted fortified foods will contain relatively high quantities of nutrients that are associated with negative health effects, in particular, total fat, saturated and trans-fatty acids, sodium or salt, sugar(s) and alcohol. The foods most incriminated are those that nutrition policies often advise against regular consumption, such as confectionery, carbonated soft drinks, sugar-based beverages and desserts, high-salt and high-fat snacks and alcoholic beverages.

At present, the concern about the proliferation of fortified foods is largely based on predictions about future market evolution, which are supported by the observation that manufacturers often use the fact that a food is fortified as a promotional tool. Those who support a liberal approach to the regulation of voluntary fortification cite the lack of evidence from any industrialized country that has a well-developed nutrition education system for such an evolution and past experience with a liberal approach to the addition of micronutrients. According to manufacturers' data, voluntarily fortified foods currently represent 1–6% of the total food supply in such countries, a percentage that has remained stable in recent years. There is also little concrete evidence of any negative effect of fortified foods on the overall balance of population micronutrient intake. Such findings suggest that the key factors to consider when deciding the extent of permissions for voluntary fortification are the strength and sustainability of nutrition education programmes, the level of consumers' nutritional knowledge and the potential for consumer confusion.

The nutritional profile of candidate foods, in particular their content of total fat, saturated and trans-fatty acids, sugar(s), sodium or salt, is clearly one criteria that could be used to select appropriate foods for voluntary fortification. However, a flexible approach that also considers the nutritional merits of a candidate food will avoid the inadvertent exclusion of nutritionally valuable foods from potential fortification. When reviewing candidate foods with respect to their nutritional value, reference should be made to the recently published report of the Joint FAO/WHO Expert Consultation on Diet, Nutrition and the Prevention of Chronic Diseases (*386*). However, it is recognized that final decisions about the suitability of foods for fortification will very much depend on the dietary profile and nutritional status of the population and so will vary from country to country. In contrast to the requirements for mandatory fortification (see section 11.3.1.1), the range of foods eligible for voluntary fortification can either be considered to be prohibited unless permitted (i.e. a positive list), or permitted unless prohibited (i.e. a negative list). If the risks to health from unsafe fortification are considerable, it is probably preferable to establish a positive rather than a negative list of foods.

11.4.1.2 The range of micronutrients and their specific chemical forms

A review of the balance between the public health significance and public health risk of individual micronutrients is generally considered to be a suitable basis for drawing up a list of micronutrients that would be appropriate to add to foods through voluntary fortification. Globally, the micronutrients of greatest public health significance are iron, vitamin A and iodine. A number of other micronutrients also offer broad public health benefits or potential benefits to smaller population groups (see Chapter 4). There may be some micronutrients, however, whose addition to foods may not necessarily confer any further public health benefit because of the surfeit of that micronutrient in the existing food supply, in which case, fortification serves only to promote the "image" of the product. Some would argue that one micronutrient more or less would not have any significant impact on consumer perception of the product, and that therefore these micronutrients should be approved, providing there were no safety concerns.

Ideally, the public health risks of individual micronutrients should be assessed in terms of the magnitude of the difference between some measure of nutrient adequacy and an upper safe intake limit. In recent years, a number of scientific bodies have proposed various risk classification systems for micronutrients, many of which have much in common (*93*). For example, thiamine is commonly rated as low risk whereas selenium is rated as high risk. The classification of micronutrients as moderate to high risk does not preclude their regulatory approval, particularly as these same micronutrients may provide significant benefits; however, it does signal the need for their addition to foods to be carefully regulated. It may also be necessary to make provision for a small number of constituents, such as vanadium, whose status as essential nutrients is uncertain at the present time. In this regard, it should be noted that the definition of fortification given in the Codex General Principles for the Addition of Essential Nutrients to Foods (*385*) refers specifically to the addition of essential nutrients. The overriding consideration must, however, be to ensure the adequate nutritional balance of the diet.

Having decided on the range of approved micronutrients, regulators are advised to include these in regulation in the form of a restrictive list. Further refinements of the permissions or prohibitions on particular food-micronutrient combinations can then be developed from this primary list. A related restrictive list of particular micronutrient fortificant compounds (i.e. the vitamin preparations and mineral salts that are used as sources of vitamins and minerals), would also be required. Regulators should bear in mind that the potential range of foods that can be voluntarily fortified is large, and so too is the range of food production methods. Therefore, the list of approved chemical compounds will need to be as large as the basic criteria for selection (i.e. bioavailability, safety) will allow. Purity criteria for these compounds will also need to be stipulated. These can be developed at the national level but the task is arduous and resource intensive. Purity criteria have been set for most substances at the international level and so reference to texts such as the *Food Chemicals Codex* (*387*) and the *British pharmacopoeia* (*388*) could be made instead.

11.4.1.3 Legal minimum and maximum levels

There are two issues to be considered here: firstly, the setting of minimum and maximum levels and, secondly, the amount of food that will be used as a reference for these levels (i.e. mg per kg or per serving).

Minimum micronutrient levels should set such that fortification results in products that contain a meaningful amount of the micronutrient, that is to say, amounts that would be expected to contribute a benefit when that product was consumed in quantities that would normally be expected as part of an overall adequate and varied diet. An alternative approach, which provides greater flexibility for manufacturers (and also importers), is to establish *minimum claim criteria*. When deciding which is the more suitable approach, regulators should take into account the health benefits that are likely to be gained from voluntary fortification.

The setting of maximum levels is a more complex matter because of the necessity to simultaneously eliminate potential risks to public health from excess intakes of certain nutrients and to preserve the balance of the nutritional composition of the diet. Decisions about the appropriate maximum limits for micronutrients in foods eligible for voluntary fortification should be based on dietary intake assessments that take account of intakes from all dietary sources of the micronutrient under consideration, including that from unfortified foods and dietary supplements. However, this does not necessarily mean that maximum amounts need to be established for all micronutrients according to their risk profile: not only would this be difficult to do for the full range of micronutrients, but the risk of excess intake varies with the micronutrient and with the level of deficiency (and so will be different for different populations). Neither does it mean that the maximum amounts need to be set at the estimated highest safe level in each fortified food category. Allowance would need to be made for the applicability of the upper limits (particularly for the at-risk group), the assumptions made in the dietary assessment (e.g. that supplement use would not become more prevalent), and the magnitude of future intakes of micronutrients from fortified food.

A risk-based approach for setting maximum fortification limits is becoming more commonly accepted, particularly with the development of reference values for upper safe intakes, the approach followed by others is that officially recommended nutrient intakes, i.e. a population measure of dietary adequacy, variously abbreviated in different countries as the DRI, the RDI, the RNI or the DRV, are better guiding criteria. The reasoning behind the latter suggestion stems from acknowledgement of the absence of need for higher intakes and greater compatibility with the amounts of micronutrients found naturally in foods.

It is apparent from the preceding discussion that it would be unwise to allow the addition of those micronutrients that have a narrow margin of safety in significant quantities to all or even a wide range of foods. Therefore, the range of foods to which they may be added should be prioritized or restricted in some way; this can be done on the basis of their nature and importance in the diet of the general population or of certain population groups. Regulators who administer systems in which the foods are restrictively listed and may be incrementally approved through petition should give consideration ahead of time, if possible, to the most appropriate food sources of these micronutrients.

Maximum levels can be established in regulation either for all added micronutrients, or just for those micronutrients that are associated with a known risk, according to the level of risk. As in the case of minimum levels, the concept of *maximum claim levels* may be advantageous. The rationale behind the use of maximum claims is that they allow regulators to set restrictions on the maximum micronutrient levels that are proportionate to the level of risk and, in the absence of a tolerance system, they allow manufacturers (and particularly importers) more latitude in deciding the micronutrient composition of foods lawfully offered for sale. However, for domestic manufacturers, commercial reality also imposes its own constraints in that the manufacturer gains no market advantage by adding considerably more fortificant than the amount that can be claimed.

As indicated above, the quantitative basis for setting minimum and maximum micronutrient levels is a very important consideration. There are three possibilities that would uniformly apply to all eligible foods. These are:

— maximum concentration per unit weight or volume (e.g. per 100 g or ml);

— maximum micronutrient density per unit energy (i.e. per 100 kcal or kJ);

— maximum quantity per nominated serving or reference quantity (e.g. g or ml per serving).

The use of weight- or energy-based criteria requires making assumptions about respective amounts of solids and liquids, or energy ingested by an average consumer in one day. Since these are likely to be broadly similar across national populations, the potential exists for agreement at the regional or international level, providing the basic approach is acceptable. On the down side, both the weight- and energy-based criteria would cause some products to be unduly favoured or penalized (e.g. energy-rich or low-energy foods, foods used in small quantities) so that exceptions would need to be made accordingly. The per serving basis has the attraction of being more relevant for consumers, especially if the label nutrient declaration is made on the same basis. However, it necessitates agreement on the serving size, which is more likely to vary among countries according to cultural food patterns. Agreement on serving size would thus be more difficult to reach at an international level, and therefore setting levels on this basis would be more likely to create problems for international trade.

11.4.2 Labelling and advertising

As previously mentioned, claims regarding the nutritional properties of fortified food, or its nutritional and, where permitted, health benefits for consumers are frequently made by manufacturers as a means of promoting their products; this is particularly true of voluntarily fortified foods. Examples of nutritional property claims are those which refer to a food "containing" or being a "source" or "high source" of a particular nutrient and those which compare the nutrient content of a food with one or more foods. Health-related claims include nutrient function and reduction of disease risk claims, i.e. they refer to the relationship between a nutrient (or a special ingredient contained in the food) and normal physiological functions of the body or to the reduction in risk of a disease, including nutrient deficiency diseases.

11.4.2.1 Nutrition and health-related claims

Appropriate regulation of claims ensures that the information manufacturers convey to consumers about their products is truthful and not misleading.

The Codex Guidelines for Use of Nutrition Claims (*343*) provides guidance to governments on the conditions for nutrition and health-related claims and establishes the general principle that these claims should be consistent with and support national nutrition policy. At the time of writing, conditions for the use of health claims are under discussion. Regulating claims about the reduction of risk of disease is an especially challenging task and should be tackled with extreme caution. Regulators should bear in mind that anything less than a case-by-case assessment and detailed evaluation of adequately substantiated requests from manufacturers to use disease reduction claims would need to be carefully considered.

The Codex Guidelines for Use of Nutrition Claims (*343*) recommend that claims should be substantiated by generally acceptable scientific data, although the meaning of "generally acceptable scientific data" can give rise to different interpretations. A list of health claims that are considered to be well established and generally acceptable would be a useful tool both for the responsible manufacturer and for food controlling authorities. Ideally, a procedure that allows updates to be made within an agreed time frame should be integral to such a list.

As an alternative to a list of approved health claims, nutrition and health-related claims may be controlled by setting qualifying and disqualifying criteria that are based on other aspects of the food. Currently-held views on this topic have much in common with those previously described in relation to the range of candidate foods for voluntary fortification. Although it is reasonable to expect that all eligible voluntarily fortified foods should also be eligible to carry nutrition and health-related claims, this approach may introduce discrepancies between the criteria that apply to fortified foods and those that apply to unfortified foods, particularly if foods not permitted direct fortification are made from fortified ingredients. It is therefore useful to consider whether the qualifying criteria for claims for fortified foods should differ from those that would apply to unfortified foods (whose claims are based on a natural micronutrient content), and if so, on what basis.

11.4.2.2 Micronutrient declaration

Because of the positive perception of fortification by the consumer, manufacturers usually wish to promote this aspect of their products by making nutrient content and/or other related claims about their product. This generally triggers nutrition labelling of the food. Even in the absence of a claim, manufacturers may choose to declare micronutrient contents in nutrition labelling.

Provision of (usually quantitative) information about nutrient contents is normally required under the rules on nutrition labelling; this coupled with information about the micronutrient(s) with which the product is fortified, would be a minimum requirement. For those consumers who read and understand nutrition labelling, the declaration of the fortificant micronutrient content in the nutrition information panel could potentially enhance the "image" of the food. It should therefore be considered whether more comprehensive nutrition information should be given for fortified foods in order to provide more balanced information about the product.

The Codex Guidelines on Nutrition Labelling (*342*) provides guidance to governments on nutrition labelling.

11.4.2.3 Other relevant considerations

The labelling and advertising of fortified products should not attribute to them undue nutritional merits. It should also avoid conveying the impression that a normal balanced and varied diet would not provide adequate quantities of nutrients, although regulations should allow for the possibility of scientifically substantiated exceptions to this. Allowing additional advice on the need for a balanced diet is an another option to consider.

11.4.3 Trade considerations

Voluntary fortification regulation, despite being less restrictive than that governing mandatory fortification, may nevertheless limit trade in fortified foods between countries, particularly in cases where the micronutrient concentrations of fortified foods do not conform to the regulatory provisions of the importing country, or where fortification of a food category is not permitted or is prohibited in the importing country. Different labelling regulations, including those governing nutrition labelling and claims, may mean that product labels would have to be adapted to local requirements. If a common language exists, for reasons of cost and efficiency, it would be preferable to harmonize regional regulations. This would bring the added bonus of minimizing such impediments to trade.

References

1. *Iron deficiency anaemia: assessment, prevention, and control. A guide for programme managers.* Geneva, World Health Organization, 2001 (WHO/NHD/01.3).
2. de Benoist B et al., eds. *Iodine status worldwide. WHO Global Database on Iodine Deficiency.* Geneva, World Health Organization, 2004.
3. *Global Prevalence of Vitamin A Deficiency. Micronutrient Deficiency Information System working paper No. 2.* Geneva, World Health Organization, 1995 (WHO/NUT/95.3.).
4. *The World Health Report 2002: reducing risks, promoting healthy life: overview.* Geneva, World Health Organization, 2002 (WHO/WHR/02.1).
5. *Indicators for assessing vitamin A deficiency and their application in monitoring and evaluating intervention programmes.* Geneva, World Health Organization, 1996 (WHO/NUT/96.10).
6. *Assessment of iodine deficiency disorders and monitoring their elimination. A guide for programme managers.* 2nd ed. Geneva, World Health Organization, 2001.
7. Allen LH. *Ending hidden hunger: the history of micronutrient deficiency control.* Washington, DC, The World Bank, 2002 (Background Paper for the World Bank/UNICEF Nutrition Assessment).
8. Hetzel BS, Pandav CS. *S.O.S. for a Billion. The Conquest of Iodine Deficiency Disorders.* Oxford, Oxford University Press, 1994.
9. Hetzel BS. Iodine deficiency disorders and their eradiaction. *Lancet*, 1983, 2:1126–1129.
10. Cobra C et al. Infant survival is improved by oral iodine supplementation. *Journal of Nutrition*, 1997, 127:574–578.
11. Thilly CH et al. Impaired fetal and postnatal development and high perinatal deathrate in a severe iodine deficient area. In: Stockigt JR et al., eds. *Thyroid Research VIII*. Canberra, Australian Academy of Science, 1980: 20–23.
12. Beaton GH et al. *Effectiveness of vitamin A supplementation in the control of young child morbidity and mortality in developing countries.* Geneva, Administrative Committee on Coordination – Sub-Committee on Nutrition, 1992 (ACC/SCN Nutrition policy paper No. 13).
13. Sommer A et al. Impact of vitamin A supplementation on childhood mortality. A randomized controlled community trial. *Lancet*, 1986, 1:1169–1173.
14. Haas JD, Brownlie T. Iron deficiency and reduced work capacity: a critical review of the research to determine a causal relationship. *Journal of Nutrition*, 2001, 131 (2S-2):676S–688S.
15. Pollitt E. The developmental and probabilistic nature of the functional consequences of iron-deficiency anemia in children. *Journal of Nutrition*, 2001, 131:669S–675S.

16. Stoltzfus RJ. Iron-deficiency anemia: reexamining the nature and magnitude of the public health problem. Summary: implications for research and programs. *Journal of Nutrition*, 2001, 131:697S–701S.
17. Brown KH et al. Effect of supplemental zinc on the growth and serum zinc concentrations of prepubertal children: a meta-analysis of randomized controlled trials. *American Journal of Clinical Nutrition*, 2002, 75:1062–1071.
18. Bhutta ZA et al. Prevention of diarrhea and pneumonia by zinc supplementation in children in developing countries: pooled analysis of randomized controlled trials. Zinc Investigators' Collaborative Group. *Journal of Pediatrics*, 1999, 135:689–697.
19. Black RE. Therapeutic and preventive effects of zinc on serious childhood infectious diseases in developing countries. *American Journal of Clinical Nutrition*, 1998, 68 (2 Suppl):476S–479S.
20. Resolution WHA 43.2. Prevention and control of iodine deficiency disorders. In: *Forty-third World Health Assembly, Geneva 14 May 1990*. Geneva, World Health Organization, 1990.
21. Demment MW, Allen LH, eds. Animal Source Foods to Improve Micronutrient Nutrition and Human Function in Developing Countries. Proceedings of the conference held in Washington, DC, 2002 June 24–26. *Journal of Nutrition*, 2003, 133 (11 Suppl 2):3875S–4061S.
22. de Pee S, Bloem MW, Kiess L. Evaluating food-based programmes for their reduction of vitamin A deficiency and its consequences. *Food and Nutrition Bulletin*, 2000, 21:232–238.
23. Gibson RS et al. Dietary strategies to combat micronutrient deficiencies of iron, zinc, and vitamin A in developing countries: Development, implementation, monitoring, and evaluation. *Food and Nutrition Bulletin*, 2000, 21:219–231.
24. Ruel MT. *Can food-based strategies help reduce vitamin A and iron deficiencies? A review of recent evidence*. Washington, DC, International Food Policy Research Institute, 2001.
25. Burgi H, Supersaxo Z, Selz B. Iodine deficiency diseases in Switzerland one hundred years after Theodor Kocher's survey: a historical review with some new goitre prevalence data. *Acta Endocrinologica*, 1990, 123:577–590.
26. Marine D, Kimball OP. Prevention of simple goiter in man. *Archives of Internal Medicine*, 1920, 25:661–672.
27. Darnton-Hill I, Nalubola R. Fortification strategies to meet micronutrient needs: successes and failures. *Proceedings of the Nutrition Society*, 2002, 61:231–241.
28. Thuy PV et al. Regular consumption of NaFeEDTA-fortified fish sauce improves iron status and reduces the prevalence of anemia in anemic Vietnamese women. *American Journal of Clinical Nutrition*, 2003, 78:284–290.
29. Mannar V, Boy Gallego E. Iron fortification: country level experiences and lessons learned. *Journal of Nutrition*, 2002, 132 (4 Suppl):856S–858S.
30. Ballot DE et al. Fortification of curry powder with NaFe(111)EDTA in an iron-deficient population: report of a controlled iron-fortification trial. *American Journal of Clinical Nutrition*, 1989, 49:162–169.
31. Muhilal et al. Vitamin A-fortified monosodium glutamate and health, growth, and survival of children: a controlled field trial. *American Journal of Clinical Nutrition*, 1988, 48:1271–1276.
32. Solon FS et al. Evaluation of the effect of vitamin A-fortified margarine on the vitamin A status of preschool Filipino children. *European Journal of Clinical Nutrition*, 1996, 50:720–723.

33. Solon FS et al. Efficacy of a vitamin A-fortified wheat-flour bun on the vitamin A status of Filipino schoolchildren. *American Journal of Clinical Nutrition*, 2000, 72:738–744.
34. van Stuijvenberg ME et al. Long-term evaluation of a micronutrient-fortified biscuit used for addressing micronutrient deficiencies in primary school children. *Public Health Nutrition*, 2001, 4:1201–1209.
35. Latham MC et al. Micronutrient dietary supplements – a new fourth approach. *Archivos Latinoamericanos de Nutricion*, 2001, 51 (1 Suppl 1):37–41.
36. Abrams SA et al. A micronutrient-fortified beverage enhances the nutritional status of children in Botswana. *Journal of Nutrition*, 2003, 133:1834–1840.
37. Yip R et al. Declining prevalence of anemia in childhood in a middle-class setting: a pediatric success story? *Pediatrics*, 1987, 80:330–334.
38. Fomon S. Infant feeding in the 20th century: formula and beikost. *Journal of Nutrition*, 2001, 131:409S–420S.
39. Layrisse M et al. Early response to the effect of iron fortification in the Venezuelan population. *American Journal of Clinical Nutrition*, 1996, 64:903–907.
40. Stekel A et al. Prevention of iron deficiency by milk fortification. II. A field trial with a full-fat acidified milk. *American Journal of Clinical Nutrition*, 1988, 47:265–269.
41. Hertrampf E. Iron fortification in the Americas. *Nutrition Reviews*, 2002, 60:S22–S25.
42. *Guidelines for iron fortification of cereal food staples*. Washington, DC, Sharing United States Technology to Aid in the Improvement of Nutrition, 2001.
43. Zimmermann MB et al. Addition of microencapsulated iron to iodized salt improves the efficacy of iodine in goitrous, iron-deficient children: a randomized, double-blind, controlled trial. *European Journal of Endocrinology*, 2002, 147:747–753.
44. Zimmermann MB et al. Dual fortification of salt with iodine and microencapsulated iron: a randomized, double-blind, controlled trial in Moroccan schoolchildren. *American Journal of Clinical Nutrition*, 2003, 77:425–432.
45. Arroyave G et al. *Evaluation of sugar fortification with vitamin A at the national level*. Washington, DC, Pan American Health Organization, 1979 (Scientific publication No. 384).
46. Arroyave G, Mejia LA, Aguilar JR. The effect of vitamin A fortification of sugar on the serum vitamin A levels of preschool Guatemalan children: a longitudinal evaluation. *American Journal of Clinical Nutrition*, 1981, 34:41–49.
47. Arroyave G et al. Effectos del consumo de azucar fortifacada con retinol, por la madre embarazada y lactante cuya dieta habitual es baja en vitamin A. Estudio de la madre y del nino. [Effects of the intake of sugar fortified with retinol, by the pregnant women and infant whose diet is usually low in vitamin A. Study of the mother and child]. *Archivos Latinoamericanos de Nutricion*, 1974, 24:485–512.
48. Honein MA et al. Impact of folic acid fortification of the US food supply on the occurrence of neural tube defects. *Journal of the American Medical Association*, 2001, 285:2981–2986.
49. Jacques PF et al. The effect of folic acid fortification on plasma folate and total homocysteine concentrations. *New England Journal of Medicine*, 1999, 340:1449–1454.
50. Lewis CJ et al. Estimated folate intakes: data updated to reflect food fortification, increased bioavailability, and dietary supplement use. *American Journal of Clinical Nutrition*, 1999, 70:198–207.

51. Ray JG et al. Association of neural tube defects and folic acid food fortification in Canada. *Lancet*, 2002, 360:2047–2048.
52. Hirsch S et al. The Chilean flour folic acid fortification program reduces serum homocysteine levels and masks vitamin B-12 deficiency in elderly people. *Journal of Nutrition*, 2002, 132:289–291.
53. Ray JG et al. Persistence of vitamin B12 insufficiency among elderly women after folic acid food fortification. *Clinical Biochemistry*, 2003, 36:387–391.
54. Park YK et al. Effectiveness of food fortification in the United States: the case of pellagra. *American Journal of Public Health*, 2000, 90:727–738.
55. Welch TR, Bergstrom WH, Tsang RC. Vitamin D-deficient rickets: the reemergence of a once-conquered disease. *Journal of Pediatrics*, 2000, 137:143–145.
56. Nesby-O'Dell S et al. Hypovitaminosis D prevalence and determinants among African American and white women of reproductive age: third National Health and Nutrition Examination Survey, 1988–1994. *American Journal of Clinical Nutrition*, 2002, 76:187–192.
57. Keane EM et al. Vitamin D-fortified liquid milk: benefits for the elderly community-based population. *Calcified Tissue International*, 1998, 62:300–302.
58. Kinyamu HK et al. Dietary calcium and vitamin D intake in elderly women: effect on serum parathyroid hormone and vitamin D metabolites. *American Journal of Clinical Nutrition*, 1998, 67:342–348.
59. *Enriching lives: overcoming vitamin and mineral malnutrition in developing countries.* Washington, DC, World Bank, 1994.
60. Horton S. Opportunities for investment in nutrition in low-income Asia. *Asian Development Review*, 1999, 17:246–273.
61. Codex Alimentarius Commission. *General Principles for the Addition of Essential Nutrients to Foods CAC/GL 09-1987 (amended 1989, 1991).* Rome, Joint FAO/WHO Food Standards Programme, Codex Alimentarius Commision, 1987 (http://www.codexalimentarius.net/download/standards/299/CXG_009e.pdf, accessed 7 October 2005).
62. Beaton GH. *Fortification of foods for refugee feeding. Final report to the Canadian International Development Agency.* Ontario, GHB Consulting, 1995.
63. Department of Health. *Nutrition and bone health. Report of the subgroup on bone health, working group on the nutritional status of the population of the Committee on Medical Aspects of Food and Nutrition Policy.* London, The Stationery Office, 1998.
64. Gibson SA. Iron intake and iron status of preschool children: associations with breakfast cereals, vitamin C and meat. *Public Health Nutrition*, 1999, 2:521–528.
65. Nestel P et al. Complementary food supplements to achieve micronutrient adequacy for infants and young children. *Journal of Pediatric Gastroenterology and Nutrition*, 2003, 36:316–328.
66. Zlotkin S et al. Treatment of anemia with microencapsulated ferrous fumarate plus ascorbic acid supplied as sprinkles to complementary (weaning) foods. *American Journal of Clinical Nutrition*, 2001, 74:791–795.
67. Briend A. Highly nutrient-dense spreads: a new approach to delivering multiple micronutrients to high-risk groups. *British Journal of Nutrition*, 2001, 85 (Suppl 2):175–179.
68. Ministry of Health and Child Welfare and CARE International. *Report of Sub-Regional Workshop on Fortification at Hammermill Level; 2000 Nov 13–16; Harare, Zimbabwe.* Harare, CARE International Zimbabwe, 2000.

69. Beyer P et al. Golden Rice: introducing the beta-carotene biosynthesis pathway into rice endosperm by genetic engineering to defeat vitamin A deficiency. *Journal of Nutrition*, 2002, 132:506S–510S.
70. Ye X et al. Engineering the provitamin A (beta-carotene) biosynthetic pathway into (carotenoid-free) rice endosperm. *Science*, 2000, 287:303–305.
71. Lucca P, Hurrell R, Potrykus I. Fighting iron deficiency anemia with iron-rich rice. *Journal of the American College of Nutrition*, 2002, 21 (3 Suppl):184S–190S.
72. *Safety aspects of genetically modified foods of plant origin. Report of a Joint FAO/WHO Expert Consultation on Foods Derived from Biotechnology, WHO Headquaters, Geneva, Switzerland, 29 May to 2 June 2000*. Geneva, World Health Organization, 2000 (WHO/SDE/PHE/FOS/00.6).
73. Allen LH, Gillespie SR. *What works? A review of the efficacy and effectiveness of nutrition interventions*. Geneva, Administrative Committee on Coordination – Sub-Committee on Nutrition, 2001 (ACC/SCN State-of-the-Art Series, Nutrition Policy Discussion Paper No. 19).
74. *Assessing the iron status of populations: report of a Joint World Health Organization/ Centers for Disease Control and Prevention Technical Consultation on the Assessment of Iron Status at the Population Level, Geneva, Switzerland, 6–8 April 2004*. Geneva, World Health Organization, 2005.
75. Staubli Asobayire F et al. Prevalence of iron deficiency with and without concurrent anemia in population groups with high prevalences of malaria and other infections: a study in Cote d'Ivoire. *American Journal of Clinical Nutrition*, 2001, 74:776–782.
76. Menendez C, Fleming AF, Alonso PL. Malaria-related anaemia. *Parasitology Today*, 2000, 16:469–476.
77. Allen LH, Casterline-Sabel JE. Prevalence and causes of nutritional anemias. In: Ramakrishnan U, ed. *Nutritional Anemias*. Boca Raton, FL, CRC Press, 2000: 17–21.
78. *Requirements of vitamin A, iron, folate and vitamin B12. Report of a Joint FAO/WHO Expert Consultation*. Rome, Food and Agriculture Organization of the United Nations, 1988 (FAO Food and Nutrition Series, No. 23).
79. De Maeyer EM et al. *Preventing and controlling iron deficiency anaemia through primary health care. A guide for health administrators and programme managers*. Geneva, World Health Organization, 1989.
80. Brownlie T et al. Marginal iron deficiency without anemia impairs aerobic adaptation among previously untrained women. *American Journal of Clinical Nutrition*, 2002, 75:734–742.
81. Brabin BJ, Hakimi M, Pelletier D. An analysis of anemia and pregnancy-related maternal mortality. *Journal of Nutrition*, 2001, 131 (2S-2):604S–614S.
82. Brabin BJ, Premji Z, Verhoeff F. An analysis of anemia and child mortality. *Journal of Nutrition*, 2001, 131 (2S-2):636S–645S.
83. Cogswell ME et al. Iron supplementation during pregnancy, anemia, and birth weight: a randomized controlled trial. *American Journal of Clinical Nutrition*, 2003, 78:773–781.
84. Rosales FJ et al. Iron deficiency in young rats alters the distribution of vitamin A between plasma and liver and between hepatic retinol and retinyl esters. *Journal of Nutrition*, 1999, 129:1223–1228.
85. Munoz EC et al. Iron and zinc supplementation improves indicators of vitamin A status of Mexican preschoolers. *American Journal of Clinical Nutrition*, 2000, 71:789–794.

86. Zimmermann MB et al. Persistence of goiter despite oral iodine supplementation in goitrous children with iron deficiency anemia in Cote d'Ivoire. *American Journal of Clinical Nutrition*, 2000, 71:88–93.
87. Zimmermann MB. Iron status influences the efficacy of iodine prophylaxis in goitrous children in Cote d'Ivoire. *International Journal of Vitamin and Nutrition Research*, 2002, 72:19–25.
88. Sommer A, Davidson FR. Assessment and control of vitamin A deficiency: the Annecy Accords. *Journal of Nutrition*, 2002, 132 (9 Suppl):2845S–2850S.
89. West KP Jr. Extent of vitamin A deficiency among preschool children and women of reproductive age. *Journal of Nutrition*, 2002, 132 (9 Suppl):2857S–2866S.
90. Allen LH, Haskell M. Vitamin A requirements of infants under six months of age. *Food and Nutrition Bulletin*, 2001, 22:214–234.
91. Food and Nutrition Board, Institute of Medicine. *Dietary reference intakes for vitamin A, vitamin K, arsenic, boron, chromium, copper, iodine, iron, manganese, molybdenum, nickel, silicon, vanadium, and zinc.* Washington, DC, National Academy Press, 2001.
92. Miller M et al. Why do children become vitamin A deficient? *Journal of Nutrition*, 2002, 132 (9 Suppl):2867S–2880S.
93. *Vitamin and mineral requirements in human nutrition. Report of a Joint FAO/WHO Expert Consultation on Human Vitamin and Mineral Requirements, Bangkok, Thailand, 21–30 September 1998.* 2nd ed. Geneva, World Health Organization, 2004.
94. de Pee S, West CE. Dietary carotenoids and their role in combating vitamin A deficiency: a review of the literature. *European Journal of Clinical Nutrition*, 1996, 50 (Suppl 3):S38–S53.
95. Rodriguez MS, Irwin MI. A conspectus of research on vitamin A requirements of man. *Journal of Nutrition*, 1972, 102:909–968.
96. Castenmiller JJ, West CE. Bioavailability and bioconversion of carotenoids. *Annual Review of Nutrition*, 1998, 18:19–38.
97. West KP Jr. et al. Double blind, cluster randomised trial of low dose supplementation with vitamin A or beta carotene on mortality related to pregnancy in Nepal. The NNIPS-2 Study Group. *British Medical Journal*, 1999, 318:570–575.
98. Christian P et al. Night blindness during pregnancy and subsequent mortality among women in Nepal: effects of vitamin A and beta-carotene supplementation. *American Journal of Epidemiology*, 2000, 152:542–547.
99. Suharno D et al. Supplementation with vitamin A and iron for nutritional anaemia in pregnant women in West Java, Indonesia. *Lancet*, 1993, 342:1325–1328.
100. Delange F. The disorders induced by iodine deficiency. *Thyroid*, 1994, 4:107–128.
101. Delange F. Cassava and the thyroid. In: Gaitan E, ed. *Environmental goitrogenesis.* Boca Raton, FL, CRC Press, 1989: 173–194.
102. Delange F. Endemic cretinism. In: Braverman LE, Utiger RD, eds. *The thyroid. A fundamental and clinical text.* Philadelphia, Lippincott, 2000: 743–754.
103. Stanbury JB, ed. *The damaged brain of iodine deficiency: cognitive, behavioral, neuromotor, educative aspects.* New York, Cognizant Communication Corporation, 1994.
104. Bleichrodt N, Born MA. A meta-analysis of research on iodine and its relationship to cognitive development. In: Stanbury J, ed. *The damaged brain of iodine deficiency: cognitive, behavioral, neuromotor, and educative aspects.* New York, Cognizant Communication Corporation, 1994: 195–200.
105. Boyages SC. Clinical review 49: Iodine deficiency disorders. *Journal of Clinical Endocrinology and Metabolism*, 1993, 77:587–591.

106. Delange F et al. Iodine deficiency in the world: where do we stand at the turn of the century? *Thyroid*, 2001, 11:437–447.
107. Osendarp SJ, West CE, Black RE. The need for maternal zinc supplementation in developing countries: an unresolved issue. *Journal of Nutrition*, 2003, 133:817S–827S.
108. Sian L et al. Zinc homeostasis during lactation in a population with a low zinc intake. *American Journal of Clinical Nutrition*, 2002, 75:99–103.
109. Holt C, Brown KH, eds. International Zinc Nutrition Consultative Group (IZiNCG) Technical Document #1. Assessment of the risk of zinc deficiency in populations and options for its control. *Food and Nutrition Bulletin*, 2004, 25 (Suppl 2):S94–S203.
110. Sandström B. Dietary pattern and zinc supply. In: Mills CF, ed. *Zinc in human biology*. New York, Springer-Verlag, 1989: 350–365.
111. Sandström B, Lonnerdal B. Promoters and antagonists of zinc absorption. In: Mills CF, ed. *Zinc in human biology*. New York, Springer-Verlag, 1989: 57–78.
112. Sandström B et al. Effect of protein level and protein source on zinc absorption in humans. *Journal of Nutrition*, 1989, 119:48–53.
113. Sian L et al. Zinc absorption and intestinal losses of endogenous zinc in young Chinese women with marginal zinc intakes. *American Journal of Clinical Nutrition*, 1996, 63:348–353.
114. Petterson DS, Sandström B, Cederblad Å. Absorption of zinc from lupin (*Lupinus angustifolius*)-based foods. *British Journal of Nutrition*, 1994, 72:865–871.
115. Davidsson L et al. Dietary fiber in weaning cereals: a study of the effect on stool characteristics and absorption of energy, nitrogen, and minerals in healthy infants. *Journal of Pediatric Gastroenterology and Nutrition*, 1996, 22:167–179.
116. Manary MJ et al. Zinc homeostasis in Malawian children consuming a high-phytate, maize-based diet. *American Journal of Clinical Nutrition*, 2002, 75:1057–1061.
117. Hambidge M. Human zinc deficiency. *Journal of Nutrition*, 2000, 130 (5S Suppl): 1344S–1349S.
118. Shankar AH et al. The influence of zinc supplementation on morbidity due to Plasmodium falciparum: a randomized trial in preschool children in Papua New Guinea. *American Journal of Tropical Medicine and Hygiene*, 2000, 62:663–669.
119. Muller O et al. Effect of zinc supplementation on malaria and other causes of morbidity in west African children: randomised double blind placebo controlled trial. *British Medical Journal*, 2001, 322:1567.
120. Caulfield LE et al. Potential contribution of maternal zinc supplementation during pregnancy to maternal and child survival. *American Journal of Clinical Nutrition*, 1998, 68 (2 Suppl):499S–508S.
121. Brenton DP, Jackson MJ, Young A. Two pregnancies in a patient with acrodermatitis enteropathica treated with zinc sulphate. *Lancet*, 1981, 2:500–502.
122. King JC. Determinants of maternal zinc status during pregnancy. *American Journal of Clinical Nutrition*, 2000, 71 (5 Suppl):1334S–1343S.
123. Merialdi M et al. Adding zinc to prenatal iron and folate tablets improves fetal neurobehavioral development. *American Journal of Obstetrics and Gynecology*, 1999, 180:483–490.
124. Caulfield LE et al. Maternal zinc supplementation does not affect size at birth or pregnancy duration in Peru. *Journal of Nutrition*, 1999, 129:1563–1568.

125. Sazawal S et al. Zinc supplementation in infants born small for gestational age reduces mortality: a prospective, randomized, controlled trial. *Pediatrics*, 2001, 108:1280–1286.
126. Domellof M et al. Iron, zinc, and copper concentrations in breast milk are independent of maternal mineral status. *American Journal of Clinical Nutrition*, 2004, 79:111–115.
127. Krebs NF et al. Zinc supplementation during lactation: effects on maternal status and milk zinc concentrations. *American Journal of Clinical Nutrition*, 1995, 61:1030–1036.
128. Food and Nutrition Board, Institute of Medicine. *Dietary reference intakes for thiamin, riboflavin, niacin, vitamin B6, folate, vitamin B12, pantothenic acid, biotin, and choline*. Washington, DC, National Academy Press, 2000.
129. Rucker RB et al. *Handbook of vitamins*. 3rd ed. New York, Marcel Dekker, 2001.
130. *Review of the magnitude of Folate and Vitamin B12 deficiencies worldwide*. McLean E, de Benoist B, Allen LH, 2005.
131. Krishnaswamy K, Madhavan Nair K. Importance of folate in human nutrition. *British Journal of Nutrition*, 2001, 85 (Suppl 2):115–124.
132. Hertrampf E et al. Consumption of folic acid-fortified bread improves folate status in women of reproductive age in Chile. *Journal of Nutrition*, 2003, 133:3166–3169.
133. Villapando S et al. Vitamins A and C and folate status in Mexican children under 12 years and women 12–49 years: A probabilistic national survey. *Salud Publica de Mexico*, 2003, 45 (Suppl 4):S508–S519.
134. Koebnick C et al. Folate status during pregnancy in women is improved by long-term high vegetable intake compared with the average western diet. *Journal of Nutrition*, 2001, 131:733–739.
135. Charoenlarp P et al. A WHO collaborative study on iron supplementation in Burma and in Thailand. *American Journal of Clinical Nutrition*, 1988, 47:280–297.
136. Berry RJ et al. Prevention of neural-tube defects with folic acid in China. *New England Journal of Medicine*, 1999, 341:1485–1490.
137. Werler MM, Shapiro S, Mitchell AA. Periconceptional folic acid exposure and risk of occurrent neural tube defects. *Journal of the American Medical Association*, 1993, 269:1257–1261.
138. Botto LD et al. Neural-tube defects. *New England Journal of Medicine*, 1999, 341:1509–1519.
139. Shibuya K, Murray CJL. Congenital anomalies. In: Murray CJL, Lopez AD, eds. *Health dimensions of sex and reproduction*. Boston, Harvard University Press, 1998: 455–512.
140. Moyers S, Bailey LB. Fetal malformations and folate metabolism: review of recent evidence. *Nutrition Reviews*, 2001, 59:215–224.
141. de Onis M, Villar J, Gulmezoglu M. Nutritional interventions to prevent intrauterine growth retardation: evidence from randomized controlled trials. *European Journal of Clinical Nutrition*, 1998, 52 (Suppl 1):S83–S93.
142. Wald NJ et al. Homocysteine and ischemic heart disease: results of a prospective study with implications regarding prevention. *Archives of Internal Medicine*, 1998, 158:862–867.
143. Perry IJ et al. Prospective study of serum total homocysteine concentration and risk of stroke in middle-aged British men. *Lancet*, 1995, 346:1395–1398.
144. De Bree A et al. Homocysteine determinants and the evidence to what extent homocysteine determines the risk of coronary heart disease. *Pharmacological Reviews*, 2002, 54:599–618.

145. Wald DS, Law M, Morris JK. Homocysteine and cardiovascular disease: evidence on causality from a meta-analysis. *British Medical Journal*, 2002, 325:1202–1206.
146. Malouf M, Grimley EJ, Areosa SA. Folic acid with or without vitamin B12 for cognition and dementia. *The Cochrane Database of Systematic Reviews*, 2003, Issue 4. Art. No.: CD004514. DOI: 10.1002/14651858.CD004514.
147. Vollset SE et al. Plasma total homocysteine, pregnancy complications, and adverse pregnancy outcomes: the Hordaland Homocysteine study. *American Journal of Clinical Nutrition*, 2000, 71:962–988.
148. Erickson JD et al. Folate status in women of childbearing age, by race/ethnicity – United States, 1999–2000. *Morbidity and Mortality Weekly Report*, 2002, 51:808–810.
149. Lawrence JM et al. Trends in serum folate after food fortification. *Lancet*, 1999, 354:915–916.
150. Allen LH. Folate and vitamin B12 status in the Americas. *Nutrition Reviews*, 2004, 62 (6 Pt 2):S29–S33.
151. Refsum H et al. Hyperhomocysteinemia and elevated methylmalonic acid indicate a high prevalence of cobalamin deficiency in Asian Indians. *American Journal of Clinical Nutrition*, 2001, 74:233–241.
152. Siekmann JH et al. Kenyan school children have multiple micronutrient deficiencies, but increased plasma vitamin B-12 is the only detectable micronutrient response to meat or milk supplementation. *Journal of Nutrition*, 2003, 133:3972S–3980S.
153. Krajcovicova-Kudlackova M et al. Homocysteine levels in vegetarians versus omnivores. *Annals of Nutrition & Metabolism*, 2000, 44:135–138.
154. Healton EB et al. Neurologic aspects of cobalamin deficiency. *Medicine (Baltimore)*, 1991, 70:229–245.
155. Allen LH et al. Cognitive and neuromotor performance of Guatemalan schoolers with deficient, marginal and normal plasma B-12. *FASEB Journal*, 1999, 13:A544.
156. Allen LH. Impact of vitamin B-12 deficiency during lactation on maternal and infant health. *Advances in Experimental Medicine and Biology*, 2002, 503:57–67.
157. Martin DC et al. Time dependency of cognitive recovery with cobalamin replacement: report of a pilot study. *Journal of the American Geriatrics Society*, 1992, 40:168–172.
158. *Thiamine deficiency and its prevention and control in major emergencies*. Geneva, World Health Organization, 1999 (WHO/NHD/99.13).
159. Djoenaidi W, Notermans SL, Verbeek AL. Subclinical beriberi polyneuropathy in the low income group: an investigation with special tools on possible patients with suspected complaints. *European Journal of Clinical Nutrition*, 1996, 50:549–555.
160. Bovet P et al. Blood thiamin status and determinants in the population of Seychelles (Indian Ocean). *Journal of Epidemiology and Community Health*, 1998, 52:237–242.
161. Butterworth RF. Maternal thiamine deficiency: still a problem in some world communities. *American Journal of Clinical Nutrition*, 2001, 74:712–713.
162. McGready R et al. Postpartum thiamine deficiency in a Karen displaced population. *American Journal of Clinical Nutrition*, 2001, 74:808–813.
163. Tang CM et al. Outbreak of beri-beri in The Gambia. *Lancet*, 1989, 2:206–207.
164. Macias-Matos C et al. Biochemical evidence of thiamine depletion during the Cuban neuropathy epidemic, 1992–1993. *American Journal of Clinical Nutrition*, 1996, 64:347–353.
165. Bates C et al. Reply to D.A. Gans. *American Journal of Clinical Nutrition*, 1997, 65:1091.

166. Lonsdale D. Thiamine deficiency and sudden deaths. *Lancet*, 1990, 336:376.
167. Combs GF Jr. *The vitamins: fundamental aspects in nutrition and health*. 2nd ed. San Diego, CA, Academic Press, 1992.
168. Bhuvaneswaran C, Sreenivasan A. Problems of thiamine deficiency states and their amelioration. *Annals of the New York Academy of Sciences*, 1962, 98:576–601.
169. Vimokesant SL et al. Effects of betel nut and fermented fish on the thiamin status of northeastern Thais. *American Journal of Clinical Nutrition*, 1975, 28:1458–1463.
170. Hustad S et al. Riboflavin, flavin mononucleotide, and flavin adenine dinucleotide in human plasma and erythrocytes at baseline and after low-dose riboflavin supplementation. *Clinical Chemistry*, 2002, 48:1571–1577.
171. Graham JM et al. Riboflavin status of pregnant Nepali women; comparison of erythrocyte riboflavin with erythrocyte reductase activity coefficient (EGRAC) methods. *FASEB Journal*, 2002, 16:A276-A277.
172. Allen LH. Micronutrients. In: Flores R, Gillespie S, eds. *Health and nutrition: emerging and reemerging issues in developing countries*. Washington, DC, International Food Policy Research Institute, 2001: 10. (2020 Vision Focus No. 5).
173. Reddy VA et al. Riboflavin, folate and vitamin C status of Gambian women during pregnancy: a comparison between urban and rural communities. *Transactions of the Royal Society of Tropical Medicine and Hygiene*, 1987, 81:1033–1037.
174. Boisvert WA et al. Prevalence of riboflavin deficiency among Guatemalan elderly people and its relationship to milk intake. *American Journal of Clinical Nutrition*, 1993, 58:85–90.
175. Campbell TC et al. Questioning riboflavin recommendations on the basis of a survey in China. *American Journal of Clinical Nutrition*, 1990, 51:436–445.
176. Allen LH et al. Supplementation of anemic lactating Guatemalan women with riboflavin improves erythrocyte riboflavin concentrations and ferritin response to iron treatment. Journal of Nutrition. In press.
177. Powers HJ et al. The relative effectiveness of iron and iron with riboflavin in correcting a microcytic anaemia in men and children in rural Gambia. *Human Nutrition: Clinical Nutrition*, 1983, 37:413–425.
178. *Pellagra and its prevention and control in major emergencies*. Geneva, World Health Organization, 2000 (WHO/NHD/00.10).
179. Malfait P et al. An outbreak of pellagra related to changes in dietary niacin among Mozambican refugees in Malawi. *International Journal of Epidemiology*, 1993, 22:504–511.
180. Setiawan B, Giraud DW, Driskell JA. Vitamin B-6 inadequacy is prevalent in rural and urban Indonesian children. *Journal of Nutrition*, 2000, 130:553–558.
181. McCullough AL et al. Vitamin B-6 status of Egyptian mothers: relation to infant behavior and maternal-infant interactions. *American Journal of Clinical Nutrition*, 1990, 51:1067–1074.
182. Fairfield KM, Fletcher RH. Vitamins for chronic disease prevention in adults: scientific review. *Journal of the American Medical Association*, 2002, 287:3116–3126.
183. Chang SJ, Kirksey A. Pyridoxine supplementation of lactating mothers: relation to maternal nutrition status and vitamin B-6 concentrations in milk. *American Journal of Clinical Nutrition*, 1990, 51:826–831.
184. *Scurvy and its prevention and control in major emergencies*. Geneva, World Health Organization, 1999 (WHO/NHD/99.11).

185. Centers for Disease Control and Prevention (CDC). Nutrition and health status of displaced persons – Sudan, 1988–1989. *Morbidity and Mortality Weekly Report*, 1989, 38:848–855.
186. Desenclos JC et al. Epidemiological patterns of scurvy among Ethiopian refugees. *Bulletin of the World Health Organization*, 1989, 67:309–316.
187. Toole MJ. Micronutrient deficiencies in refugees. *Lancet*, 1992, 339:1214–1216.
188. Grusin H, Kincaid-Smith PS. Scurvy in adult Africans – a clinical, haematological, and pathological study. *American Journal of Clinical Nutrition*, 1954, 2:323–335.
189. Hampl JS, Taylor CS, Johnston CS. NHANES III data indicate that American subgroups have a high risk of vitamin C deficiency. *Journal of the American Dietetic Association*, 2000, 100:A-59 (Abstract).
190. Sauberlich HE, Skala OH, Dowdy RP. *Laboratory tests for the assessment of nutritional status*. Cleveland, OH, CRC Press, 1974.
191. Severs D, Williams T, Davies JW. Infantile scurvy – a public health problem. *Canadian Journal of Public Health*, 1961, 52:214–220.
192. Turner E, Pitt D, Thomson R. Scurvy yesterday and today. *Medical Journal of Australia*, 1959, 46:243–246.
193. Food and Nutrition Board, Institute of Medicine. *Dietary reference intakes for calcium, phosphorus, magnesium, vitamin D, and fluoride*. Washington, DC, National Academy Press, 1999.
194. Specker BL et al. Prospective study of vitamin D supplementation and rickets in China. *Journal of Pediatrics*, 1992, 120:733–739.
195. Zeghoud F et al. Subclinical vitamin D deficiency in neonates: definition and response to vitamin D supplements. *American Journal of Clinical Nutrition*, 1997, 65:771–778.
196. Dagnelie PC et al. High prevalence of rickets in infants on macrobiotic diets. *American Journal of Clinical Nutrition*, 1990, 51:202–208.
197. Lebrun JB et al. Vitamin D deficiency in a Manitoba community. *Canadian Journal of Public Health*, 1993, 84:394–396.
198. Yan L et al. Vitamin D status and parathyroid hormone concentrations in Chinese women and men from north-east of the People's Republic of China. *European Journal of Clinical Nutrition*, 2000, 54:68–72.
199. Du X et al. Vitamin D deficiency and associated factors in adolescent girls in Beijing. *American Journal of Clinical Nutrition*, 2001, 74:494–500.
200. Goswami R et al. Prevalence and significance of low 25-hydroxyvitamin D concentrations in healthy subjects in Delhi. *American Journal of Clinical Nutrition*, 2000, 72:472–475.
201. El-Sonbaty MR, Abdul-Ghaffar NU. Vitamin D deficiency in veiled Kuwaiti women. *European Journal of Clinical Nutrition*, 1996, 50:315–318.
202. Kreiter SR et al. Nutritional rickets in African American breast-fed infants. *Journal of Pediatrics*, 2000, 137:153–157.
203. Thacher TD et al. A comparison of calcium, vitamin D, or both for nutritional rickets in Nigerian children. *New England Journal of Medicine*, 1999, 341:563–568.
204. Dawson-Hughes B et al. Effect of vitamin D supplementation on wintertime and overall bone loss in healthy postmenopausal women. *Annals of Internal Medicine*, 1991, 115:505–512.
205. Lee WT et al. Bone mineral content of two populations of Chinese children with different calcium intakes. *Bone and Mineral*, 1993, 23:195–206.

206. Dibba B et al. Effect of calcium supplementation on bone mineral accretion in Gambian children accustomed to a low-calcium diet. *American Journal of Clinical Nutrition*, 2000, 71:544–549.
207. Yang GQ et al. The role of selenium in Keshan disease. *Advances in Nutritional Research*, 1984, 6:203–231.
208. Food and Nutrition Board, Institute of Medicine. *Dietary reference Intakes for Vitamin C, Vitamin E, Selenium, and Carotenoids.* Washington, DC, National Academy Press, 2000.
209. Fox TE, Fairweather-Tait S. Selenium. In: Hurrell RF, ed. *The mineral fortification of foods.* Leatherhead, Surrey, Leatherhead Publishing, 1999: 112–153.
210. *Trace Elements in Human Nutrition and Health.* Geneva, World Health Organization, 1996.
211. Ge K, Yang G. The epidemiology of selenium deficiency in the etiological study of endemic diseases in China. *American Journal of Clinical Nutrition*, 1993, 57 (2 Suppl):259S–263S.
212. Chen XS et al. Studies on the relations of selenium and Keshan disease. *Biological Trace Element Research*, 1980, 2:91–107.
213. Zhang WH et al. Selenium, iodine and fungal contamination in Yulin District (People's Republic of China) endemic for Kashin-Beck disease. *International Orthopaedics*, 2001, 25:188–190.
214. Moreno-Reyes R et al. Kashin-Beck disease and iodine deficiency in Tibet. *International Orthopaedics*, 2001, 25:164–166.
215. Vanderpas JB et al. Selenium deficiency mitigates hypothyroxinemia in iodine-deficient subjects. *American Journal of Clinical Nutrition*, 1993, 57 (2 Suppl): 271S–275S.
216. Giray B et al. Status of selenium and antioxidant enzymes of goitrous children is lower than healthy controls and nongoitrous children with high iodine deficiency. *Biological Trace Element Research*, 2001, 82:35–52.
217. Aro A, Alfthan G, Varo P. Effects of supplementation of fertilizers on human selenium status in Finland. *Analyst*, 1995, 120:841–843.
218. Cheng YY, Qian PC. The effect of selenium-fortified table salt in the prevention of Keshan disease on a population of 1.05 million. *Biomedical and Environmental Sciences*, 1990, 3:422–428.
219. *Fluorides and oral health. Report of a WHO Expert Committee on Oral Health Status and Fluoride Use.* Geneva, World Health Organization, 1994 (WHO Technical Report Series, No. 846).
220. Hillier S et al. Fluoride in drinking water and risk of hip fracture in the UK: a case-control study. *Lancet*, 2000, 355:265–269.
221. Demos LL et al. Water fluoridation, osteoporosis, fractures – recent developments. *Australian Dental Journal*, 2001, 46:80–87.
222. Phipps KR et al. Community water fluoridation, bone mineral density, and fractures: prospective study of effects in older women. *British Medical Journal*, 2000, 321:860–864.
223. Semba RD et al. Impact of vitamin A supplementation on hematological indicators of iron metabolism and protein status in children. *Nutrition Research*, 1992, 12:469–478.
224. Hurrell RF. How to ensure adequate iron absorption from iron-fortified food. *Nutrition Reviews*, 2002, 60 (7 Pt 2):S7–S15.
225. Hurrell RF. Iron. In: Hurrell RF, ed. *The mineral fortification of food.* Leatherhead, Surrey, Leatherhead Publishing, 1999: 54–93.

226. Swain JH, Newman SM, Hunt JR. Bioavailability of elemental iron powders to rats is less than bakery-grade ferrous sulfate and predicted by iron solubility and particle surface area. *Journal of Nutrition*, 2003, 133:3546–3552.
227. Hurrell RF et al. Ferrous fumarate fortification of a chocolate drink powder. *British Journal of Nutrition*, 1991, 65:271–283.
228. Theuer RC et al. Effect of processing on availability of iron salts in liquid infants formula products – experimental milk-based formulas. *Journal of Agricultural and Food Chemistry*, 1973, 21:482–485.
229. Hurrell RF et al. The usefulness of elemental iron for cereal flour fortification: a SUSTAIN Task Force report. *Nutrition Reviews*, 2002, 60:391–406.
230. Lee PW, Eisen WB, German RM, eds. *Handbook of powder metal technologies and applications*. Materials Park, OH, American Society of Metals, 1998.
231. International Nutritional Anemia Consultative Group (INACG). *Iron EDTA for food fortification*. Washington, DC, International Life Sciences Institute, 1993.
232. Hurrell RF et al. An evaluation of EDTA compounds for iron fortification of cereal-based foods. *British Journal of Nutrition*, 2000, 84:903–910.
233. Davidsson L et al. Iron bioavailability from iron-fortified Guatemalan meals based on corn tortillas and black bean paste. *American Journal of Clinical Nutrition*, 2002, 75:535–539.
234. Fairweather-Tait SJ et al. Iron absorption from a breakfast cereal: effects of EDTA compounds and ascorbic acid. *International Journal of Vitamin and Nutrition Research*, 2001, 71:117–122.
235. Barclay D et al. Cereal products having low phytic acid content. Societe des Produits Nestlé S.A. Federal Institute of Technology Zurich. International Patent Application PCT/EP00/05140, publication No. WO/00/72700, 2000.
236. Egli I. *Traditional food processing methods to increase mineral bioavailability from cereal and legume based weaning foods* [Dissertation]. Swiss Federal Institute of Technology, Zurich, 2001.
237. Dary O, Freire W, Kim S. Iron compounds for food fortification: guidelines for Latin America and the Caribbean 2002. *Nutrition Reviews*, 2002, 60:S50–S61.
238. *Evaluation of certain food additives and contaminants. Fifty-third report of the Joint FAO/WHO Expert Committee on Food Additives*. Geneva, World Health Organization, 2000 (WHO Technical Series No. 896).
239. Allen LH. Advantages and limitations of iron amino acid chelates as iron fortificants. *Nutrition Reviews*, 2002, 60 (Suppl 1):S18–S21.
240. Bovell-Benjamin AC, Viteri FE, Allen LH. Iron absorption from ferrous bisglycinate and ferric trisglycinate in whole maize is regulated by iron status. *American Journal of Clinical Nutrition*, 2000, 71:1563–1569.
241. Fidler MC et al. A micronised, dispersible ferric pyrophosphate with high relative bioavailability in man. *British Journal of Nutrition*, 2004, 91:107–112.
242. Zimmermann MB et al. Comparison of the efficacy of wheat-based snacks fortified with ferrous sulfate, electrolytic iron, or hydrogen-reduced elemental iron: randomized, double-blind, controlled trial in Thai women. *American Journal of Clinical Nutrition*, 2005, 82:1276–1282.
243. Dary O. Lessons learned with iron fortification in Central America. *Nutrition Reviews*, 2002, 60 (7 Pt 2):S30–S33.
244. Sarker SA et al. Helicobacter pylori infection, iron absorption, and gastric acid secretion in Bangladeshi children. *American Journal of Clinical Nutrition*, 2004, 80:149–153.

245. Wang CF, King RL. Chemical and sensory evaluation of iron-fortified milk. *Journal of Food Science*, 1973, 38:938–940.
246. Moretti D et al. Development and Evaluation of Iron-fortified Extruded Rice Grains. *Journal of Food Science*, 2005, 70:S330–S336.
247. Douglas FW et al. Color, flavor, and iron bioavailability in iron-fortified chocolate milk. *Journal of Dairy Science*, 1981, 64:1785–1793.
248. Davidsson L et al. Influence of ascorbic acid on iron absorption from an iron-fortified, chocolate-flavored milk drink in Jamaican children. *American Journal of Clinical Nutrition*, 1998, 67:873–877.
249. Fidler MC et al. Iron absorption from fish sauce and soy sauce fortified with sodium iron EDTA. *American Journal of Clinical Nutrition*, 2003, 78:274–278.
250. Huo J et al. Therapeutic effects of NaFeEDTA-fortified soy sauce in anaemic children in China. *Asia Pacific Journal of Clinical Nutrition*, 2002, 11:123–127.
251. Oppenheimer SJ. Iron and its relation to immunity and infectious disease. *Journal of Nutrition*, 2001, 131 (2S-2):616S–633S.
252. Heresi G et al. Effect of supplementation with an iron-fortified milk on incidence of diarrhea and respiratory infection in urban-resident infants. *Scandinavian Journal of Infectious Diseases*, 1995, 27:385–389.
253. Hemminki E et al. Impact of iron fortification of milk formulas on infants growth and health. *Nutrition Research*, 1995, 15:491–503.
254. Power HM et al. Iron fortification of infant milk formula: the effect on iron status and immune function. *Annals of Tropical Paediatrics*, 1991, 11:57–66.
255. Brunser O et al. Chronic iron intake and diarrhoeal disease in infants. A field study in a less-developed country. *European Journal of Clinical Nutrition*, 1993, 47:317–326.
256. Danesh J, Appleby P. Coronary heart disease and iron status: meta-analyses of prospective studies. *Circulation*, 1999, 99:852–854.
257. Lund EK et al. Oral ferrous sulfate supplements increase the free radical-generating capacity of feces from healthy volunteers. *American Journal of Clinical Nutrition*, 1999, 69:250–255.
258. Stevens RG et al. Body iron stores and the risk of cancer. *New England Journal of Medicine*, 1988, 319:1047–1052.
259. Arya SS, Thakur BR. Effect of water activity on vitamin A degradation in wheat flour (atta). *Journal of Food Processing and Preservation*, 1990, 14:123–134.
260. Favaro RMD et al. Studies on fortification of refined soybean oil with all-trans-retinyl palmitate in Brazil: stability during cooking and storage. *Journal of Food Composition and Analysis*, 1991, 4:237–244.
261. *Fortification Basics: Sugar.* Arlington, VA, Opportunities for Micronutrient Interventions, 1997.
262. Olson JA. Vitamin A. In: Ziegler EE, Filer LJ, eds. *Present knowledge in nutrition.* Washington, DC, International Life Sciences Institute Press, 1996: 109–119.
263. Dary O, Mora JO. Food fortification to reduce vitamin A deficiency: International Vitamin A Consultative Group recommendations. *Journal of Nutrition*, 2002, 132 (9 Suppl):2927S–2933S.
264. Johnson LE. Oils, fats and margarine: overview of technology. In: Micronutrient Initiative, ed. *Food fortification to end micronutrient malnutrition. State of the Art.* Ottawa, Micronutrient Initiative, 1998: 22–26.
265. Bloch CE. Effects of deficiency in vitamins in infancy. *American Journal of Diseases of Children*, 1931, 42:271.

266. Aykroyd WR et al. Medical Resurvey of Nutrition in Newfoundland 1948. *Canadian Medical Association Journal*, 1949, 60:329–352.
267. Sridhar KK. Tackling micronutrient malnutrition: Two case studies in India. In: Micronutrient Initiative, ed. *Food fortification to end micronutrient malnutrition. State of the Art*. Ottawa, Micronutrient Initiative, 1998: 32–36.
268. Atwood SJ et al. Stability of vitamin A in fortified vegetable oil and corn soy blend used in child feeding programs in India. *Journal of Food Composition and Analysis*, 1995, 8:32–44.
269. Opportunities for Micronutrient Interventions (OMNI). *Fortification of wheat flour with vitamin A: an update*. Washington, D.C., US Agency for International Development, 1998.
270. *Final Report of the Micronutrient Assessment Project*. Washington, DC, Sharing United States Technology to Aid in the Improvement of Nutrition, 1999.
271. Chavez JF. Enrichment of precooked corn flour and wheat flour in Venezuela: A successful experience. In: Micronutrient Initiative, ed. *Food fortification to end micronutrient malnutrition. State of the Art*. Ottawa, Micronutrient Initiative, 1998: 62–65.
272. Dary O. Sugar fortification with vitamin A: A Central American contribution to the developing world. In: Micronutrient Initiative, ed. *Food fortification to end micronutrient malnutrition. State of the Art*. Ottawa, Micronutrient Initiative, 1998: 95–98.
273. Arroyave G. The program of fortification of sugar with vitamin A in Guatemala: some factors bearing on its implementation and maintenance. In: Scrimshaw NS, Wallerstein MT, eds. *Nutrition policy implementation. Issues and experience*. New York, Plenum Press, 1982: 75–88.
274. Krause VM, Delisle H, Solomons NW. Fortified foods contribute one half of recommended vitamin A intake in poor urban Guatemalan toddlers. *Journal of Nutrition*, 1998, 128:860–864.
275. Dary O, Guamuch M, Nestel P. Recovery of retinol in soft-drink beverages made with fortified unrefined and refined sugar: implications for national fortification programs. *Journal of Food Composition and Analysis*, 1998, 11:212–220.
276. Rosado JL et al. Development, production, and quality control of nutritionnal supplements for a national supplementation programme in Mexico. *Food and Nutrition Bulletin*, 2000, 21:30–34.
277. Tartanac F. Incaparina and other Incaparina-based foods: Experience of INCAP in Central America. *Food and Nutrition Bulletin*, 2000, 21:49–54.
278. Lopez de Romana D. Experience with complementary feeding in the FONCODES project. *Food and Nutrition Bulletin*, 2000, 21:43–48.
279. Chavasit V, Tontisirin K. Triple fortification: instant noodles in Thailand. In: Micronutrient Initiative, ed. *Food fortification to end micronutrient malnutrition. State of the Art*. Ottawa, Micronutrient Initiative, 1998: 72–76.
280. Bynum D. Fortification of dairy products with micronutrients to end malnutrition. In: Micronutrient Initiative, ed. *Food fortification to end micronutrient malnutrition. State of the Art*. Ottawa, Micronutrient Initiative, 1998: 38–42.
281. Allen LH, Haskell M. Estimating the potential for vitamin A toxicity in women and young children. *Journal of Nutrition*, 2002, 132 (9 Suppl):2907S–2919S.
282. *Evaluation of certain food additives and contaminants. Thirty-seventh report of the Joint FAO/WHO Expert Committee on Food Additives*. Geneva, World Health Organization, 1991 (WHO Technical Series No. 806).

283. *Recommended iodine levels in salt and guidelines for monitoring their adequacy and effectiveness.* Geneva, World Health Organization, 1996 (WHO/NUT/96.13).
284. *Progress towards the elimination of iodine deficiency disorders (IDD).* Geneva, World Health Organization, 1999 (WHO/NHD/99.4).
285. Codex Alimentarius Commision. *Codex Standard for Food Grade Salt. CODEX STAN 150-1985, revised 1997, amended 2001.* Rome, Joint FAO/WHO Food Standards Programme, Codex Alimentarius Commision, 1985 (http://www.codexalimentarius.net/download/standards/3/CXS_150e.pdf, accessed 7 October 2005).
286. Burgi H. Iodization of salt and food. Technical and legal aspects. In: Delange F, Dunn JT, Glinoer D, eds. *Iodine deficiency in Europe. A continuing concern.* New York, Plenum Press, 1993: 261–266.
287. Mannar V, Dunn JT. *Salt iodization for the elimination of iodine deficiency.* The Netherlands, International Council for Control of Iodine Deficiency Disorders, 1995.
288. Diosady LL et al. Stability of iodine in iodized salt used for correction of iodine-deficiency disorders. II. *Food and Nutrition Bulletin,* 1998, 19:240–250.
289. *The state of the world's children.* New York, United Nations Children's Fund, 2003.
290. Delange F, Hetzel BS. The iodine deficiency disorders. In: Hennemann G, DeGroot L, eds. *The thyroid and its diseases.* MA, Endocrine Education, Inc, 2003: (http://www.thyroidmanager.org, accessed 22 March 2005).
291. Gerasimov G et al. Bread iodization for iodine deficient regions of Russia and other newly independant states. *IDD Newsletter,* 1997, 13:12–13.
292. Suwanik R, Pleehachinda R, Pattanachak C, et al. Simple technology provides effective IDD control at the village level in Thailand. *IDD Newsletter,* 1989, 5:1–6.
293. Fisch A et al. A new approach to combatting iodine deficiency in developing countries: the controlled release of iodine in water by a silicone elastomer. *American Journal of Public Health,* 1993, 83:540–545.
294. Elnagar B et al. Control of iodine deficiency using iodination of water in a goitre endemic area. *International Journal of Food Sciences and Nutrition,* 1997, 48:119–127.
295. Foo LC et al. Iodization of village water supply in the control of endemic iodine deficiency in rural Sarawak, Malaysia. *Biomedical and Environmental Sciences,* 1996, 9:236–241.
296. Anonymous. Iodized water to eliminate iodine deficiency. *IDD Newsletter,* 1997, 13:33–39.
297. Cao XY et al. Iodination of irrigation water as a method of supplying iodine to a severely iodine-deficient population in Xinjiang, China. *Lancet,* 1994, 344:107–110.
298. Phillips DI. Iodine, milk, and the elimination of endemic goiter in Britain: the story of an accidental public health triumph. *Journal of Epidemiology and Community Health,* 1997, 51:391–393.
299. Eltom M et al. The use of sugar as a vehicle for iodine fortification in endemic iodine deficiency. *International Journal of Food Sciences and Nutrition,* 1995, 46:281–289.
300. Sinawat S. Fish sauce fortification in Thailand. In: Micronutrient Initiative, ed. *Food fortification to end micronutrient malnutrition. State of the Art.* Ottawa, Micronutrient Initiative, 1998: 102–104.
301. Burgi H, Schaffner TH, Seiler JP. The toxicology of iodate: a review of the literature. *Thyroid,* 2001, 11:449–456.

302. Stanbury JB et al. Iodine-induced hyperthyroidism: occurrence and epidemiology. *Thyroid*, 1998, 8:83–100.
303. Bourdoux PP et al. Iodine induced thyrotoxicosis in Kivu, Zaire. *Lancet*, 1996, 347:552–553.
304. Todd CH et al. Increase in thyrotoxicosis associated with iodine supplements in Zimbabwe. *Lancet*, 1995, 346:1563–1564.
305. Delange F, de Benoist B, Alnwick D. Risks of iodine-induced hyperthyroidism after correction of iodine deficiency by iodized salt. *Thyroid*, 1999, 9:545–556.
306. Todd CH. *Hyperthyroidism and other thyroid disorders: a practical handbook for recognition and management*. Geneva, World Health Organization, 1999 (WHO/AFRO/NUT/99.1).
307. Laurberg P et al. Thyroid disorders in mild iodine deficiency. *Thyroid*, 2000, 10:951–963.
308. Diaz M et al. Bioavailability of zinc sulfate and zinc oxide added to corn tortilla. A study using stable isotopes. *FASEB Journal*, 2001, 15:A578.5 (Abstract).
309. Lopez de Romana D, Lonnerdal B, Brown KH. Absorption of zinc from wheat products fortified with iron and either zinc sulfate or zinc oxide. *American Journal of Clinical Nutrition*, 2003, 78:279–283.
310. Hurrell RF et al. Degradation of phytic acid in cereal porridges improves iron absorption by human subjects. *American Journal of Clinical Nutrition*, 2003, 77:1213–1219.
311. Davidsson L, Kastenmayer P, Hurrell RF. Sodium iron EDTA [NaFe(III)EDTA] as a food fortificant: the effect on the absorption and retention of zinc and calcium in women. *American Journal of Clinical Nutrition*, 1994, 60:231–237.
312. Hambidge KM et al. Zinc nutritional status of young middle-income children and effects of consuming zinc-fortified breakfast cereals. *American Journal of Clinical Nutrition*, 1979, 32:2532–2539.
313. Kilic I et al. The effect of zinc-supplemented bread consumption on school children with asymptomatic zinc deficiency. *Journal of Pediatric Gastroenterology and Nutrition*, 1998, 26:167–171.
314. Lopez de Romana D, Brown KH, Guinard JX. Sensory trial to assess the acceptability of zinc fortificants added to iron-fortified wheat products. *Journal of Food Science*, 2002, 67:461–465.
315. Pfeiffer CM et al. Absorption of folate from fortified cereal-grain products and of supplemental folate consumed with or without food determined by using a dual-label stable-isotope protocol. *American Journal of Clinical Nutrition*, 1997, 66:1388–1397.
316. *Fortification Basics: Stability*. Arlington, VA, Opportunities for Micronutrient Interventions, 1998.
317. Bauernfeind JC, DeRitter E. Foods considered for nutrient addition: cereal grain products. In: Bauernfeind JC, Lachance PA, eds. *Nutrient additions to food: nutritional, technological and regulatory aspects*. Trumbull, CT, Food and Nutrition Press, 1991: 143–209.
318. Bowley A, ed. *Mandatory food enrichment*. Basel, Roche Vitamins Europe Ltd, 2003 (Nutriview Special Issue 1–12).
319. *Opinion of the Scientific Committee on Food on the tolerable upper intake levels of nicotinic acid and nicotinamide (niacin)*. Brussels, European Commission, 2002 (SCF/CS/NUT/UPPLEV/39).

320. Flynn A, Cashman K. Calcium. In: Hurrell RF, ed. *The mineral fortification of foods*. Leatherhead, Surrey, Leatherhead Publishing, 1999: 18–53.
321. Ranhotra GS, Lee C, Gelroth JA. Expanded cereal fortification – bioavailability and functionality (breadmaking) of various calcium sources. *Nutrition Reports International*, 1980, 22:469–475.
322. Van Dael P et al. Comparison of selenite and selenate apparent absorption and retention in infants using stable isotope methodology. *Pediatric Research*, 2002, 51:71–75.
323. Estupinan-Day SR et al. Salt fluoridation and dental caries in Jamaica. *Community Dentistry and Oral Epidemiology*, 2001, 29:247–252.
324. Stephen KW et al. Effect of fluoridated salt intake in infancy: a blind caries and fluorosis study in 8th grade Hungarian pupils. *Community Dentistry and Oral Epidemiology*, 1999, 27:210–215.
325. National Program of Salt Fluoridation. *Salt fluoridation program in Costa Rica*. Tres Rios, Instituto Costarricense de Investigación y Enseñanza en Nutrición y Salud (INCIENSA), 2002.
326. Stephen KW, Banoczy J, Pakhomov GN, eds. *Milk fluoridation for the prevention of dental caries*. Geneva, World Health Organization, 1996 (WHO/ORH/MF/DOC96.1).
327. Woodward SM et al. School milk as a vehicle for fluoride in the United Kingdom. An interim report. *Community Dental Health*, 2001, 18:150–156.
328. Marino R, Villa A, Guerrero S. A community trial of fluoridated powdered milk in Chile. *Community Dentistry and Oral Epidemiology*, 2001, 29:435–442.
329. Bian JY et al. Effect of fluoridated milk on caries in primary teeth: 21-month results. *Community Dentistry and Oral Epidemiology*, 2003, 31:241–245.
330. Stephen KW et al. Five-year double-blind fluoridated milk study in Scotland. *Community Dentistry and Oral Epidemiology*, 1984, 12:223–229.
331. Ketley CE, West JL, Lennon MA. The use of school milk as a vehicle for fluoride in Knowsley, UK; an evaluation of effectiveness. *Community Dental Health*, 2003, 20:83–88.
332. Food and Nutrition Board, Institute of Medicine. *Dietary reference intakes: applications in dietary planning*. Washington, DC, National Academy Press, 2003.
333. Food and Nutrition Board, Institute of Medicine. *Dietary reference intakes: applications in dietary assessment*. Washington, DC, National Academy Press, 2000.
334. Department of Health. *Dietary Reference Values of food energy and nutrients for the United Kingdom*. London, Her Majesty's Stationery Office, 1991.
335. Scientific Committee for Food. *Nutrient and energy intakes for the European Community. Reports of the Scientific Committee for Food*. Luxembourg, Commission of the European Community, 1992 (31st Series).
336. Nusser SM et al. A semiparametric transformation approach to estimating usual daily intake distributions. *Journal of the American Statistical Association*, 1996, 91:1440–1449.
337. Guenther PM, Kott PS, Carriquiry AL. Development of an approach for estimating usual nutrient intake distributions at the population level. *Journal of Nutrition*, 1997, 127:1106–1112.
338. Nyambose J, Koski KG, Tucker KL. High intra/interindividual variance ratios for energy and nutrient intakes of pregnant women in rural Malawi show that many days are required to estimate usual intake. *Journal of Nutrition*, 2002, 132:1313–1318.

339. *Technical consultation on recommended levels of folic acid and vitamin B12 fortification in the Americas.* Washington, DC, Pan American Health Organization, 2003.
340. *Complementary feeding of young children in developing countries: a review of current scientific knowledge.* Geneva, World Health Organization, 1998 (WHO/NUT/98.1).
341. Codex Alimentarius Commission. *Guidelines on Formulated Supplementary Foods for Older Infants and Young Children CAC/GL 08-1991.* Joint FAO/WHO Food Standards Programme, Codex Alimentarius Commision, 1991 (http://www.codexalimentarius.net/download/standards/298/CXG_008e.pdf, accessed 7 October 2005).
342. Codex Alimentarius Commission. *Codex Guidelines on Nutrition Labelling CAC/GL 02-1985, (revised 1993).* Joint FAO/WHO Food Standard Programme, Codex Alimentarius Commision, 1985 (http://www.codexalimentarius.net/download/standards/34/CXG_002e.pdf, accessed 7 October 2005).
343. Codex Alimentarius Commission. *Guidelines for Use of Nutrition Claims CAC/GL 23-1997, (revised 2004).* Joint FAO/WHO Food Standards Programme, Codex Alimentarius Commision, 1997 (http://www.codexalimentarius.net/download/standards/351/CXG_023e.pdf, accessed 7 October 2005).
344. Habicht JP, Victora CG, Vaughan JP. Evaluation designs for adequacy, plausibility and probability of public health programme performance and impact. *International Journal of Epidemiology*, 1999, 28:10–18.
345. Codex Alimentarius Commission. *Codex Alimentarius, Volume 13 – Methods of analysis and sampling.* 2nd ed. Rome, Joint FAO/WHO Food Standard Programme, Codex Alimentarius Commision, 1994.
346. Nestel P, Nalubola R, Mayfield E, eds. *Quality assurance as applied to micronutrient fortification: guidelines for technicians, supervisors and workers, concerned with nutrition.* Washington, DC, International Life Sciences Institute Press, 2002.
347. Pandav CS et al. Validation of spot-testing kits to determine iodine content in salt. *Bulletin of the World Health Organization*, 2000, 78:975–980.
348. Sullivan KM, May S, Maberly G. *Urinary iodine assessment: a manual on survey and laboratory methods.* Atlanta, GA, Program Against Micronutrient Malnutrition, 2000 (2nd ed.).
349. Sullivan KM et al., eds. *Monitoring universal salt iodization programs.* Atlanta, GA, Program Against Micronutrient Malnutrition, 1995.
350. Valadez JJ. *Assessing child survival programs in developing countries: testing lot quality assurance sampling.* Boston, MA, Harvard University Press, 1991.
351. Binkin N et al. Rapid nutrition surveys – how many clusters are enough? *Disasters*, 1992, 16:97–103.
352. Valadez JJ et al. Using lot quality assurance sampling to assess measurements for growth monitoring in a developing country's primary health care system. *International Journal of Epidemiology*, 1996, 25:381–387.
353. Valadez JJ et al. *A trainers guide for baseline surveys and regular monitoring: using LQAS for assessing field programs in community health in developing countries.* Washington, DC, NGO Networks for Health, 2001.
354. World Bank. *World Development Report 1993: Investing in health.* New York, Oxford University Press, 1993.
355. Murray CJL, Lopez AD, eds. *The global burden of disease: a comprehensive assessment of mortality and disability from diseases, injuries, and risk factors in 1990 and projected to 2020.* Cambridge, MA, Harvard University Press, 1996.

356. Nestel P, Nalubola R. *Manual for wheat flour fortification with iron. Part 1: Guidelines for the development, implementation, monitoring, and evaluation of a program for wheat flour fortification with iron.* Arlington, VA, Micronutrient Operational Strategies and Technologies, United States Agency for International Development, 2000.
357. Levin HM et al. Micronutrient deficiency disorders. In: Jamison DT et al., eds. *Disease control priorities in developing countries.* New York, Oxford University Press, 1993: 421–451.
358. Population Health and Nutrition Department. *Bangladesh: food and nutrition sector review mission: cost-effectiveness of food and nutrition intervention programs.* Washington, DC, World Bank, 1985 (No. 4974-BD).
359. Mason JB et al. *The Micronutrient Report. Current progress and trends in the control of vitamin A, iodine, and iron deficiencies.* Ottawa, Micronutrient Initiative, 2001.
360. Gillespie S. *Major issues in the control of iron deficiency.* Ottawa, The Micronutrient Initiative, 1998.
361. Horton S, Ross J. The economics of iron deficiency. *Food Policy*, 2003, 28:51–75.
362. Ross JS. *Relative risk of child mortality due to vitamin A deficiency. PROFILES 3 Working Series No. 2.* Washington, DC, Academy for Education Development, 1995 (PROFILES 3 Working Series, No.2).
363. Clugston GA et al. Iodine deficiency disorders in South East Asia. In: Hetzel BS, Dunn JT, Stanbury JB, eds. *The prevention and control of iodine deficiency disorders.* Amsterdam, Elsevier, 1987: 273–308.
364. Stoltzfus RJ, Mullany L, Black RE. Iron deficiency anaemia. *Comparative quantification of health risks: the global and regional burden of disease due to 25 selected major risk factors.* Cambridge, Harvard University Press (in press), 2004.
365. Ross J, Horton S. *Economic consequences of iron deficiency.* Ottawa, Micronutrient Initiative, 1998.
366. *Yearbook of labour statistics.* 55th ed. Geneva, International Labour Organization, 1997.
367. Arkin E, Maibach E, Parvanta C. General public: communicating to persuade. In: Nelson DE et al., eds. *Communicating public health information effectively: a guide for practitioners.* Washington, DC, American Public Health Association, 2002: 59–72.
368. Cotento I. Nutrition education: definitions. *Journal of Nutrition Education*, 1995, 27:279.
369. Roper WL. Health communication takes on new dimensions at CDC. *Public Health Reports*, 1993, 108:179–183.
370. Lefebvre RC, Flora JA. Social marketing and public health intervention. *Health Education Quarterly*, 1988, 15:299–315.
371. Jernigan DH, Wright PA. Media advocacy: lessons from community experiences. *Journal of Public Health Policy*, 1996, 17:306–330.
372. Manoncourt E. Participation and social mobilization. *Promotion & Education*, 1996, 3:3–4, 44.
373. Rothschild ML. Carrots, sticks, and promises: A conceptual framework for the management of public health and social issue behaviors. *Journal of Marketing*, 1999, 63:24–37.
374. Parvanta C. Health and nutrition communication. *Public Health Reviews*, 2000, 28:197–208.
375. Brownson RC, Malone BR. Communicating public health information to policy makers. In: Nelson DE et al., eds. *Communicating public health effectively: a guide for practitioners.* Washington, DC, American Public Health Association, 2002: 97–114.

376. Smitasiri S et al. *Social marketing vitamin A-rich foods in Thailand*. Nakhon Pathom, Institute of Nutrition, Mahidol University, 1993.
377. Centers for Disease Control and Prevention (CDC). *CDCynergy 2001. Micronutrients edition. Your guide to effective health communications*. Atlanta, GA, United State Department of Health and Human Services, 2001 (http://www.cdc.gov/nccdphp/ dnpa/impact/tools/cdcynergy.htm, accessed 15 October 2005).
378. Alcalay R, Bell RA. *Promoting nutrition and physical activity through social marketing: current practices and recommendations*. Davis, CA, Center for Advanced Studies in Nutrition and Social Marketing, University of California, 2000.
379. Saadé C, Tucker H. *Beyond pharmacies: new perspectives in ORS marketing*. Arlington, VA, PRITECH Project, Management Sciences for Health, 1992.
380. Slater S, Saadé C. *Mobilizing the commercial sector for public health objectives: a practical guide*. Washington, DC, Basic Support for Institutionalizing Child Survival (BASICS), 1996.
381. *The results of the Uruguay Round of multilateral trade negotiations – the legal texts*. Geneva, World Trade Organization, 1995 (http://www.wto.org/english/docs_e/legal_e/legal_e.htm, accessed 19 April 2005).
382. Codex Alimentarius Commission. *Procedural manual*. 12th ed. Rome, Food and Agriculture Organization of the United Nations, 2001.
383. Codex Alimentarius Commission. *Codex General Standard for the Labelling of Prepackaged Foods CODEX STAN 1-1985 (revised 1985, 1991, 1999, 2001)*. Rome, Joint FAO/WHO Food Standard Programme, Codex Alimentarius Commision, 1985 (CODEX STAN 01-1985, amended 2001) (http://www.codexalimentarius.net/download/standards/32/CXS_001e.pdf, accessed 7th October 2005).
384. *WTO agreements and public health: a joint study by the WHO and WTO secretariat*. Geneva, World Health Organization, 2002.
385. *General Principles for the Addition of Essential Nutrients to Foods CAC/GL 09-1987 (amended 1989, 1991)*. Rome, Joint FAO/WHO Food Standards Programme, Codex Alimentarius Commision, 1987 (http://www.codexalimentarius.net/download/standards/299/CXG_009e.pdf, accessed 7 October 2005).
386. *Diet, nutrition and the prevention of chronic diseases. Report of Joint WHO/FAO Expert Consultation*. Geneva, World Health Organization, 2003 (WHO Technical Report Series No. 916).
387. Institute of Medicine. *Food Chemicals Codex*. 5th ed. Washington, DC, National Academy Press, 2003.
388. British Pharmacopoeial Commission. *The British Pharmacopoeia 2003*. London, Her Majesty's Stationery Office, 2003.

Further reading

Part I.   The role of food fortification in the control of micronutrient malnutrition (Chapters 1 and 2)

Dexter PB. *Rice fortification for developing countries*. Arlington, VA, Opportunities for Micronutrient Interventions, 1998 (No. 15) (http://www.mostproject.org/PDF/rice4.pdf, accessed 7 October 2005).

Lofti M et al. *Micronutrient fortification of foods: current practices, research and opportunities*. Ottawa, Micronutrient Initiative, International Agricultural Centre, 1996.

Micronutrient Initiative. *Food fortification to end micronutrient malnutrition: State-of-the-Art Symposium Report, 2 August 1997, Montreal, Canada*. Ottawa, Micronutrient Initiative, International Agricultural Centre, 1998.

Part II.   Evaluating the public health significance of micronutrient malnutrition (Chapters 3 and 4)

Sommer A. *Vitamin A deficiency and its consequences : a field guide to detection and control*. 3rd ed. Geneva, World Health Organization, 1995.

Part III.   Fortificants: physical characteristics, selection and use with specific food vehicles (Chapters 5 and 6)

Arroyave G and Dary O. *Manual for Sugar Fortification with Vitamin A. Part 1: Technical and operational guidelines for preparing vitamin A premix and fortified sugar*. Arlington, VA, Opportunities for Micronutrient Interventions, 1996 (2nd) (http://www.mostproject.org/PDF/1final.pdf, accessed 7 October 2005).

Hurrell RF, ed. *The mineral fortification of foods*. Leatherhead, Surrey, Leatherhead Publishings, 1999.

Fortification basics: milk. Arlington, VA, Micronutrient Operational Strategies and Technologies, The United States Agency for International Developement Micronutrient Program, 1999 (http://www.mostproject.org/Updates_Feb05/Milk.pdf accessed 7 October 2005).

Fortification basics: maize flour/ meal. Arlington, VA, Micronutrient Operational Strategies and Technologies, The United States Agency for International Developement Micronutrient Program,1999 (http://www.mostproject.org/Updates_Feb05/Maize_Corn.pdf, accessed 7 October 2005).

Fortification Basics: instant noodles. Arlington, VA, Micronutrient Operational Strategies and Technologies, The United States Agency for International Developement Micronutrient Program,1999 (http://www.mostproject.org/Updates_Feb05/noodles.pdf, accessed 7 October 2005).

Mora JO et al. *Vitamin A Sugar Fortification in Central America: Experience and Lessons Learned.* Arlington, VA, Micronutrient Operational Strategies and Technologies, The United States Agency for International Developement Micronutrient Program, 2000 (http://www.mostproject.org/PDF/sugarlessonsEnglish.pdf, accessed 7 October 2005).

Nalubola R and Nestel P. *Wheat flour fortification with vitamin A.* Arlington, VA, Opportunities for Micronutrient Interventions, 1998.

Manual for Wheat Flour Fortification with Iron. Part 2: Technical and operational guidelines. Arlington, VA, Micronutrient Operational Strategies and Technologies, The United States Agency for International Developement Micronutrient Program, 2000 (http://www.mostproject.org/PDF/2.pdf, accessed 7 October 2005).

Fortification basics: Wheat flour. Arlington, VA, Opportunities for Micronutrient Interventions, 1997 (http://www.mostproject.org/Updates_Feb05/Wheat.pdf, accessed 7 October 2005).

Fortification Basics: sugar. Arlington, VA, Opportunities for Micronutrient Interventions, 1997 (http://www.mostproject.org/Updates_Feb05/Sugar.pdf, accessed 7 October 2005).

Fortification basics: Oils and margarine. Arlington, VA, Opportunities for Micronutrient Interventions, 1997 (http://www.mostproject.org/Updates_Feb05/Oils.pdf, accessed 7 October 2005).

Fortification Basics: choosing a vehicle. Arlington, VA, Opportunities for Micronutrient Interventions, 1997 (http://www.mostproject.org/Updates_Feb05/Vehicles.pdf, accessed 7 October 2005).

Fortification Basics: stability. Arlington, VA, Opportunities for Micronutrient Interventions, 1998 (http://www.mostproject.org/Updates_Feb05/Stability.pdf, accessed 7 October 2005).

Part IV. Implementing effective and sustainable food fortification programmes (Chapters 7–11)

Monitoring and evaluation (Chapter 8)

Dary O, Arroyave G. *Manual for Sugar Fortification with Vitamin A. Part 2: Guidelines for the development, implementation, monitoring and evaluation of a vitamin A sugar fortification program.* 2nd ed. Arlington, VA, Opportunities for Micronutrient Interventions, 1996 (http://www.mostproject.org/PDF/2final.pdf, accessed 7 October 2005).

Dary O et al. *Manual for Sugar Fortification with Vitamin A. Part 3: Analytical methods for the control and evaluation of sugar fortification with vitamin A.* 2nd ed. Arlington, VA, Opportunities for Micronutrient Interventions, 1996 (http://www.mostproject.org/PDF/3final.pdf, accessed 7 October 2005).

Nalubola R, Nestel P. *Manual for Wheat Flour Fortification with Iron. Part 3: Analytical methods for monitoring wheat flour fortification with iron.* Arlington, Virginia, Micronutrient Operational Strategies and Technologies, The United States Agency for International Developement Micronutrient Program, 2000 (http://www.mostproject.org/PDF/3.pdf, accessed 7 October 2005).

Nestel P, Nalubola R, Mayfield E. *Quality assurance as applied to micronutrient fortification.* Washington, DC, International Life Sciences Institute Press, 2002 (http://www.ilsi.org/file/QAtext.pdf, accessed 7 October 2005).

Fortification basics: principles of assay procedures. Arlington, VA, Opportunities for Micronutrient Interventions, 1998 (http://www.mostproject.org/Updates_Feb05/Assay.pdf, accessed 7 October 2005).

National food law (Chapter 11)

Bauernfeind JC, Lachance PA. *Nutrient additions to food. Nutritional, technological and regulatory aspects.* Trumbull, CT, Food and Nutrition Press Inc., 1991.

Nathan R. *Regulation of fortified foods to address micronutrient malnutrition: legislation, regulations, and enforcement.* Ottawa, Micronutrient Initiative, 1999 (http://www.micronutrient.org/idpas/pdf/315RegulationOfFortified.pdf, accessed 7 October 2005).

ANNEXES

ANNEX A

Indicators for assessing progress towards the sustainable elimination of iodine deficiency disorders

The international community has endorsed the goal of the sustainable elimination of iodine deficiency as a public health problem. In order to measure progress made towards this goal, various indicators have been developed (*1*). These indicators can be conveniently grouped into three categories, namely indicators related to salt iodization itself, those that reflect the population's iodine status and thirdly, those that provide a measure of the sustainability of the salt iodization programme. Success criteria for each of these sets of indicators have also been established; these can to be used to assess whether the sustainable elimination of iodine deficiency as a public health problem has been achieved (see **Table A.1**).

TABLE A.1
Indicators for monitoring progress towards the sustainable elimination of iodine deficiency as a public health problem

Indicator	Success criteria/goals
Salt iodization	
Proportion of households using adequately iodized salt[a]	>90%
Urinary iodine[b]	
Proportion of the population having urinary iodine below 100 µg/l	<50%
Proportion of the population having urinary iodine below 50 µg/l	<20%
Programmatic indicators	
An effective, functional national multidisciplinary body responsible to the government for the national programme for the elimination of iodine deficiency disorders, with a chairman appointed by the ministry of health.	At least 8 of the 10 programmatic indicators listed should exist
Evidence of political commitment to universal salt iodization and the elimination of iodine deficiency disorders.	
Appointment of a responsible executive officer for the iodine deficiency disorders elimination programme.	
Legislation or regulations on universal salt iodization (ideally regulations should cover both human and agricultural salt).	
Commitment to assessment and reassessment of progress in the elimination of iodine deficiency disorders, with access to laboratories able to provide accurate data on salt and urinary iodine.	

TABLE A.1 Continued

Indicator	Success criteria/goals
Programme of public education and social mobilization on the importance of iodine deficiency disorders and the consumption of iodized salt.	
Regular monitoring of salt iodine at the factory, retail and household levels.	
Regular monitoring of urinary iodine in school-aged children, with appropriate sampling for higher risk areas.	
Cooperation from the salt industry in maintenance of quality control.	
A system for the recording of results or regular monitoring procedures, particularly for salt iodine, urinary iodine and, if available, neonatal thyroid stimulating hormone, with mandatory public reporting.	

[a] Adequately iodized salt is salt that contains at least 15 ppm iodine. Additional conditions for the use of salt as a vehicle for eliminating iodine deficiency disorders are:
- Local production and/or importation of iodized salt in a quantity that is sufficient to satisfy the potential human demand (about 4–5 kg per person per year).
- At the point of production (or importation), 95% of salt destined for human consumption must be iodized according to government standards for iodine content.
- Salt iodine concentrations at the point of production or importation, and at the wholesale and retail levels, must be determined by titration; at the household level, it may be determined by either titration or certified kits.

[b] Data (national or regional) should have been collected within the last 2 years.

Source: adapted from reference (1).

Reference

1. *Assessment of iodine deficiency disorders and monitoring their elimination. A guide for programme managers.* 2nd ed. Geneva, World Health Organization, 2001 (WHO/NHD/01.1).

ANNEX B
The international resource laboratory for iodine network

The International Resource Laboratory for Iodine network (IRLI), launched in 2001, is sponsored by the Centers for Disease Control and Prevention (CDC), the International Council for Control of Iodine Deficiency Disorders (ICCIDD), the Micronutrient Initiative (MI), the United Nations Children's Fund (UNICEF) and the World Health Organization (WHO). Its purpose is to support the national public health and industry monitoring that contributes to sustaining progress towards achieving universal salt iodization and the elimination of iodine deficiency[1].

The global IRLI network works to strengthen the capacity of participating laboratories to accurately measure iodine in urine and salt. Its main activities include:

(i) training and technology transfer to national laboratories;

(ii) formation of regional iodine networks;

(iii) development of technical standards and external quality assurance/proficiency testing programmes;

(iv) collaboration with the salt industry and other sectors when appropriate;

(v) information sharing among regional networks and communications with the IRLI Coordinating Committee and other interested parties;

(vi) seeking necessary resources to sustain the operation of regional networks.

As of 2004?? membership of the International Resource Laboratory for Iodine network extended to 12 countries, as follows:

Australia

Institute of Clinical Pathology and Medical Research
Westmead Hospital
Darcy Road

---

[1] More information on the IRLI network can be obtained by e-mailing: **iodinelab@cdc.gov**.

Westmead
New South Wales 2145
http://www.wsahs.nsw.gov.au/icpmr

Belgium

Centre Hospitalier Universitaire Saint-Pierre
322 Rue Haute
1000 Brussels
e-mail: Daniella_GNAT@stpierre-bru.be

Bulgaria

National Center of Hygiene, Medical Ecology and Nutrition
15 Dimiter Nestorov Street
Floor 6, Laboratory 5–6
Sofia 1431
http://www.nchmen.government.bg

Cameroon

Faculty of Medicine and Biomedical Sciences
BP 1364
Sciences – FMBS
Yaounde
e-mail: WHO.YAO@camnet.cm

China

National Reference Laboratory for Iodine Deficiency Disorders
Disease Control Department
Ministry of Health
PO Box No 5
Changping
Beijing 102206
e-mail: nrl@cnidd.org

Guatemala

Food Safety and Fortification Area
Instituto de Nutrición de Centro América y Panamá (INCAP)
Calzada Roosevelt, Zona 11
Apartado Postal 1188
Guatemala City
http://www.incap.ops-oms.org

India

All India Institute of Medical Sciences
Centre for Community Medicine
Room 28
New Delhi – 110 029
e-mail: cpandav@now-india.net.in

Indonesia

Laboratorium Biotehnologi Kedokteran/GAKY
Diponegoro Medical Faculty
Gedung Serba Guna Lantai 2
Jalan Dr Sutomo No. 14
Kedokteran
Semarang
e-mail: hertanto@indosat.net.id

Kazakhstan

The Kazakh Nutrition Institute
Klochkov Str. 66
Almaty 480008
e-mail: nutrit@nursat.kz

Peru

Unidad de Endocrinologia y Metabolismo
Instituto de Investigaciones de la Altura
Universidad Peruana Cayetano Heredia
Av. Honorio Delgado 430
San Martin de Porres
Lima 1
e-mail: epretell@terra.com.pe

Russia

Institute of Endocrinology
Dm Ulyanova, 11
Moscow
e-mail: iod@endocrincentr.ru

South Africa

Nutritional Intervention Research Unit
Medical Research Council
PO Box 19070
Tygerberg 7505
Cape Town
e-mail: pieter.jooste@mrc.ac.za

ANNEX C
Conversion factors for calculating Estimated Average Requirements (EARs) from FAO/WHO Recommended Nutrient Intakes (RNIs)

The recommended method for setting fortificant levels in foods is the Estimated Average Requirement cut-point method (1). Estimated Average Requirements (EARs) for use in such computations can be derived from published Recommended Nutrient Intakes (RNIs), by the application of the conversion factors listed in the table below. The EAR is obtained by dividing the RNI (or an equivalent dietary reference value) for a given population subgroup by the corresponding conversion factor (**Table C.1**).

The conversion is equivalent to subtracting 2 standard deviations of the average nutrient requirement for a population subgroup. The conversion factors listed here are based on standard deviations derived by the United States Food and Nutrition Board of the Institute of Medicine (FNB/IOM) and which are used by the Board to calculate its Recommended Dietary Allowances (RDAs).

TABLE C.1
Conversion factors for calculating Estimated Average Requirements (EARs) from FAO/WHO Recommended Nutrient Intakes (RNIs)

Nutrient	Children				Males			Females				Pregnant	Lactating
	1–3 years	4–6 years	7–9 years	10–18 years	19–65 years	>65 years	10–18 years	19–50 years	51–65 years	>65 years			
Vitamin A	1.4	1.4	1.4	1.4	1.4	1.4	1.4	1.4	1.4	1.4		1.4	1.4
Vitamin D[a]	–	–	–	–	–	–	–	–	–	–		–	–
Vitamin E	1.25	1.25	1.25	1.25	1.3	1.3	1.25	1.2	1.2	1.2		1.2	1.2
Vitamin C	1.2	1.2	1.2	1.2	1.2	1.2	1.2	1.3	1.3	1.2		1.2	1.2
Thiamine (vitamin B$_1$)	1.25	1.25	1.25	1.2	1.2	1.2	1.2	1.2	1.2	1.2		1.2	1.2
Ribiflavin (vitamin B$_2$)	1.25	1.25	1.25	1.2	1.2	1.2	1.1	1.2	1.2	1.2		1.2	1.2
Niacin	1.3	1.3	1.3	1.3	1.3	1.3	1.3	1.3	1.3	1.3		1.3	1.3
Vitamin B$_6$	1.25	1.25	1.25	1.2	1.2	1.2	1.2	1.2	1.2	1.2		1.2	1.2
Folate	1.25	1.25	1.25	1.25	1.25	1.25	1.25	1.25	1.25	1.25		1.25	1.25
Vitamin B$_{12}$	1.3	1.2	1.2	1.2	1.2	1.2	1.2	1.2	1.2	1.2		1.2	1.2
Iron[b]	–	–	–	1.4	1.3	1.3	1.6	–	1.6	1.6		1.2	1.4
Zinc	1.2	1.2	1.2	1.2	1.2	1.2	1.2	1.2	1.2	1.2		1.2	1.2
Calcium[c]	1.2	1.2	1.2	1.2	1.2	1.2	1.2	1.2	1.2	1.2		1.2	1.2
Selenium	1.2	1.3	1.2	1.2	1.2	1.2	1.2	1.2	1.2	1.2		1.2	1.2
Iodine	1.4	1.4	1.4	1.4	1.4	1.4	1.4	1.4	1.4	1.4		1.4	1.4
Fluoride[a]	–	–	–	–	–	–	–	–	–	–		–	–

[a] Conversion factors are not given for vitamin D and fluoride because there is insufficient information to support the derivation of an EAR for these micronutrients. The recommended intakes are usually expressed as Adequate Intakes (AIs), or represented by the usual intake of healthy people.
[b] Conversion factors are not provided for children ≤9 years or for menstruating women aged 19–50 years, and should not be used for women aged 14–18 years who are menstruating, due to the high variability and the skewed nature of the distribution of the requirements for iron in these population groups.
[c] Conversion factors to be applied to calcium requirements set by the United Kingdom Department of Health (i.e. Reference Nutrient Intakes), which are conceptually similar to the FAO/WHO RNIs. (2)

Source: reference (1).

References

1. Food and Nutrition Board, Institute of Medicine. *Dietary reference intakes: applications in dietary planning.* Washington, DC, National Academy Press, 2003
2. Department of Health. *Dietary Reference Values of food energy and nutrients for the United Kingdom.* London, Her Majesty's Stationery Office, 1991.

ANNEX D

A procedure for estimating feasible fortification levels for a mass fortification programme

1. Introduction

Mass fortification is the term used to describe the addition of micronutrients to foods that are widely consumed, such as staples, condiments and several other commodities. This can be a very efficient way of supplying micronutrients to a large proportion of the target population for a number of reasons. Firstly, mass fortification does not require changes in dietary habits and secondly, programmes can be based on existing food distribution networks. In addition, staples and condiments tend to be consumed throughout the year, and when fortified on an industrial scale, the increase in the cost of the product due to fortification is usually relatively small. On the downside, because staples and condiments are also consumed in large amounts by non-target groups, when fortified, some individuals could be put at risk of increasing their nutrient intakes to levels that are close to, or exceed, the Tolerable Upper Intake Level (UL). This can be a potential problem for nutrients such as vitamin A, vitamin D, vitamin C, niacin (when using nicotinic acid as the fortificant), folic acid, iron, zinc, calcium, iodine and fluoride.

In practice, the amount of fortificant micronutrient that can be added to a food is often dictated by safety concerns for those at the top end of consumption of the chosen food vehicle. In addition, some micronutrients, including β-carotene, vitamin C, riboflavin (vitamin B_2), iron, zinc, calcium and iodine, can only be added in amounts up to a certain threshold, beyond which the sensory properties of the food vehicle are negatively affected. Fortification levels can also be restricted by the cost of the added micronutrients; high fortificant costs might mean that programmes are unaffordable or at risk of not being implemented as planned. Vitamin A (non-oily), vitamin D, vitamin C, niacin and some compounds of iron and calcium are among those nutrients whose addition to food are most likely to be limited by cost constraints. In sum, such limitations on the magnitude of micronutrient additions need to be balanced against the desire to achieve a particular nutritional goal.

For this reason, when planning a mass fortification programme, or more specifically, when deciding on the level of fortification, it is advisable to first determine the probable safety, technological and cost constraints on the amount of micronutrient that can be added to a given food vehicle. Having established a limiting level for each of these factors, the "lowest" value of the three then becomes what is referred to as the *Feasible Fortification Level* (FFL). A methodology for determining the FFL is described in section 2 below, and its application illustrated by means of a worked example in section 3.

> The **Feasible Fortification Level (FFL)** is that which is determined, subject to cost and technological constraints, as the level that will provide the greatest number of at-risk individual with an adequate micronutrient intake without causing an unacceptable risk of excess intake in the whole population.

The FFL is a useful concept in that it can be used to estimate the additional intake that would result from the consumption of a given amount of a fortified food, to decide the final formulation of a micronutrient premix, and to estimate the cost of fortification for each micronutrient added. The FFL is used as the basis for various production and regulatory parameters that are commonly associated with food fortification. Production parameters are applied at food processing factories, and include the *Target Fortification Level* (TFL), the *Maximum Fortification Level* (MFL), and the *Minimum Fortification Level* (mFL). The latter is used in national food regulation to establish the *Legal Minimum Level* (LmL). Another important regulatory parameter is the *Maximum Tolerable Level* (MTL), which is invoked in food law for those nutrients whose intake might approach the UL as a result of fortification (see section 2.4). **Figure D1** illustrates the relationship between the production and regulatory parameters defined here.

> The **Target Fortification Level (TFL)** is the average micronutrient concentration of a fortified food product measured at the factory. Food factories should aim to produce products that contain this target level. It is calculated by adding the natural intrinsic concentration of each micronutrient in the unfortified food vehicle to the FFL.

> The **Minimum Fortification Level (mFL)** is given by reducing the TFL by an amount equivalent to two coefficients of variation in the measured micronutrient content of a fortified food at the factory. This level represents the lower limit of the micronutrient content to be achieved by the fortification process.

FIGURE D1

Relationship between the various production and regulatory parameters associated with mass fortification

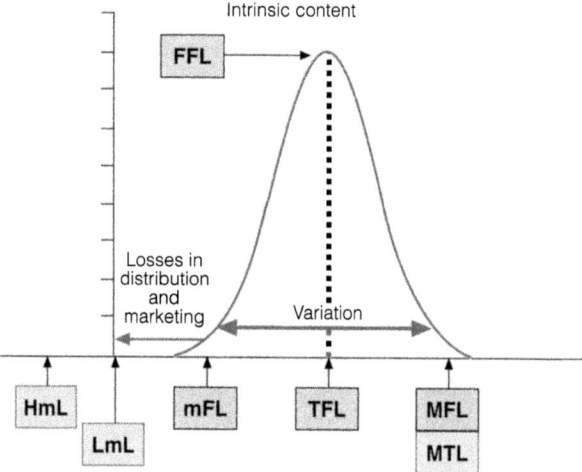

FFL = Feasible Fortification Level; mFL = Minimum Fortification Level (a production parameter); TFL = Target Fortification Level (a production parameter); MFL = Maximum Fortification Level (a production parameter); LmL = Legal Minimum Level (a regulatory parameter), MTL = Maximum Tolerable Level (a regulatory parameter).

The graph also shows the Household Minimum Level (HmL), which may be lower than the LmL, on account of losses during storage in the home (i.e. before the food is consumed). This parameter is sometimes used to monitor the utilization, coverage and consumption of fortified foods by consumers.

The **Maximum Fortification Level (MFL)** is given by increasing the TFL by an amount equivalent to two coefficients of variation of the measured micronutrient content of a fortified food at the factory. This level represents the upper limit of the micronutrient content to be achieved by the fortification process.

The **Legal Minimum Level (LmL)** is the minimum micronutrient content of a fortified food as defined in regulations and standards; it is the amount that should appear on the label of a fortified food. The LmL is obtained by reducing the mFL by an amount equivalent to the average loss of micronutrient during distribution and storage, within the stated shelf-life of the product.

The Maximum Tolerable Level (MTL) is the maximum micronutrient content that a fortified food can present as it is established in food law; its purpose is to minimize the risk of excess intake of certain micronutrients. The MTL should coincide with the MFL for those micronutrients for which there is a risk of excess intake.

2. Selecting fortification levels on the basis of safety, technological and cost constraints

2.1 Limits to micronutrient additions

2.1.1 The safety limit

Micronutrient intake is a function of the amount of food consumed and also the micronutrient content of the food. Since adult males tend to have the highest food consumption rates of staple foods (and thus the highest micronutrient intakes if a staple were to be mass fortified), this group has the greatest risk of excessive micronutrient intakes. In order to assess the risk of excessive intakes, it is necessary to determine the 95th percentile of consumption of the food to be fortified, as well as the usual nutrient intake from all dietary sources (including dietary supplements if they supply nutrient forms that are of concern from a safety point of view) for those individuals most at risk – in this case, adult males.

Based on these assumptions, the safety limit for a micronutrient addition can be calculated using Equation 1. Note that if more than one food is being considered for mass fortification, the safety limit should be divided among all of them. If the food vehicles to be fortified are interchangeable in the diet (e.g. wheat flour and maize flour, cereals and pastas) the usual intake of the interchangeable foods can be combined in order to estimate a common safety limit, and in turn, a common Feasible Fortification Level.

Equation 1

$$\text{Safety limit}^1 (\text{mg/kg}) = \frac{[\text{UL}(\text{mg}) - \text{amount of micronutrient from diet (mg) and any supplements (mg)}]}{[\text{95th percentile of consumption (kg)}]}$$

2.1.2 The technological limit

A food can only be fortified up to a level that does not change its organoleptic (i.e. colour, flavour, odour) and physical properties, measured just after fortifi-

---

[1] A more accurate calculation may consider losses during distribution and storage, as well as losses during food preparation. However, because losses vary hugely according to conditions and situations, and because allowance is often made to compensate for these losses (i.e. an overage), it is usually acceptable to use this simplified approach.

cation and over the shelf-life of the food. This level should be determined experimentally both for the food and for products for which the fortified food is an important ingredient. Ideally, a range of micronutrient levels – and, if more than one micronutrient is involved, combinations of micronutrient levels – should be tested by individuals with expertise in the sensory analysis of foods in order to determine what amount of each nutrient is technically compatible with a given food matrix. Each combination of micronutrient(s) and food matrix will have its own set of technological maxima. Technological limits are not necessarily fixed; as a result of technological innovation (e.g. the development of new fortificants that have fewer colour, odour and reactive problems), it may well be possible to raise the technological maximum at a future date.

2.1.3 The cost limit

Of the three, the cost limit is generally the more flexible and adjustable parameter, being dependent on value judgements about what is an acceptable price increase for fortified food products. Most ongoing food fortification programmes operate with price increases in the range 0.25–2.0%.

It is recommended that fortification programme managers discuss with industry at an early stage of programme development what an acceptable increment in production costs and product price would be, i.e. one that would make any mass fortification programme both feasible and sustainable. If more than one micronutrient is to be added, then their combined cost should fall within this predefined permitted increment.

When conducted on a relatively large-scale industrial basis, by far the largest share of the incremental cost of fortification (90% or more) can be attributed to the cost of the fortificant itself. This being the case, the cost limit can be calculated according to Equation 2, where the cost of the fortificant micronutrient(s) is used to substitute for the cost of the entire fortification programme. This approximation does not apply to some rice fortification processes, which rely on the use of rice premixes in low dilution rates (1:100 or 1:200). In this case, the cost of manufacturing of the premix exceeds that of the fortificant compounds.

Equation 2

$$\text{Cost limit}^1 (mg/kg) = \frac{[\text{Food price (US\$ per kg)} \times \text{price increment (\%100)} \times \text{proportion of micronutrient in fortificant (\%100)} \times 10^6]}{[\text{Fortificant price (US\$ per kg)}]}$$

---

[1] A more accurate calculation may consider losses during distribution and storage, as well as losses during food preparation. However, because losses vary hugely according to conditions and situations, and because allowance is often made to compensate for these losses (i.e. an overage), it is usually acceptable to use this simplified approach.

2.2 Estimating the Feasible Fortification Level (FFL)

As stated in the introduction, whichever one of the three limits defined and calculated as above, i.e. the safety, the technological and the cost limit is the lowest becomes the FFL. Each micronutrient in a given food matrix will have its own FFL.

Once the FFL has been defined, it is possible to estimate for each micronutrient the additional intake that would be supplied to the target population, as well as the probable cost of the fortification process (based on the cost of the fortificants), and the final formulation of the premix (by multiplying the FFL by the dilution factor).

2.3 Estimating production parameters: the Target Fortification Level (TFL), the Minimum Fortification Level (mFL) and the Maximum Fortification Level (MFL)

The TFL is given by the sum of the calculated FFL and the natural intrinsic content of the micronutrient in the unfortified food. The value of the TFL should be used at the factory level as the target average micronutrient content of a fortified food, and thus as the reference value for quality control specifications.

The mFL is derived from the TFL according to Equation 3, that is to say, the TFL is reduced by an amount that is proportional to two times the coefficient of variation (CV) of the measured nutrient content of a food that has been fortified by a given process (when that process is performing adequately). The variability in the micronutrient content of a fortified food depends on the nature of the food vehicle and the amount of micronutrient added. Generally speaking, the inherent variability in the fortification process is lowest for liquids and greatest for coarse solids. For liquids, a CV of 10% is typical; for fine solids, such as cereal flours, the addition of niacin, iron, zinc and calcium has a CV of 15%, which rises to 25% for most other micronutrients. The variability for coarse solids, such as sugar and unrefined salt, is higher still, generally speaking around 30–50%.

Equation 3

$$\text{mFL (mg/kg)} = \text{TFL} \times [1 - (2 \times \text{CV in the nutrient content of the fortification process (\%/100)})]$$

The MFL is calculated in a similar way, the only difference being that twice the CV of the micronutrient content achieved by the fortification process when performing adequately is *added* to the TFL (Equation 4):

Equation 4

$$\text{MFL (mg/kg)} = \text{TFL} \times [1 + (2 \times \text{CV in the nutrient content during the fortification process } (\%/100))]$$

2.4 Estimating regulatory parameters: the Legal Minimum Level (LmL) and the Maximum Tolerable Level (MTL)

Irrespective of whether mass fortification is mandatory or voluntary, from a public health perspective, fortification levels should be prescribed in national standards and regulations. Such regulations may mention the technological parameters described in section 2.3, but it is essential that they refer to those levels that should feature on food labels and which should be used for inspection and enforcement purposes, i.e. the LmL and the MTL.

The LmL is calculated by subtracting from the mFL the expected losses of micronutrients during the distribution and storage of fortified products. Equation 5 summarizes the calculation:

Equation 5

$$\text{LmL (mg/kg)} = [\text{mFL (mg/kg)} (1 - \text{proportion of losses during storage and distribution})]$$

It may be necessary to specify a time frame after fortification, during which time nutritional claims must be upheld. In general, most mineral contents, with the exception of iodine in raw salt, should remain more or less constant, but vitamin contents are more liable to change with time, depending on the product. However, such losses rarely exceed 50%, even for the most sensitive nutrients (e.g. vitamin A, folic acid) during the shelf-life of the fortified food.

The MTL is simply the legal expression of the MFL for those nutrients for which there may be a safety concern, for example, vitamin A, vitamin D, folic acid, niacin (as nicotinic acid) iron, zinc, calcium and iodine. For other nutrients it may not be necessary to specify this parameter in regulations, something which reduces the complexity of the enforcement system required.

3. Selecting a fortification level based on the FFL: an example calculation

A government of a country is aware that most of its population has a diet rich in cereals but poor in foods of animal origin. Consequently, the general population is at risk of deficiencies in vitamin A, riboflavin (vitamin B_2), folate, vitamin B_{12}, iron and zinc. The government is considering introducing a mass fortification programme to counteract the risk of multiple micronutrient deficiencies and to this end has requested its public health nutritionists to investigate the feasibility of supplying 70% of the Estimated Average Requirements (EARs) of these micronutrients via fortified foods and to recommend suitable fortification levels for achieving this nutritional goal.

3.1 Selecting appropriate food vehicles and determining the significance of food fortification in public health terms

Data on the level of consumption among the target population of four widely consumed staples, sugar, oil, wheat flour and rice, are summarized in **Table D.1**.

On the grounds that they are consumed by at least 50% of the population, sugar, oil and wheat flour were singled out as being the most appropriate vehicles for mass fortification. Although rice is also consumed in large amounts by the population, much of the supply is produced at small-scale, local mills, and thus much more difficult to fortify.

Although reasonable coverage can be achieved by the fortification of the three nominated food vehicles, there was nevertheless some concern that up to 30% of the target population might not benefit from the planned fortification programme. The sector of the population falling into this category is that which resides in rural areas and whose accessibility to industrially-processed foods is likely to be limited. Since it is technically possible to add vitamin A to all three vehicles, coverage is likely to be the greatest for this vitamin. However, for some of the other nutrients under consideration, which can only be easily added to one of the three proposed vehicles (i.e. wheat flour), coverage is likely to be significantly lower. It was concluded that the potential coverage made vitamin A fortification of all three products worthwhile, but that it would be necessary to provide micronutrient supplements in various forms (e.g. tablets, powders, beverages) to ensure an adequate micronutrient intake by that fraction of the population not covered by mass fortification (in particular those living in rural areas). It was recommended that supplements be distributed both commercially and through social programmes, and that they should provide the equivalent of 70% of the EAR for the micronutrients of concern. The proposed composition

TABLE D.1
Consumption profile of selected industrially-produced staples

Food	Consumers (% of population)	Consumption[a] (g/day)		
		P-5th	P-50th	P-95th
Sugar	70	10	20	60
Oil	60	5	10	25
Wheat flour	50	100	200	600
Rice[b]	10	100	250	700

[a] Expressed as percentiles of consumption.
[b] Refers to rice produced at larger-scale industrial facilities only.

TABLE D.2
Recommended composition of dietary supplements to complement fortified foods

Micronutrient	Daily equivalent dose[a]
Vitamin A	300 µg
vitamin B_2 (riboflavin)	0.8 mg
Folic acid	200 µg[b]
Vitamin B_{12}	1.4 µg[c]
Iron	10 mg
Zinc	4 mg

[a] These doses are given as equivalent doses so that they can be used to formulate a daily as well as a discontinuous dose (e.g. a weekly dose). The aim is to supply at least 70% EAR for adult males, which is used as the reference average for the family.
[b] 200 µg folic acid is equivalent to 340 µg Dietary Folate Equivalents (200 × 1.7), which means that a dietary supplement containing this dose would contribute 106% of the Estimated Average Requirement (EAR) for this particular nutrient.
[c] This dosage could provide up to 140% of the Estimated Average Requirement (EAR) of vitamin B_{12} in view of the higher bioavailability of the synthetic form relative to natural dietary sources.

of the dietary supplements (expressed as daily equivalent doses) are presented in **Table D.2**.

3.2 Analysing the safety, technological and cost limits to vitamin A fortification

The calculation of a safety limit for vitamin A fortification needs to take account of the fact that this micronutrient is to be added to more than one food (in this case three). Thus as a first step in the calculation, it is necessary to adjust the UL that will be used for the estimation of the safety limit for each food as follows:

$$\text{UL per food} = [\text{UL} - (\text{diet and supplement intake})]/3$$

The intake of vitamin A (in the retinol form) from dietary sources by the target population was estimated to be around 600 µg per day. This value represents the high end of consumption (i.e. the 95th percentile of intakes). Given that the UL for vitamin A is 3 000 µg and assuming a further daily intake of vitamin from supplements of 300 µg (see **Table D.2**), then:

$$\text{UL per food} = [3\,000 - (600 + 300)]/3,$$

that is:

TABLE D.3
Safety limits for vitamin A

Food	95th percentile of consumption (g/day)	Safety limit (mg/kg)
Sugar	60	12
Oil	25	28
Wheat flour	300	1.2

$$\text{UL per food} = 700\,\mu g.$$

Then, using Equation 1, it is possible to calculate a safety limit for each food. The results are given in **Table D.3**.

The question then arises whether or not it is technologically feasible to add these levels of vitamin A to the chosen food vehicles. According to the country's food technologists it is, and thus it was concluded that vitamin A fortification is unlikely to be limited by technological considerations in this scenario.

As food technologists warned that price increases in food products due to fortification in excess of 2% for sugar and oil, and 0.3% for wheat flour, might meet with opposition from the food industry, it was considered instructive at this point to estimate the increase in price that would result from fortification of the three products at the safety limits of vitamin A addition. **Table D.4** summarizes the results of such calculations.

On the basis of these computations, it is evident that the addition of vitamin A to sugar at a level of 12 mg/kg is barely cost compatible. On the other hand, of the three food vehicles, sugar has the best penetration (see **Table D.1**). On balance, it was decided to proceed with the fortification of sugar, despite the fact that the relative high cost might make the implementation of this intervention much more difficult.

3.2.1 Assessing the nutritional implications of the fortification with vitamin A at the Feasible Fortification Levels

The probable additional intakes of vitamin A due to fortification at the safety limits calculated above, at the 5th, 50th and 95th percentiles of consumption of each food, are shown in **Table D.5**. In each case, the additional intake is expressed as a percentage of the EAR, which for adult males is 429 µg per day.

According to the figures given in **Table D.5**, use of a three-food strategy would provide an additional intake somewhere between 28%[1] and 499% of the

---

[1] This value corresponds to the additional intake of vitamin A at the 5th percentile consumption of fortified sugar, which is the food with the widest consumption (70% of the population).

TABLE D.4
Cost analysis of fortification with vitamin A at the estimated safety limits for sugar, oil and wheat flour

Food	Level of vitamin A addition (mg/kg)	Cost analysis		
		Cost of fortification (US$ per MT[a])	Product price (US$/kg)	Price increment (%)
Sugar	12	11.00	0.50	2.0
Oil	28	6.00	0.70	0.9
Wheat flour	1.2	0.67	0.45	0.15

[a] MT stands for metric ton or 1000 kg.

TABLE D.5
Additional intake of vitamin A at various levels of consumption of fortified foods

Food	Level of vitamin A addition (mg/kg)	Additional intake (as a % of the EAR[a])		
		P-5th	P-50th	P-95th
Sugar	12	28	56	168
Oil	28	33	65	163
Wheat flour	1.2	28	56	168
TOTAL		89	177	499

EAR, Estimated Average Requirement.
[a] Based on the EAR of vitamin A for adult males (429 µg/day). This value is used to represent the "average" intake for the family.

EAR for adult males (i.e. the extreme values of this combined strategy). This finding provides justification for the decision to proceed with the vitamin A fortification of sugar (despite the cost) as without it, the programme is unlikely to attain its nutritional goal of supplying 70% of the EAR to most individuals in the population.

The above analysis also demonstrates the benefits of fortifying three vehicles with lower amounts of vitamin A rather than just one with a relatively high amount. Adopting the latter approach would not only result in an unacceptably high cost increment, but also increases the risk of those individuals at the high end of consumption of the single vehicle reaching the UL without significantly improving the intake of those individuals at the low end of consumption. Furthermore, the coverage of the intervention would be limited to those consuming the single chosen food vehicle.

Taking into account all of the above considerations, it was decided to select the safety limits of vitamin A fortification as the FFLs, i.e. for sugar, 12 mg/kg, for oil, 28 mg/kg and for wheat flour: 1.2 mg/kg.

TABLE D.6
Production parameters for vitamin A fortification

Food	FFL (mg/kg)	Intrinsic vitamin A content (mg/kg)	TFL[a] (mg/kg)	CV[b] (%)	mFL[c] (mg/kg)	MFL[d] (mg/kg)
Sugar	12	0.0	12	33	4	20
Oil	28	0.0	28	10	22	34
Wheat flour	1.2	0.0	1.2	25	0.6	1.8

FFL, Feasible Fortification Level; TFL, Target Fortification Level; CV, coefficient of variation; mFL, Minimum Fortification Level; MFL, Maximum Fortification Level.
[a] The Target Fortification Level is given by adding the intrinsic vitamin A content of the food vehicles to the FFL.
[b] The coefficient of variation (CV) is a measure of the reproducibility of the fortification process.
[c] Calculated using Equation 3.
[d] Calculated using Equation 4.

TABLE D.7
Regulatory parameters for vitamin A fortification

Food	FFL (mg/kg)	Losses during distribution and storage (%)	LmL[a] (mg/kg)	MTL[b] (mg/kg)
Sugar	12	30	3	20
Oil	28	30	15	34
Wheat flour	1.2	25	0.5	1.8

FFL, Feasible Fortification Level; LmL, Legal minimum Level; MTL, Maximum Tolerable Level.
[a] Calculated using Equation 5.
[b] In this case, this is the same as the Maximum Fortification Level (MFL) given in **Table D.6**.

3.2.2 Establishing the production parameters

Having selected the FFLs, and using the definitions and equations given in section 2.3, the next task is to establish the production parameters for vitamin A additions at the factory level. These parameters are given in **Table D.6**.

3.2.3 Establishing the regulatory parameters

Regulatory parameters, the LmL and the MTL, for vitamin A fortification are summarized in **Table D.7**. These will form the basis of label claims and government enforcement activities. In the case of vitamin A fortification, it is necessary to set a MTL because of the need to make sure that individuals within the population (i.e. those at the high end of consumption) would not be at risk of excessive intakes of vitamin A.

3.3 Analysing the safety, technological and cost limits to wheat flour fortification

Having assessed the feasibility of vitamin A additions, the same procedure can be repeated to address the question of the incorporation of folic acid, vitamin

B_{12}, riboflavin (vitamin B_2), iron and zinc to wheat flour. Table D.8 provides a summary of the main features of this analysis, which reveals that folic acid addition is limited by safety concerns, vitamin B_{12} addition by cost, and vitamin B_2, iron and zinc additions by the risk of organoleptic changes in the sensorial and physical properties of the wheat flour.

3.3.1 Assessing the nutritional implications of the fortification of wheat flour, and adjusting the Feasible Fortification Levels

The nutritional implications of fortifying wheat flour at the FFLs calculated in **Table D.8** (i.e. as determined by safety, technological and cost constraints) are summarized in **Table D.9**. This is expressed in terms of the additional intakes that will result from the consumption of fortified wheat flour at three levels of consumption, the 5th percentile (i.e.100 g per day), the 50th percentile (i.e. 200 g per day) and the 95 percentile (i.e. 600 g per day). Intakes are given as absolute amounts and as a percentage of the EAR for adult males. Please note that this consumption pattern is high, and although it is typical of the Middle East and Central Asian countries, it may not be the case for other countries of the world. Each region or country should make their own calculations based on their own conditions in order to select the most appropriate fortification levels.

The calculations show that addition of folic acid to wheat flour would achieve the goal of supplying 70% of the EAR to nearly all consumers of wheat flour (that is to say, to 50% of the population). The case of vitamin B_{12} is also favourable, in fact, particularly so. Its level can be reduced to 0.010 mg/kg (from 0.040 mg/kg), which will help to reduce overall cost of the programme while still satisfying the nutritional target (i.e. an additional intake of 100% of the biological requirements (EAR) of this nutrient for almost all individuals who consume wheat flour).

In contrast, the addition of vitamin B_2 at a level of 4.5 mg per kg is not sufficient to meet nutritional goals, and therefore other sources of this nutrient (e.g. dietary supplements) would have to be supplied to the target population. The same is true of iron, and, in the case of reproductive-age women the deficit is likely to be even worse, since their iron requirements are greater than those used in the present calculation.

Although fortification with zinc at a level of 40 mg/kg would be expected to attain the EAR goal, in the interests of avoiding possible problems with iron absorption (zinc additions at these levels could inhibit the absorption of iron), it was considered prudent to reduce the level to 20 mg/kg. This would maintain a suitable balance with the additional iron intake. Any future interventions should pair zinc and iron additions in a way that complements the impact of wheat flour fortification.

D. A PROCEDURE FOR ESTIMATING FEASIBLE FORTIFICATION LEVELS

TABLE D.8
Safety, technological and cost limits for wheat flour fortification[a]

Nutrient	Fortificant	Cost of fortificant (US$/kg)	Proportion of nutrient in fortificant	UL (mg/day)[b]	Intake from the diet and supplements (mg/day)[c]	Limits (mg/kg)			FFL[g] (mg/kg)
						Safety[d]	Technological[e]	Cost[f]	
Folate	Folic acid	90.00	0.90	1	0.2	1.3	NA	13.5	1.3
Vitamin B_{12}	Vitamin B_{12}, 0.1% water soluble	38.00	0.001	NA	NA	NA	NA	0.040	0.040
Vitamin B_2	Riboflavin	38.00	1.00	NA	NA	NA	4.5	36	4.5
Iron	Ferrous sulphate, dried	2.52	0.32	45	10	58	30	171	30
Zinc	Zinc oxide	3.35	0.80	45	4	68	40	322	40

UL, Tolerable Upper Intake Level; FFL, Feasible Fortification Level; NA, not applicable.

[a] Assumes that the per capita consumption of wheat flour is 100–600 g/day, and that the price of wheat flour is US$ 0.45/kg. This high level of consumption is typical of countries in the Middle East and Central Asia. Other countries should calculate their safety values according to their own consumption figures.
[b] Values are for adult males; this group is considered to be at greatest risk of reaching the UL through the consumption of fortified wheat flour.
[c] Intakes are specified only for those micronutrients for which there may be a safety concern (the main source of which, in this case, will be dietary supplements).
[d] Calculated using Equation 1.
[e] Technological compatibility is determined experimentally to confirm the absence of undesirable changes in the food vehicle due to the addition of fortificants.
[f] Calculated using Equation 2. It was predetermined that each nutrient should not increase the price of wheat flour by more than 0.3%.
[g] The Feasible Fortification Level (FFL) is the lowest of the three limits.

TABLE D.9
Nutritional implications of wheat flour fortification[a]

Nutrient	Fortificant	FFL (mg/kg)	EAR[b] (mg/day)	Absolute additional intakes (mg/day)			Additional intakes (as a % of the EAR)		
				P-5th	P-50th	P-95th	P-5th	P-50th	P-95th
Folate[c]	Folic acid	1.3	0.32	0.130	0.260	0.780	69	138	414
Vitamin B$_{12}$[d]	Vitamin B$_{12}$, 0.1% water soluble	0.040	0.002	0.0040	0.0080	0.0240	400	800	2400
	Vitamin B$_{12}$, 0.1% water soluble	0.010[e]	0.002	0.001	0.002	0.006	100	200	600
Vitamin B$_2$	Riboflavin	4.5	1.1	0.45	0.9	2.7	41	82	245
Iron[f]	Ferrous sulphate, dried	30	10	3	6	18	28	56	167
Zinc	Zinc oxide	40	5.8	4	8	24	69	138	414
	Zinc oxide	20[g]	5.8	2	4	8	34	69	207

FFL, Feasible Fortification Level; EAR, Estimated Average Requirement.
[a] Assumes that the per capita consumption of wheat flour is 100 g/day at the 5th percentile of consumption, 200 g/day at the 50th percentile and 600 g/day at the 95th percentile.
[b] Based on the values for the EAR for adult males. These values are used to represent the "average" intake for the family.
[c] The calculation of the additional intake as a percentage of the EAR takes account of the higher bioavailability of folic acid as compared with dietary folate (1 μg folic acid = 1.7 Dietary Folate Equivalents (DFEs) or 1.7 μg food folate).
[d] The calculation of the additional intake as a percentage of the EAR takes account of the higher bioavailability of the synthetic form of vitamin B$_{12}$ as compared with dietary sources (% EAR multiplied by 2).
[e] The FFL has been adjusted downwards because the original value provided much more than was necessary to attain the nutritional goal of an additional intake of 70% of the EAR.
[f] If the average consumption of wheat flour is less than 150 g/day, ferrous fumarate may be used in place of ferrous sulfate as the fortificant in order to achieve the nutritional goal of an additional intake of around 50% EAR. However, it is important to note that this change increases iron fortification costs four-fold.
[g] The FFL has been adjusted downwards because it was important to keep the nutritional balance of the diet.

TABLE D.10
Production and regulatory parameters for wheat flour fortification

Nutrient	Fortificant	Accepted FFL[a] (mg/kg)	Intrinsic content (mg/kg)	CV[b] (%)	Production parameters			Regulatory parameters	
					MFL[c] (mg/kg)	TFL[d] (mg/kg)	mFL[e] (mg/kg)	LmL[f] (mg/kg)	MTL[g] (mg/kg)
Folate	Folic acid	1.3	0.2	25	0.8	1.5	2.3	0.6	2.3
Vitamin B_{12}	Vitamin B_{12}, 0.1% water soluble	0.010	0.000	25	0.005	0.010	0.015	0.005	NA
Vitamin B_2	Riboflavin	4.5	0.5	25	2.5	5.0	7.5	2.3	NA
Iron	Ferrous sulphate, dried	30	10	15	28	40	52	28	52
Zinc	Zinc oxide	20	10	15	21	30	39	21	39
Vitamin A	250-SD	1.2	0	25	0.6	1.2	1.8	0.5	1.8

FFL, Feasible Fortification Level; CV, coefficient of variation; mFL, Minimum Fortification Level; TFL, Target Fortification Level; MFL, Maximum Fortification Level; LmL, Legal minimum Level; MTL, Maximum Tolerable Level; NA, not applicable.

[a] The level of fortification that was finally selected, having adjusted the original FFLs for some micronutrients. The composition of a fortification premix for use with wheat flours is obtained by multiplying the FFL by the dilution factor.
[b] The coefficient of variation (CV) is a measure of the reproducibility of the fortification process.
[c] Calculated using Equation 3.
[d] The Target Fortification Level is given by summing the intrinsic micronutrient content of the unfortified wheat flour and the FFL. Factories should aim to produce foods that, on average, contain this amount of micronutrient.
[e] Calculated using Equation 4.
[f] Calculated using Equation 5.
[g] Relevant only for those micronutrients with safety concerns; equivalent, in this case, to the MFL.

GUIDELINES ON FOOD FORTIFICATION WITH MICRONUTRIENTS

3.3.2 Establishing production and regulatory parameters

Based on the slightly revised FFLs, production and regulatory parameters for the fortification of wheat flour with folate, vitamins B_2 and B_{12}, iron and zinc are calculated in the same way as for vitamin A (see section 3.2.2 and 3.2.3). These are given in Table D.10. For completeness, **Table D.10** also includes the corresponding parameters for vitamin A, calculated earlier (**Tables D.6 and D.7**).

3.4 Concluding comments and recommendations

The above analysis establishes that fortification of wheat flour at the levels proposed (the "accepted" FFLs) would provide appropriate amounts of essential micronutrients to the majority of consumers. Moreover, the cost of the addition

TABLE D.11
Final formulation for the fortification of refined wheat flour and estimated associated costs for a hypothetical country[a]

Nutrient	Fortificant	Accepted FFL (mg/kg)	Regulatory parameters		Estimated costs of fortification	
			LmL[b]	MTL[c]	(US$ per MT[d])	(% of total cost)
Folate	Folic acid	1.3	0.6	2.3	0.13	5.6
Vitamin B_{12}	Vitamin B_{12}, 0.1% water soluble	0.010	0.005	NA	0.38	16.2
Vitamin B_2	Riboflavin	4.5	2.3	NA	0.17	7.3
Iron	Ferrous sulphate, dried	30	28	52	0.24	10.1
Zinc	Zinc oxide	20	21	39	0.08	3.6
Vitamin A	250-SD	1.2	0.5	1.8	0.67	28.7
Vitamin B_1	Thiamine mononitrate	6	2.8	NA	0.18	7.6
Vitamin B_6	Pyridoxin	5	2.4	NA	0.17	7.3
Niacin	Niacinamide	50	40	NA	0.45	13.6
Total					2.34	100.0
Price increment due to fortification (%)					0.5	

FFL, Feasible Fortification Level; LmL, Legal minimum Level; MTL, Maximum Tolerable Level; NA, not applicable.

[a] Assumes an average per capita consumption of wheat flour of 200 g/day (the 95th percentile of consumption is 600 g/day), and that the price of wheat flour is US$ 0.45 per kg. This high level of consumption is typical of countries in the Middle East and Central Asia. Other countries should calculate their fortification formulas according to their own consumption figures.
[b] The Legal Minimum Level (LmL) is the level of fortificant which should appear on the label and is the level to be enforced. It includes the intrinsic nutrient content of the unfortified wheat flour.
[c] The Maximum Tolerable Level is specified for those micronutrients for which there is safety concern; its purpose in food law is to assure that almost all wheat flour consumers do not reach the Upper Tolerable Intake Level for the nutrients for which this parameter is specified.
[d] MT stands for metric ton or 1000 kg.

TABLE D.12
Estimating the overall cost of the proposed fortification programme and the annual investment required

Food vehicle	Consumer base (% of the population)	Cost of fortification (US$ per MT[g])	Annual demand (MT[g])	Per capita consumption[a] (kg/year)	Per capita consumption[b] (g/day)	Consumption per consumer[c] (g/day)	Total cost[d] (Million of US$ per year)	Annual investment per person[e] (US$)	Annual investment per consumer[f] (US$)
Sugar	70	11.00	100 000	10	27	39	1.10	0.110	0.157
Oil	60	6.00	30 000	3	8	13	0.18	0.018	0.030
Wheat flour	50	2.34	500 000	50	137	274	1.17	0.117	0.234
Total							2.45	0.245	0.421

[a] The annual per capita consumption (in kg) is calculated by dividing the annual demand by the total population, which for the purposes of this example is assumed to be 10 million persons (i.e. annual demand (in MT) × 1000/10 000 000).

[b] The daily per capita consumption (in g) is calculated by dividing the annual per capita consumption by the number of days in the year (i.e. annual per capita consumption (in kg) × 1000/365).

[c] The daily consumption per consumer is calculated by dividing the daily per capita consumption (in g) by the proportion of population that consumes the food. Ideally the daily consumption per consumer calculated in this way should equate to between the 50th and 95th percentile of daily consumption as determined by dietary surveys.

[d] The total annual cost of fortification is calculated as the product of the fortification cost per MT (in US$) and the annual total demand (in MT).

[e] The annual investment per person (in US$) is calculated as the annual total cost (in US$) divided by the total population (in this example, 10 million persons).

[f] The annual investment per consumer (in US$) is calculated as the annual investment per person (in US$) divided by the proportion of the population that consumes the food.

[g] MT stands for metric ton or 1000 kg.

of vitamin A, vitamin B_2 (riboflavin), folate (folic acid), vitamin B_{12}, iron and zinc, was within acceptable limts.

Given that the process of milling eliminates many of the B vitamins that are necessary for the metabolic transformation of starch and protein, and that the costs associated with the addition of these vitamins are relatively small, it was decided to include some of the other the B vitamins in the nutrient premix. **Table D.11** thus shows the final formulation of the fortified wheat flour, as well as an estimate of the associated costs.

Estimates of the overall cost of the fortification programme to the country, as well as the annual investment required per person and per consumer, are given in **Table D.12**. These figures indicate that the health benefits that can be expected from the proposal to fortify selected foods make the investment an excellent option for the country.

ANNEX E
A quality control monitoring system for fortified vegetable oils: an example from Morocco

1. Background

In 2002, the Moroccan Ministry of Health launched a programme to fortify vegetable oils with vitamins A and D. Prior to its implementation, a National Food Fortification Committee (NFFC), hosted by the Ministry of Health, was established to serve as a forum for the supervision, follow up and evaluation of the oil fortification programme in Morocco. This Committee comprised food industry representatives, university researchers, staff members of government technical standards and inspection units, and representatives from each of the sponsoring agencies.

The Committee's first task was to conduct a feasibility study of soybean oil fortification. One of the objectives of this study was to determine an appropriate level of fortification, bearing in mind the overages that would be required to compensate for losses of vitamins A and D_3 during storage and culinary treatment (i.e. cooking and frying). Fortificant levels for vitamins A and D_3 were subsequently set at 30 IU/g and 3.0 IU/g, respectively, with tolerances at the product distribution stage in the range of 70–150% of these levels. It was also established that fortified vegetable oils would need to be commercialized in opaque containers.

2. Design of the QC/QA system

Having completed its feasibility study, the Committee reviewed and subsequently approved the proposed quality control and quality assurance (QC/QA) procedures for the oil fortification programme. These procedures, which were based on good manufacturing practice (GMP), were set out in the form of a technical manual. The technical manual provides comprehensive guidance on a full range of monitoring, inspection and auditing activities but places particular emphasis on quality control, recognizing this as being a key component of the fortification programme. In a measure designed to encourage compliance among producers, fortified oils that had been produced according to the prescribed internal quality control procedures were identified as having been done so by means of a Ministry of Health logo.

2.1 Hazard analysis and critical control point

The hazard analysis and critical control point (HACCP) approach was used as the basis of the system that was developed for monitoring the quality of fortified oils produced in Morocco. The usefulness of this approach for ensuring the safety of processed foods is acknowledged by both the Codex Alimentarius Commission and the World Health Organization (WHO). It can also be applied to the management of the quality of food products as this relates to the manufacturing process; this makes the HACCP approach complementary to other quality control systems such as the ISO 9001:2000[1].

HACCP analysis is a tool that is used to identify specific hazards (i.e. biological, chemical or physical hazards), as well as preventive measures for eliminating or controlling those hazards. In the case of fortified vegetable oils, microbiological hazards are unlikely to be a major concern, largely because of the absence of water in such products. The potential hazards are more likely to be chemical in nature, for example, contamination by polyaromatic hydrocarbons or by migration products from the packaging materials. Quality hazards may arise due to problems with the refined vegetable oil used as the vehicle for fortification (e.g. high rates of peroxidation, defects in the flavour characteristics) or with the fortificant compounds that are added (e.g. lumping, colour, odour).

The seven principles of HACCP, as adopted by Codex (*1*), establish a framework for developing a HACCP-based system that is specific to a given combination of food product and production line. Such a system identifies hazards at a series of critical control points (CCP), and then for each CCP, identifies critical limits and appropriate monitoring and control measures. The system is managed through daily review and analysis of the records for each CCP.

It is generally recommended that a HACCP system is periodically evaluated by an external auditor. In addition, the system should be revised whenever a modification is made to the production process, for example, in the wake of customer complaints or customer surveys that report a product defect.

2.2 Critical control points in the production of fortified vegetable oils

Application of the HACCP methodology to the production of fortified oils in Morocco identified the following CCPs; in each case, the appropriate preventive measure or action is described:

---

[1] ISO 9001:2000 is a norm of the International Standards Organization for the certification of quality management systems in the food industry. It signifies adherence to effective quality systems to ensure compliance with statutory and regulatory requirements applicable to products, and the existence of management reviews, quality objectives and process management focused on continuous improvement.

1. Receiving of the refined vegetable oils (the food vehicle)

   Action. Each lot should be tested using approved methods to confirm compliance with Moroccan specifications.

2. Quality of the fortificant premix

   Action. A quality assurance certificate should be obtained from the provider of the premix, and periodic analyses should be conducted to verify the vitamin content as well as the organoleptic properties of the premix (e.g. colour, texture, odour).

3. Storage of the fortificant premix

   Action. The premix should be re-assayed periodically for vitamin content to ensure that it continues to meet the required concentrations until the end of its shelf-life.

4. Addition of the fortificant premix

   Action. The premix use inventory should be assessed, that is to say, the amount of premix used should be compared with the amount of fortified vegetable oil produced (this is the simplest method). Alternatively, the metering pump should be calibrated by weekly testing and its in-line accuracy recorded.

2.3 Quality control and feedback systems for implementing corrective actions

The following quality control procedures and feedback mechanisms were established as part of the quality control monitoring system developed for the oil fortification process:

1. Product sampling and frequency

   Procedure: Three to five samples of fortified vegetable oil (collected after packaging) should be taken daily from each production line and the levels of vitamins A and D_3 measured. Levels should be within 95–150% of the declared content. One "composite sample" should be prepared daily from each production line and kept in an opaque airtight container for up to 3 months. These composite samples may be tested for their vitamin contents by government inspectors. Four samples should be analysed monthly by an external laboratory, and the results obtained used to verify the quality of the process.

- Labelling of fortified vegetable oils
  Procedure: Fortified vegetable oils must be identified with a label, which should specify, as a mimimum, the product brand, the batch number, the address of the responsible entity, the date of production and durability, as well as the declared levels of vitamins A and D_3. Fortified vegetable oils should be designated using the product's usual name followed by the words "vitamins A & D_3 fortified", or "vitamins A & D_3 enriched". Any expression of a therapeutic nature of the product on the labels is not allowed, but functional nutritional allegations for the vitamins A and D_3 are permitted.

- Distribution of fortified vegetable oils
  Procedure: Producers should be required to keep detailed records about the quantities of fortified oils they distribute to wholesalers and retailers. This is to facilitate the monitoring of the turnover of fortified oils and the assurance of the declared levels of vitamins A and D_3. Every 3 months, about 10 samples should be taken from retailers and households for testing. Whenever deviations from the admitted tolerances in vitamin A and D_3 contents are observed (−30% to +50%), an internal technical audit should be carried out to determine the cause(s) of such deviations.

- Documentation
  Procedure: All results of quality assurance activities should be recorded and made available to government inspectors upon request. A recall procedure should be established to deal with cases of overdosed vegetable oils (i.e. those containing high amounts of vitamins A and D_3) that might pose a threat to consumer health.

- Inspection and technical audits
  Procedure: Technical auditing, rather than sample testing, forms the mainstay of the inspection activities. At the factory level government inspection activities should concentrate on the internal quality control and assurance procedures adopted by individual manufacturers of fortified vegetable oils. Due vigilance must be given to corrective measures taken by producers to solve any limitations or errors. Attention should also be paid to the production equipment, conditions of the premix storage and addition, analysis and labelling of fortified vegetable oils, and product storage conditions. Warnings must be issued to manufacturers in cases of negligence and deviations from the established procedures. If no corrective measures are taken by manufacturers to ensure compliance, an external technical audit should then be carried out.

  — During each visit, between three and five samples of packaged product should be taken and sent to the Official Laboratory of Analysis and

Chemical Research (OLACR) in Casablanca for analysis. Vitamin A and D_3 contents should lie between 95% and 150% of the declared levels.

At the level of the wholesaler and retailer, inspection activities are mainly concerned with labelling, turnover of fortified oils according to the "FIFO" (first in-first out) principle, and the conditions of storage and handling of these products.

- Training activities

  Procedure: One-day training sessions should be scheduled for fortified oil production managers and government inspectors. The areas that should be covered during these sessions are as follows: techniques of vegetable oil refining; methods for vitamin A and D_3 analysis; techniques of vegetable oil sampling; factors affecting the stability of vitamins A and D_3 in vegetable oils; and the principles of the HACCP approach and its application to fortified vegetable oils.

Reference

1. Hazard analysis and critical control point (HACCP) system and guidelines for its application. *Codex Alimentarius -Food hygiene- Basis texts- Second editions*. Rome, Food and Agriculture Organization of the United Nations, 1997: Annex.

ANNEX F
The Codex Alimentarius and the World Trade Organization Agreements

1. The Codex Alimentarius

The Codex Alimentarius, which means "food law" or "code" in Latin, is a comprehensive collection of internationally adopted and uniformly presented food standards and related texts (including guidelines) that are commonly referred to as the "Codex texts". The Codex texts address a wide range of general matters that apply to all processed, semi-processed and raw foods distributed to consumers, such as food hygiene, food additives, pesticide residues, contaminants, labelling and presentation, and methods of analysis and sampling. The texts also deal with various matters that are specific to individual commodities; for instance, commodity standards, guidelines and related texts have been developed for commodity groups such as milk, meat, cereals, and foods for special dietary uses. The complete Codex Alimentarius is available via the Codex web site[1].

The ongoing revision and development of the Codex Alimentarius is the responsibility of the Codex Alimentarius Commission, which was established in the early 1963 as an intergovernmental body by the Food and Agriculture Organization of the United Nations (FAO) and the World Health Organization (WHO). Membership is open to all Member countries of FAO and/or WHO.

The Codex texts are developed or revised though 29 subsidiary bodies comprising regional, commodity and general committees, all of which are intergovernmental in nature and most of which are currently active. The committees of most relevance to fortification and related issues are the Codex Committee on Nutrition and Foods for Special Dietary Uses (CCNFSDU), which is hosted by Germany, and the Codex Committee on Food Labelling (CCFL), hosted by Canada. The terms of reference for the CCNFSDU is to advise on general nutrition issues and to draft general provisions concerning the nutritional aspects of all foods, develop standards, guidelines and related texts for foods for special dietary uses (1). The remit of the Codex Committee on Food Labelling is to study problems related to the labelling and advertising of foods, to draft provisions on labelling that are applicable to all foods and to endorse draft provisions on labelling prepared by other Codex Committees.

---

[1] www.codexalimentarius.net.

1.1 Codex texts relevant to food fortification

The part of the Codex Alimentarius of greatest direct relevance to food fortification is the General Principles for the Addition of Essential Nutrients to Foods (CAC/GL 07-1987, amended 1989, 1991) (2). This section, which covers the addition of essential nutrients for the purposes of restoration, nutritional equivalence of substitute foods as well as fortification, provides guidance to governments with regard to the planning and implementation of national food fortification programmes.

More specifically, the Codex General Principles for the Addition of Essential Nutrients to Foods by:

— providing guidance to those responsible for developing guidelines and legal texts pertaining to the addition of essential nutrients to foods; and by

— establishing a uniform set of principles for the rational addition of essential nutrients to foods;

seek to:

— maintain or improve the overall nutritional quality of foods;

— prevent the indiscriminate addition of essential nutrients to foods, thereby decreasing the risk of health hazard due to essential nutrient excesses, deficits or imbalances (this also helps to prevent practices that may mislead or deceive the consumer);

— facilitate acceptance in international trade of foods that contain added essential nutrients.

The General Principles state that the essential nutrient:

- should be present at a level that will not result in an excessive or an insignificant intake of the added nutrient considering the amounts from other sources in the diet;

- should not result in an adverse effect on the metabolism of any other nutrient;

- should be sufficiently stable in the food during packaging, storage, distribution and use;

- should be biologically available from the food;

- should not impart undesirable characteristics to the food, or unduly shorten its shelf-life;

- the additional cost should be reasonable for the intended consumers, and the addition of nutrients should not be used to mislead the consumer concerning the nutritional quality of the food;
- adequate technology and processing facilities should be available, as should methods of measuring and/or enforcing the levels of added nutrients.

A number of other Codex texts provide guidance and recommendations that are of relevance to fortified foods. Advice relating to the nutritional quality of foods for special dietary uses is contained in *Codex Alimentarius, Volume 4 – Foods for special dietary uses (3)*. Food labelling, nutrition labelling, and claims that can be used by governments to establish their national regulations are covered in *Codex Alimentarius – Food labelling – Complete texts (4)*.

1.2 Recommended levels of nutrients in foods for special dietary uses

A series of Codex standards propose maximum and minimum levels of selected nutrients, in particular minerals and vitamins, for various foods having special dietary uses, for example, foods for infants and children. Recommended minimum and maximum vitamin and mineral levels for infant formulas are given in the Codex Standard for Infant Formula (CODEX STAN 72-1981, amended 1997) (5), and for follow-up formulas in the Codex Standard for Follow-up Formula (CODEX STAN 156-1987, amended 1989) (6). Rather than prescribing minimum and maximum nutrient levels, the Codex Standard for Canned Baby Foods (CAC/STAN 73-1981, amended 1989) (7) prefers to leave this matter to the national regulations of the country in which the food is sold.

The Advisory List of Mineral Salts and Vitamin Compounds for Use in Foods for Infants and Children (CAC/GL 10-1979, amended 1991) (8) sets out recommendations regarding the source of any added minerals, their purity requirements, and the type of foods in which they can be used. In the case of the vitamins, the various forms are listed (with purity requirements), together with a number of specially formulated vitamin preparations, where applicable.

The Guidelines on Formulated Supplementary Foods for Older Infants and Young Children (CAC/GL 08-1991) not only provide recommendations relating to nutritional matters but also address technical aspects of the production of formulated supplementary foods (9). These Guidelines include a list of reference daily requirements for those vitamins and minerals "for which deficiency is most frequently found in the diets of older infants and young children", these being the nutrients which should be given primary consideration in the formulation of supplementary foods. However, local conditions, in particular, the nutrient contribution of locally produced staple foods to the diet and the nutritional status of the target population, should be taken into account when deciding which micronutrients to add. The Guidelines make the general recommendation that when a food is supplemented with one or more of the following nutrients (vitamins A, D, E or C, thiamine (vitamin B_1), riboflavin (vitamin B_2), niacin, B_6, folate, B_{12}, calcium, iron, iodine or zinc), the total amount added per 100 g of dry food should be at least two thirds of the reference daily requirement for that nutrient (9).

In the Codex Standard for Processed Cereal-based Foods for Infants and Children (CODEX STAN 74-1981, amended 1991) (10) maximum levels of sodium are defined for different types of products covered by the standard. It is also specified that "the addition of vitamins, minerals and iodized salt shall be in conformity with the legislation of the country in which the product is sold".

1.3 Labelling

General labelling requirements are defined in the Codex General Standard for the Labelling of Prepackaged Foods (CODEX STAN 01-1985, amended 2001) (11) and the Codex General Guidelines on Claims (CAC/GL 01-1979, revised 1991) (12). Nutritional labelling is covered by the Codex Guidelines on Nutrition Labelling (CAC/GL 02-1985, revised 1993) (13) and nutritional claims by the Guidelines for Use of Nutrition Claims (CAC/GL 23-1997, amended 2001) (14).

The Codex Guidelines on Nutrition Labelling are based on the principle that no food should be described or presented in a manner that is false, misleading or deceptive, and that any claims made should be substantiated (13). A nutrient declaration, defined in section 2.3 of the Codex Guidelines as "a standard statement or listing of the nutrient content of a food", is mandatory only when claims are made. The Guidelines include provisions for nutrient declarations, calculation and presentation. Nutrient Reference Values (NRVs) for labelling purposes are defined for 14 vitamins and minerals, as well as for protein.

The Codex Guidelines for Use of Nutrition Claims (14) were developed as a supplement to the general provisions of the General Guidelines on Claims (12), primarily to provide a basis for the harmonization of nutrition claims. Nutrition claims are widely used as a marketing tool but have the potential to cause confusion for consumers. The Codex Guidelines for Use of Nutrition Claims specify that nutrition claims must be consistent with, and support, national nutrition policy. Nutrition claims that did not support national policy should not be permitted.

The Codex texts recognize the importance of establishing a link between nutrition labelling provisions and nutrition policy as a whole. Thus the Codex texts on nutrition and labelling, by providing guidance to national governments, allow for the development of national regulations and requirements according to the specific needs of the population. Conditions have been defined for foods that are a "source" of, or are "high" in, vitamins and minerals and protein. These provisions apply to claims that are made about any foods, not just fortified foods. When such claims are made, nutrient declaration should be provided in accordance with the Guidelines on Nutrition Labelling (*13*), as mentioned above. Conditions for the use of health claims are currently under discussion by the Commission.

2. The World Trade Organization Agreements

The World Trade Organization (WTO) is the only international organization in existence that deals with the global rules of trade between nations. Its main function is to ensure that trade flows as smoothly, predictably and as freely as possible (*15*). By February 2002, 144 countries, which are collectively responsible for more than 90% of world trade, had negotiated their accession to membership of the WTO (*16*). Further information about the work of WTO and its agreements is available via the WTO web site[1].

The two WTO agreements (*17*) of most relevance to food are the Agreement on the Application of Sanitary and Phytosanitary Measures (the SPS Agreement), and the Agreement on Technical Barriers to Trade (the TBT Agreement). Under the terms of both agreements, countries may adopt provisions that limit trade for legitimate reasons; the legitimate reasons can include health considerations, provided that such measures do not unnecessarily restrict trade. However, it is the latter, the TBT Agreement, that usually has the more significant implications for food fortification regulations, whether mandatory and voluntary, and for this reason is the focus of the discussion here[2].

2.1 The Agreement on Technical Barriers to Trade: background and general provisions

In the 1970s, Contracting Parties to the General Agreement on Tariffs and Trade (GATT) expressed their dissatisfaction with the emergence of new non-tariff barriers (NTBs) to trade. A GATT working group was thus established to evaluate the impact of NTBs on international trade, and reached the conclusion that the main form of NTBs that exporters faced were in fact technical barriers. During the Tokyo Round of GATT talks held in 1979 an Agreement on Technical Barriers to Trade (also called the Standards Code) which governed the preparation, adoption and application of technical regulations, standards and conformity assessment procedures was drafted. The final form of the TBT Agreement was negotiated during the Uruguay Round in 1994 and entered into force in 1995, at the same time as the WTO.

---

[1] www.wto.org.
[2] This part of the Guidelines has been drafted by the WTO's Trade and Environment Division and remains their responsibility.

The TBT Agreement is premised on an acknowledgement of the right of WTO Members to develop technical requirements[1], and to ensure that they are complied with (through what are known as conformity assessment procedures). However, the objective of the TBT Agreement is to ensure that unnecessary obstacles to international trade are not created. This is achieved through a number of principles that govern the preparation, adoption and application of mandatory and voluntary requirements and conformity assessment procedures. These principles include:

- non-discrimination;

- the avoidance of unnecessary obstacles to international trade;

- harmonization;

- the equivalence of technical regulations and of the results of conformity assessment procedures;

- mutual recognition of conformity assessment procedures;

- transparency.

At the international level, the TBT Agreement acts as an important instrument to guard against the improper use of technical requirements and conformity assessment procedures, that is to say, as disguised forms of restrictions on trade. It also guards against the development of inefficient requirements and procedures that create avoidable obstacles to trade. In some settings, it can act as a mechanism for encouraging countries to adopt less trade restrictive approaches to meeting regulatory objectives.

2.2 Coverage and definitions of the TBT Agreement

The TBT Agreement divides technical requirements into three categories, namely technical regulations, standards and conformity assessment procedures, which are defined as follows.

- *A technical regulation:* a "Document which lays down product characteristics or their related processes and production methods, including the applicable administrative provisions, with which compliance is mandatory. It may also include or deal exclusively with terminology, symbols, packaging, marking or labelling requirements as they apply to a product, process or production method."

---

[1] The term "technical requirement" in the context of these Guidelines embraces both voluntary and mandatory product specifications.

- A *standard*: a "Document approved by a recognized body, that provides for common and repeated use, rules, guidelines or characteristics for products or related processes and production methods, with which compliance is not mandatory. It may also include or deal exclusively with terminology, symbols, packaging, marking or labelling requirements as they apply to a product, process or production method."

- A *conformity assessment procedure:* "Any procedure used, directly or indirectly, to determine that relevant requirements in technical regulations or standards are fulfilled."

While both technical regulations and standards are technical product requirements, the main difference between the two is that compliance with technical regulations is mandatory, whereas compliance with standards is voluntary. A law that stipulated that a nominated food must contain a minimum amount of a micronutrient (as is the case with mandatory fortification) is an example of a technical regulation. Voluntary fortification provisions or a labelling permission for voluntary micronutrient content claims are examples of standards.

The TBT Agreement contains provisions which ensure that technical regulations do not act as unnecessary obstacles to trade. These provisions apply to technical regulations developed by central and local governments, as well as those developed by nongovernmental bodies. WTO Members are fully responsible for ensuring the observance of all the provisions of the TBT Agreement as they relate to technical regulations. They must also formulate and implement positive measures and mechanisms in support of the observance of the provisions of the TBT Agreement by local and nongovernmental bodies.

Standards are addressed separately under a "Code of Good Practice", which is contained in Annex 3 of the TBT Agreement. Most of the principles that apply to technical regulations, also apply to standards through the Code. The Code is open to acceptance by central, local and nongovernmental standardizing bodies (at the national level), as well as by regional governmental and nongovernmental bodies. However, the TBT Agreement notes that, "The obligations of Members with respect to compliance of standardizing bodies with the provisions of the Code of Good Practice shall apply irrespective of whether or not a standardizing body has accepted the Code of Good Practice."

Conformity assessment procedures are subject to many of the same principles as those that apply to technical regulations and standards, in order to ensure that they themselves do not constitute unnecessary obstacles to international trade. WTO Members are fully responsible for ensuring observance of all provisions relating to conformity assessment under the terms of the TBT Agreement, and must formulate and implement positive measures and mechanisms in support of the observance of the provisions by local government bodies. They must also ensure that central government bodies rely on conformity assessment procedures operated by nongovernmental bodies, but only if such bodies are in compliance with the relevant provisions of the TBT Agreement.

2.3 Legitimate objectives

Under the TBT Agreement, technical regulations may be developed for one or more of the objectives considered as legitimate by the TBT Agreement. Legitimate objectives include: "inter alia, national security requirements, the prevention of deceptive practices, the protection of human health or safety, animal or plant life or health, or the environment". Fortification measures are most likely to fall under the protection of human health category. However, the prevention of deceptive practices, which refers to measures that mislead or deceive consumers (e.g. false nutritional information given on food labels), might also constitute a legitimate objective and thus WTO Members would be allowed to adopt technical regulations to guard against such practices.

The risks associated with legitimate objectives are assessed against a number of factors, including: "inter alia, available scientific and technical information, related processing technology or intended end-uses of products". Once again, the inclusion of the words "inter alia", indicates that some flexibility may be exercised in the selection of factors against which risks may be assessed.

2.4 Principles which govern the preparation, adoption and application of mandatory and voluntary requirements and conformity assessment procedures

2.4.1 Non-discrimination

The principle of non-discrimination forms the backbone of the international trading system. The TBT Agreement embraces the GATT principle of non-discrimination, and applies it to technical regulations, standards and conformity assessment procedures. In general, it is the principle that outlaws discrimination between products of WTO Member countries, and between imported and domestically produced products.

With respect to both technical regulations and standards, the TBT Agreement stipulates that the non-discrimination principle be observed throughout the various stages of their preparation, adoption and application. For instance, a WTO Member cannot adopt a technical regulation mandating that all imported food meet certain micronutrient standards, if it does not enforce such standards on its own domestically produced food. Nor can it enforce a technical regulation on one, but not on another, of its trading partners. In short, under the disciplines of the TBT Agreement and the WTO system as a whole, treatment must be no less favourable.

WTO Members must also ensure that conformity assessment procedures are not prepared, adopted or applied in a discriminatory manner. Achieving non-discrimination with respect to conformity assessment requires, among other things, ensuring suppliers' right to conformity assessment under the rules of procedure, including the option of having conformity assessment activities undertaken in situ and to receive the mark of the system. Conformity assessment systems must not distinguish between the procedures to be followed for products originating from different sources. For instance, systems cannot subject similar products to tests of varying degrees of stringency depending on their source of supply.

2.4.2 Avoidance of unnecessary obstacles to international trade

The avoidance of unnecessary obstacles to international trade is the principal objective of the TBT Agreement. With respect to both technical regulations and standards, the TBT Agreement states that WTO Members must ensure that neither technical regulations nor standards are "prepared, adopted or applied with a view to or with the effect of creating unnecessary obstacles to international trade". With respect to technical regulations, the TBT Agreement elaborates on the meaning of this phrase; it stipulates that technical regulations may not be more trade restrictive than is necessary to fulfil a legitimate objective, taking into account the risks that non-fulfilment would create.

Determining whether or not a technical regulation poses an unnecessary obstacle to international trade involves two steps. Firstly, the regulation must be designed to meet one of the legitimate objectives delineated in the TBT Agreement (see section 2.3). Secondly, the regulation must be the least trade-restrictive option available to a WTO Member that achieves that legitimate objective, taking into account the risks that would be associated with its non-fulfilment.

The TBT Agreement encourages WTO Members to develop technical regulations and standards that are based on product performance requirements, rather than on design requirements. The former creates fewer obstacles to trade, providing exporters greater leeway in terms of fulfilling the objectives of the technical requirements. For instance, it would be preferable for a country to stipulate the minimum amount of a micronutrient that must be present in a specific type of food rather than a specific process for the addition of that micronutrient.

To help avoid unnecessary obstacles to international trade, the TBT Agreement requires WTO Members to revoke technical regulations when the objectives that had given rise to their adoption no longer exist, or if changed circumstances or objectives can be addressed in a less trade-restrictive manner.

WTO Members must also ensure that unnecessary obstacles to international trade are avoided when preparing, adopting and applying conformity assessment procedures for technical regulations and standards. The TBT Agreement states that, "Conformity assessment procedures shall not be more strict or be applied more strictly than is necessary to give the importing Member adequate confidence that products conform with the applicable technical regulations or standards, taking account of the risks that non-conformity would create." In other words, conformity assessment procedures must not be applied more stringently than is necessary to ensure conformity. They must consider the risks of reduced stringency, and decide whether or not the risks outweigh the benefits of having fewer obstacles to international trade.

The TBT Agreement also urges Members to ensure that conformity assessment procedures are undertaken as expeditiously as possible, that information requirements are limited to whatever is necessary, that the confidentiality of information is respected for legitimate commercial interests, and finally that the fees charged domestically are equitable to the fees charged for foreign products.

2.4.3 Harmonization

The TBT Agreement encourages WTO Members to base their technical regulations, standards and conformity assessment procedures on international standards, guidelines and recommendations, when these exist or their completion is imminent, excepting when they are deemed to be inappropriate or ineffective. For example, it allows derogation from technical regulations and standards in the event of climatic or geographic differences, or because of fundamental technological problems. Although not specifically refered to in the TBT Agreement, the Codex Alimentarius is widely interpreted as being the relevant text or "gold standard" with respect to the development of regulations on food products.

The call for harmonization is intended to avoid undue layers of technical requirements and assessment procedures, and to encourage the wider application of those that have already been developed and approved by the international community. To support this endeavour, the TBT Agreement calls upon WTO Members to participate in the work of international standardizing and conformity assessment bodies.

2.4.4 Equivalence and mutual recognition

International harmonization is a time-consuming process, and is sometimes difficult to achieve. The principle of equivalency is thus designed to complement that of harmonization and the TBT Agreement encourages WTO Members to accept each other's regulations as equivalent until international harmonization becomes possible. More specifically, the TBT Agreement stipulates that WTO Members give positive consideration to recognizing other Members' technical regulations as being equivalent to their own, even when they differ, provided that they are satisfied that the regulations adequately fulfil their objective. Through the establishment of equivalency arrangements between countries, products that meet the regulations of the exporting country do not have to comply with the regulations of the importing country, so long as the same objectives are fulfilled by the two sets of requirements. This significantly reduces barriers to trade.

The TBT Agreement also calls upon WTO Members to ensure, whenever possible, that the results of conformity assessment procedures of other Member Countries are accepted, even when they differ from their own, provided that the procedures give the same level of confidence. The purpose of this provision is to avoid multiple product testing (in both exporting and importing country markets), and its associated costs. However, it is acknowledged that in order to achieve acceptance, negotiations may be needed, primarily to ensure the continued reliability of conformity assessment results (the accreditation of conformity assessment bodies is a factor that can be taken into account in this regard). The TBT Agreement encourages these kinds of mutual recognition agreements between WTO Members.

2.4.5 Transparency

Transparency is a central feature of the TBT Agreement, and is achieved through notification obligations, the establishment of enquiry points, and the creation of the WTO TBT Committee.

Notification obligations require WTO Members to notify their draft technical regulations, standards and conformity assessment procedures and also to allow other Members sufficient time to comment on them. Members are obliged to take comments from other countries into account.[1] Notifications provide a useful means of disseminating information, and can often help to avoid unnecessary obstacles to international trade at an early stage. The advantage of the notification system is that it provides exporters with the opportunity to learn of new requirements prior to their entry into force, to comment on these requirements (and know that their comments will be taken into account), and to prepare themselves for compliance.

The TBT Agreement stipulates that each WTO Member establish an enquiry point for responding to questions on technical regulations, standards and conformity assessment procedures (whether proposed or adopted), and for supplying relevant documents.

A TBT Committee has been established as part of the TBT Agreement to act as a forum for consultation and negotiation on all issues pertaining to the Agreement. Participation in the Committee is open to all WTO Members, and a number of international standardizing bodies are invited to attend meetings as observers.

---

[1] Draft technical regulations and conformity assessment procedures only have to be notified when an international standard, guide or recommendation, does not exist (or they are not in accordance with existing ones), and if they may a have a significant effect on the trade of other WTO Members.

References

1. Codex Alimentarius Commission. *Procedural manual.* 12th ed. Rome, Food and Agriculture Organization of the United Nations, 2001.
2. *General Principles for the Addition of Essential Nutrients to Foods CAC/GL 09-1987 (amended 1989, 1991).* Rome, Joint FAO/WHO Food Standards Programme, Codex Alimentarius Commision, 1987 (http://www.codexalimentarius.net/download/standards/299/CXG_009e.pdf, accessed 7 October 2005).
3. *Codex Alimentarius, Volume 4. Foods for special dietary uses.* 2nd ed. Rome, Joint FAO/WHO Food Standard Programme, Codex Alimentarius Commision, 1994.
4. *Codex Alimentarius – Food labelling – Complete texts.* Rome, Food and Agriculture Organization of the United Nations, 2001.
5. Codex Alimentarius Commission. *Codex Standard for Infant Formula CODEX STAN 72-1981 (amended 1983, 1985, 1987, 1997).* Joint FAO/WHO Food Standards Programme, Codex Alimentarius Commission, 1981 (http://www.codexalimentarius.net/download/standards/288/CXS_072e.pdf, accessed 7 October 2005).
6. Codex Alimentarius Commission. *Codex Standard Follow-up Formula CODEX STAN 156-1987 (amended 1989).* Joint FAO/WHO Food Standards Programme, Codex Alimentarius Commission, 1987 (http://www.codexalimentarius.net/download/standards/293/CXS_156e.pdf, accessed 7 October 2005).
7. Codex Alimentarius Commission. *Codex Standard for Canned Baby Foods CODEX STAN 73-1981 (amended 1985, 1987, 1989).* Joint FAO/WHO Food Standards Programme, Codex Alimentarius Commission, 1981 (http://www.codexalimentarius.net/download/standards/289/CXS_073e.pdf, accessed 7 October 2005).
8. Codex Alimentarius Commission. *Advisory List of Minereal Salts and Vitamin Compounds for Use in Foods for Infants and Children, CAC/GL 10-1979 (amended 1983, 1991).* Joint FAO/WHO Food Standards Programme, Codex Alimentarius Commission, 1979 (http://www.codexalimentarius.net/download/standards/300/CXG_010e.pdf, accessed 7 October 2005).
9. *Guidelines on Formulated Supplementary Foods for Older Infants and Young Children CAC/GL 08-1991.* Joint FAO/WHO Food Standards Programme, Codex Alimentarius Commision, 1991 (http://www.codexalimentarius.net/download/standards/298/CXG_008e.pdf, accessed 7 October 2005).
10. Codex Alimentarius Commission. *Codex Standard for Processed Cereal-based Foods for Infants and Children CODEX STAN 74-1981 (amended 1985, 1987, 1989, 1991).* Joint FAO/WHO Food Standards Programme, Codex Alimentarius Commission, 1981 (http://www.codexalimentarius.net/download/standards/290/CXS_074e.pdf, accessed 7 October 2005).
11. *Codex General Standard for the Labelling of Prepackaged Foods CODEX STAN 1-1985 (revised 1985, 1991, 1999, 2001).* Rome, Joint FAO/WHO Food Standard Programme, Codex Alimentarius Commision, 1985 (http://www.codexalimentarius.net/download/standards/32/CXS_001e.pdf, accessed 7th October 2005).
12. *Codex General Guidelines on Claims CAC/GL 01-1979, (revised 1991).* Joint FAO/WHO Food Standard Programme, Codex Alimentarius Commision, 1985 (http://www.codexalimentarius.net/download/standards/33/CXG_001e.pdf, accessed 7 October 2005).
13. *Codex Guidelines on Nutrition Labelling CAC/GL 02-1985, (revised 1993).* Joint FAO/WHO Food Standard Programme, Codex Alimentarius Commision, 1985 (http://www.codexalimentarius.net/download/standards/34/CXG_002e.pdf, accessed 7 October 2005).

14. *Guidelines for Use of Nutrition Claims CAC/GL 23-1997, (revised 2004)*. Joint FAO/WHO Food Standards Programme, Codex Alimentarius Commision, 1997 (http://www.codexalimentarius.net/download/standards/351/CXG_023e.pdf, accessed 7 October 2005).
15. *The WTO in brief*. Geneva, World Trade Organization, 2003 (http://www.wto.org/english/res_e/doload_e/10b_e.pdf, accessed 22/02/05).
16. *WTO agreements and public health: a joint study by the WHO and WTO secretariat*. Geneva, World Health Organization, 2002.
17. *The results of the Uruguay Round of multilateral trade negotiations – the legal texts*. Geneva, World Trade Organization, 1995 (http://www.wto.org/english/docs_e/legal_e/legal_e.htm, accessed 19/04/05).

Index

Adequate Intake (AI), 146
Advocacy, 228
  policy-makers, 228
Africa
  folate deficiency, 63
  inadequate iodine nutrition, 54
  iodine fortification, 121
  pellagra, 74
  vitamin A deficiency, 49
  vitamin C deficiency, 78
  vitamin C fortification, 130
Africa, sub-Saharan
  iron deficiency, 43
  vitamin A fortification, 14
Agreement on Technical Barriers to Trade. *See* TBT Agreement
Agreement on the Application of Sanitary and Phytosanitary Measures. *See* SPS Agreement
Americas
  inadequate iodine nutrition, 54
Anaemia, 44
  prevalence, 44
Appropriate nutrient composition of a special purpose food, 26
Ascorbic acid. *See also* vitamin C fortificants
  iron fortification, 101
Asia
  iodine fortification, 121
Australia
  mandatory fortification, 32
Average Requirement (AR), 146

Beriberi, 17, 20, 68, 71
Biofortification, 30
Bone mineral density (BMD), 85

Botswana
  multiple fortification, 17
  prevalence of vitamin B_{12} deficiency, 66
Brazil
  iron fortification, 108
Bread
  iodine fortification, 121

Calcium
  defined, 84
Calcium deficiency
  health consequences of, 86
  osteoporosis, 85
  prevalence of, 84
  rickets, 86
  risk factors for, 85
Calcium fortificants, 131
Calcium fortification
  defined, 131
  wheat flour, 131
Calcium salts, 132
Canada
  folic acid fortification, 14, 128
  mass fortification, 27
  vitamin A fortification, 19, 113
  vitamin D fortification, 20
Cancer. *See* iron intake
Causality. *See* impact evaluation:probability evaluation
Central African Republic
  iodine fortification, 121
Central America
  iron fortification, 99, 106
  vitamin A fortification, 14, 19
Cereals
  folic acid fortification, 128
  zinc fortification, 125
CCP. *See* critical control points

Children
- vitamin A deficiency, 5
- zinc deficiency, 5

Chile
- fluoride fortification, 134
- folic acid fortification, 128
- iron and vitamin C fortification, 17
- iron fortification, 101, 106
- vitamin A fortification, 20
- vitamin C fortification, 81

China
- calcium deficiency, 86
- folic acid supplementation trials, 63
- iodine fortification, 122
- iron fortification, 15, 109
- pellagra, 74
- riboflavin deficiency, 73
- selenium deficiency, 88
- selenium fortification, 89, 133
- vitamin D deficiency, 82

Cobalamin. See vitamin B_{12}

Cocoa
- iron fortification, 109

Codex Alimentarius Commission, 172, 176, 318
- Advisory List of Mineral Salts and Vitamin Compounds for Use in Foods for Infants and Children, 320
- Committee on Food Labelling (CCFL), 318
- Committee on Nutrition and Foods for Special Dietary Uses (CCNFSDU), 318
- General Principles for the Addition of Essential Nutrients to Foods, 319
- Guidelines for Use of Nutrition Claims, 321
- Guidelines on Formulated Supplementary Foods for Older Infants and Young Children, 320
- Guidelines on Nutrition Labelling, 321
- Standard for Canned Baby Foods, 320
- Standard for Infant Formula, 320
- Standard for Processed Cereal-based Foods for Infants and Children, 321
- Standard for the Labelling of Prepackaged Foods, 321

Complementary foods
- defined, 107
- fortification, 169
- iron fortification, 107
- zinc fortification, 125

Consumer marketing strategies, 238
- demand-driven, 238
- supply-driven, 238

Cost calculation
- cost of monitoring and evaluation, 211
- industry costs (t), 212
- initial investment costs, 211
- recurrent costs, 211

Costa Rica
- fluoride fortification, 134
- folic acid fortification, 128
- prevalence of vitamin B_{12} deficiency, 66

Cost–benefit analysis, 210, 215

Cost-effectiveness
- analysis, 208
- cost per death averted, 207
- cost per disability-adjusted life-year saved, 207
- cost–benefit ratio, 210
- defined, 207, 223
- sensitivity analysis, 217

Critical control points (CCP), 314–15

Cuba
- thiamine deficiency, 70

Dairy products
- iron fortification, 108

DALYs. See disability-adjusted life years

Dental caries
- prevention, 134

Dietary Reference Intakes (DRIs)
- Adequate Intake (AI), 146
- Average Requirement (AR), 146
- Estimated Average Requirement (EAR), 146
- Lower Reference Nutrient Intake, 146

Lower Threshold Intake, 146
Recommended Dietary Allowance (RDA), 146
Safe Intake, 146
Tolerable Upper Level (UL), 146
Disability-adjusted life years (DALYs), defined, 3
Djibouti
 thiamine deficiency, 70
Dominican Republic
 folic acid fortification, 128
Dual fortification
 salt, 18

EAR cut-point method. *See* Estimated Average Requirement (EAR)
Eastern Mediterranean
 inadequate iodine nutrition, 54
 prevalence of vitamin A deficiency, 49
Egypt
 vitamin B_6 deficiency, 76
El Salvador
 folic acid fortification, 128
 vitamin A fortification, 116
Enrichment
 defined, 25
Erythrocyte protoporphyrin
 as indicator for iron deficiency (t), 46
Estimated Average Requirement (EAR), 146
 EAR cut-point method, 143
Ethiopia
 thiamine deficiency, 70
Europe
 inadequate iodine nutrition, 54
 iodine fortification, 121
 pellagra, 74
European Union
 market-driven fortification, 28
 voluntary fortification, 34
Evaluation
 impact evaluation, 180

Ferric phosphate compounds, 100
Ferric pyrophosphate
 micronizing, 104
Ferric saccharate, 99

Ferritin
 as indicator for iron deficiency (t), 45
Ferrous bisglycinate, 103
Ferrous fumarate, 99
 encapsulated, 103
Ferrous sulfate, 99
 encapsulated, 103
Fertilizer
 selenium fortification, 133
Finland
 iodine fortification, 122
 selenium fortification, 89
Flour Fortification Initiative, 233
Fluoride
 defined, 89
Fluoride deficiency
 defined, 89
 health consequences of, 90
 risk factors for, 90
Fluoride fortificants, 134
Folate
 defined, 61
 dietary folate equivalents (DFE), 160
 intake levels, 160
 Pan American Health Organization (PAHO), 160
Folate deficiency
 health consequences of, 63
 prevalence of, 61–62
 risk factors for, 63
Folic acid, 126
Folic acid fortificants. *See also* vitamin B fortificants
 safety issues, 129
Folic acid fortification
 cereals, 128
 efficacy trials, 19
Food and Agriculture Organization (FAO), xviii, 41
Food-based strategies, 11
 breastfeeding, 12
 dietary diversity, 12
 dietary quality, 12
Food fortificants
 defined, 95
 iodine, 118

Food fortification
  blended foods, 169
  complementary foods, 169
  consumer perceptions, xix
  cost limit, 164
  cost-effectiveness. *See* cost effectiveness
  defined, 13, 24–25
  efficacy trials, 15
  history of, 14
  human rights, xix
  market-driven, 171
  overview, xix
  production costs, xix
  regulation of, 31
  safety, 162–63, 212
  targeted, 169
  technological limit, 162–63, 212
  voluntary. *See* voluntary fortification
Food fortification levels
  cost limit, 298
  Feasible Fortification Level (FFL), 295
  Legal Minimum Level (LmL), 296
  Maximum Fortification Level (MFL), 296
  Maximum Tolerable Level (MTL), 297
  Minimum Fortification Level (mFL), 295
  safety limit, 297
  Target Fortification Level (TFL), 295
  technological limit, 298
  Tolerable Upper Intake Level (UL), 294
Food fortification programmes
  advocacy. *See* advocacy
  biomarker, 141
  commercial monitoring, 182
  consumer marketing strategies. *See* consumer marketing strategies
  coverage methods, 195
  data collection, 178
  design and planning, 95, 178
  dietary goal, 142
  dietary intakes, 139
  dietary patterns, 139
  EAR cut-point method, 143
  evaluation, 179
  external monitoring, 180
  guidelines, *see* World Food Programme (WFP)
  household/individual monitoring, 179
  impact evaluation, 180. *See* impact evaluation
  information needs, 139
  internal monitoring, 180
  monitoring and evaluating, 178
  nutritional status, 139
  operational performance, 178
  overview, xv, xvi
  planning (*t*), 140
  probability method, 143, 157
  promotion. *See* promotion
  regulatory monitoring, 179
  skewed requirements, 157
  vitamin A, 113
Food law, 241
  claims, nutrition and health-related, 249
  composition, 244
  contain, 245
  food labelling, 247–48
  legal minimum and maximum levels, 245
  mandatory fortification, 243–44
  minimum and maximum levels, 254
  minimum claim criteria, 254
  name of food, 244
  name of micronutrient, 246
  permitted fortificant compounds, 247
  Philippines Act Promoting Salt Iodization Nationwide, 242
  voluntary fortification. *See* voluntary fortification
Food systems
  overview, xv
Food vehicles
  defined, xix, 95
  fluoride, 134
  iron fortification, 104
  limits on fortificants, 23
  salt, 110
  vitamin A, 111, 113
France
  vitamin D deficiency, 82

Gambia, The
  beriberi, 71
  calcium supplementation, 86
  riboflavin deficiency, 73
  thiamine deficiency, 70
General Agreement on Tariffs and Trade (GATT), 322
General Principles for the Addition of Essential Nutrients to Foods, 25
Germany
  prevalence of vitamin B_{12} deficiency, 66
Global Alliance for Improved Nutrition (GAIN), 11, 223
Global trade agreements, 240
  SPS Agreement, 240
  TBT Agreement, 240
  World Trade Organization (WTO), 240, 322
Goitre, 54
  goitrogens, 54
Guatemala
  folic acid fortification, 128
  riboflavin deficiency, 73
  targeted fortification, 28
  vitamin A fortification, 19, 116
  vitamin B_{12} deficiency, 67
Guinea
  thiamine deficiency, 70

HACCP. See hazard analysis and critical control point
Haemoglobin
  as indicator for iron deficiency (t), 45
Hazard analysis and critical control point (HACCP), 314
Helicobacter pylori infection. See vitamin B_{12} deficiency
Honduras
  folic acid fortification, 128
  vitamin A fortification, 116
Household and community fortification, 29
Hungary
  fluoride fortification, 134

Impact evaluation, 196
  adequacy evaluation, 197
  outcome indicators, 200
  plausibility evaluation, 197
  probability evaluation, 199
  regulatory monitoring, 204
  timing, 202
India
  folate deficiency, 63
  iron deficiency, 43
  prevalence of vitamin B_{12} deficiency, 66
  vitamin D deficiency, 83
  zinc supplementation, 61
Indonesia
  folic acid fortification, 128
  targeted fortification, 28
  thiamine deficiency, 70
  zinc fortification, 125
INFOODS, 153
Intake
  24-hour recall survey, 152
  excessive, 151
  folate, 160
  inadequate, 151
  median nutrient, 150
  target median, 147, 150
International Conference on Nutrition (ICN), xviii
International Resource Laboratory for Iodine network (IRLI), 121
International Zinc Nutrition Consultative Group (IZiNCG), 124
Iodate, 118
Iodide, 118
Iodine
  defined, 52
  WHO fortification levels in salt, 159
Iodine deficiency
  correction of, 56
  Council for Control of Iodine Deficiency Disorders (ICCIDD), 287
  DALYs, 3
  disorders, 54, 55 (t)
  Global Network for Sustained Elimination of Iodine Deficiency, The, 11, 222–23
  goitre, 52
  health consequences of, 54

International Resource Laboratory
for Iodine network (IRLI), The,
287
mental retardation, 52, 55
prevalence of, 52
risk factors for, 54
sustainable elimination, 285
Iodine fortification
bread, 121
efficacy trials, 17
iron. *See* dual fortification
safety issues, 122
water, 121
Iodine-induced hyperthyroidism (IIH),
122–23
Iodine-induced thyroiditis, 123
Iodized salt. *See* salt
Iron
bioavailability from fortificants,
100
water-soluble forms, 98
Iron deficiency
anaemia, 44
benefits of intervention, 48
DALYs, 3
defined, 43
health consequences of, 48
mortality data, 3
prevalence of, 43
risk factors, 44
transferrin. *See* transferrin
Iron fortificants, 97
alternative, 101
sensory changes, 104
Iron fortification
cocoa, 109
complementary foods, 107
curry powder, 16
dairy products, 108
efficacy trials, 15, 17
encapsulation, 110
iodine. *See* dual fortification
maize flours, 107
rice, 108
safety issues, 110
salt, 110
soy sauce, fish sauce, 109
SUSTAIN Task Force, 106
wheat flour, 105

Iron intake
cancer, 110
Iron supplementation
encapsulation, 103
Israel
vitamin D deficiency, 83
Italy
iodine fortification, 121
iron fortification, 108

Jamaica
fluoride fortification, 134
Japan
iron fortification, 108
prevalence of vitamin B_{12} deficiency,
66
selenium deficiency, 88
thiamine deficiency, 70

Kaschin-Beck Disease, 88–9
Kenya
prevalence of vitamin B_{12} deficiency,
66
vitamin B_{12} supplementation, 67
Keshan Disease, 88
Korea
selenium deficiency, 88

Lacto-ovo vegetarians
defined, 63
folate intake, 63
risk of vitamin B_{12} deficiency, 66
Latin America
prevalence of vitamin A deficiency,
49
zinc fortification, 125
Legal Minimum Level (LmL). *See* Food
fortification levels
Lower Reference Nutrient Intake,
146
Lower Threshold Intake (LTI), 146

Maize flour
iron fortification, 106
Pan American Health Organization
recommendation, 107
Malaria
anaemia, 44
effects of, 204

Malaysia
  iodine fortification, 121
Mali
  iodine fortification, 121
Mandatory fortification
  defined, 31
Market-driven fortification, 171
  defined, 26, 28
  maximum micronutrient content, 173
  safe maximum limit, 173
Mass fortification, 294
  defined, 26–27
Mass fortification programmes
  constraints, 166
  enforcement, 168
  Feasible Fortification Levels, 168
  fortification costs, 166
Maximum Fortification Level (MFL). See Food fortification levels
Maximum Tolerable Level (MTL). See Food fortification levels
Measles, 51
Mexico
  folic acid fortification, 128
  targeted fortification, 28
Micronutrient malnutrition
  at-risk ages, 3
  common forms, 3
  defined, 3
  food-based strategies. See food-based strategies
Micronutrient-poor processed foods, 5
Micronutrient-rich foods
  examples, 4
Milk
  iodine fortification, 122
  vitamin D fortification, 20, 130
  zinc fortification, 125
Millennium Development Goals, xix
Minimum Fortification Level (mFL). See Food fortification levels
Monitoring
  Household Minimum, 182
  household/individual, 179
  Maximum Tolerable Level (t), 185
  Production Minimum, 182
  Quality Audit for Evaluation of Conformity (t), 184
  regulatory, 179
  Retail or Legal Minimum, 182
Monitoring, commercial, 180, 182
  label claims, 190
  minimum durability, 190
Monitoring, external, 180, 188
  corroborating tests, 190
  inspection, 189
  Legal Minimum, 190
  Maximum Tolerable Level, 189–90
  quantitative assay, 189
  technical auditing, 189
Monitoring, household, 191
  30-cluster surveys, 192
  cross-sectional surveys, 193
  lot quality assurance sampling, 192
  market surveys, 193 (t), 195
  school surveys or censuses, 193 (t)
  sentinel sites monitoring, 192
Monitoring, internal, 180
  good manufacturing practice (GMP), 184
  quality assurance, 186
  quality control, 186–87
  semi-quantitative assays, 188
Monitoring, sampling, 187
  demanding intensity, 188
  normal intensity, 188
  relaxed intensity, 187
Multiple fortification
  efficacy trials, 16
Multiple micronutrient deficiencies
  prevalence and risk factors, 91

NaFeEDTA. See sodium iron EDTA
Nepal
  riboflavin deficiency, 73
  thiamine deficiency, 70
New Zealand
  mandatory fortification, 32
Niacin
  bioavailability of, 74
  defined, 73

Niacin deficiency
  health consequences of, 76
  pellagra, 74
  prevalence of, 74
  risk factors for, 74
Niacin fortification
  food vehicles, 128
  safety issues, 129
Niacinamide, 129
  ULs, 129
Nicaragua
  folic acid fortification, 128
  vitamin A fortification, 116
Nicotinic acid, 129
  ULs, 129
Night blindness, 49
Nutrient Reference Values (NRVs)
  defined, 172
Nutritional equivalence, 26

Osteomalacia
  vitamin D deficiency, 81
Osteoporosis, 84

Panama
  folic acid fortification, 128
Pellagra. See Niacin deficiency
Peru
  targeted fortification, 28
Philippines Act Promoting Salt Iodization Nationwide. See food law
Phytic acid
  iron absorption, 102
Potassium iodate, 118
Potassium iodide, 118
Promotion
  advocacy, 225
  nutrition education, 225
  social marketing, 225
Protein–Energy Malnutrition (PEM), 5

Recommended Dietary Allowance (RDA), 146
Recommended Nutrient Intake (RNI)
  defined, 144
Restoration, 26
Retinol, 49

Riboflavin
  bioavailability of, 73
  defined, 71
Riboflavin deficiency
  health consequences of, 73
  prevalence of, 71
  risk factors for, 73
Riboflavin fortification
  food vehicles, 128
  safety issues, 129
Rice
  iron fortification, 108
  vitamin A fortification, 116
Rice fortification (iron)
  difficulties of, 108
Rickets
  defined, 81
  vitamin D deficiency, 81

Safe Intake, 146
Salt
  fluoridation, 134
  iodine fortification, 119
  iodized, consumption rate, 120
  iodized, stability of, 120
  with iron and iodine. See dual fortification
Salt iodization, 54, 119
  history of, 14
  processing, 119–20
  recommended levels, 159
  WHO programmes, 121
Salt refining, 119
Scandinavia
  selenium deficiency, 88
Scientific Committee for Food of the European Community, 147
Scotland
  fluoride fortification, 134
Scurvy. See vitamin C deficiency
Selenium
  bioavailability of, 88
  defined, 86
Selenium deficiency
  defined, 88
  health consequences of, 88
  Kaschin-Beck Disease, 89

Keshan Disease, 88
  prevalence of, 88
  risk factors for, 88
Selenium fortificants, 133
Selenium fortification, 133
Seychelles, The
  thiamine deficiency, 70
Sicily
  iodine fortification, 121
Social marketing
  communication, 230
  defined, 229
  place, 230
  price, 230
  product positioning, 230
  promotion, 230
Sodium EDTA
  uses in iron fortification, 101
Sodium iron EDTA (NaFeEDTA), 102
Sodium selenate
  selenium fortificants, 174
South Africa
  iron fortification, 16
  multiple fortification, 16
  targeted fortification, 28
South-East Asia
  inadequate iodine nutrition, 54
  prevalence of vitamin A deficiency, 49
Soy sauce & fish sauce
  iron fortification, 109
SPS Agreement, 240, 322
Sudan
  iodine fortification, 121
Sugar
  iodine fortification, 122
  vitamin A fortification, 116
Supplementation
  defined, 13
Switzerland
  salt iodization, 14
  voluntary fortification, 35

Tanzania
  multiple fortification, 17
Targeted fortification, *see* food fortification levels, 169
  defined, 27

TBT Agreement, 240, 322
  conformity assessment procedure, 324
  non-discrimination, 325
  standard, 324
  technical regulation, 323
Technological limit
  defined, 163
  organoleptic properties, 163
Thailand
  iodine fortification, 121
  iron fortification, 105, 109
  prevalence of vitamin B_{12} deficiency, 66
  thiamine deficiency, 70
Thiamine
  defined, 68
  main sources of, 70
Thiamine deficiency
  beriberi, 68
  beriberi, dry, 71
  beriberi, wet, 71
  defined, 68
  prevalence of, 68
  risk factors, 70
  severe forms of, 71
  Wernicke–Korsakov syndrome, 71
Thiamine fortification
  food vehicles, 128
  safety issues, 128
Tolerable Upper Level (UL), 146–47
Transferrin
  receptors, 46
  saturation, 46
Turkey
  vitamin D deficiency, 83

Undernourished mothers
  fortification for, 169
United Kingdom
  fluoride fortification, 134
  prevalence of vitamin B_{12} deficiency, 66
  selenium fortification, 133
  voluntary fortification, 34
United States Food and Nutrition Board, 129

United States of America
- beriberi, 20
- calcium deficiency, 85
- dental caries, 89
- folic acid fortification, 14, 19, 128
- folic acid supplementation trials, 63
- iodine fortification, 17
- iron fortification, 17
- iron supplementation, 48
- mandatory fortification, 32
- mass fortification, 27
- pellagra, 74
- prevalence of vitamin B_{12} deficiency, 66
- rickets, 83
- salt iodization, 14
- selenium fortification, 133
- vitamin C deficiency, 79
- vitamin C fortification, 130
- vitamin D deficiency, 83
- vitamin D fortification, 20
- voluntary fortification, 33
- zinc fortification, 125

Vegetarians
- lacto-ovo vegetarians. *See* lacto-ovo vegetarians
- risk of vitamin B_{12} deficiency, 66

Venezuela
- iron fortification, 17, 99, 106–107
- prevalence of vitamin B_{12} deficiency, 66

Viet Nam
- iron fortification, 15, 109

Vitamin A
- beta carotene, 112
- retinol. *See* retinol
- sources of, 51
- Tolerable Upper Intake Levels (ULs), 117

Vitamin A deficiency
- child mortality, 51
- DALYs, 3
- defined, 49
- diarrhoea, 51
- health consequences of, 51
- maternal mortality, 52
- measles, 51
- mortality data, 3
- night blindness, 52
- pregnant women, 52
- prevalence of, 49
- risk factors for, 49

Vitamin A fortificants
- defined, 111
- forms of, 112
- retinyl acetate, 111
- retinyl palmitates, 111

Vitamin A fortification
- cereals and flours, 115
- efficacy trials, 16, 19
- margarines and oils, 113

Vitamin A supplementation
- safety issues, 117

Vitamin B fortificants, 126
- folic acid, 126

Vitamin B fortification
- food vehicles, 128

Vitamin B_6
- defined, 76

Vitamin B_6 deficiency
- health consequences of, 78
- prevalence of, 76
- risk factors for, 78

Vitamin B_9. *See* folate

Vitamin B_{12}
- defined, 64

Vitamin B_{12} deficiency
- defined, 66
- health consequences of, 67
- helicobacter pylori infection, 66
- risk factors for, 66

Vitamin C
- bioavailability of, 80
- defined, 78

Vitamin C deficiency
- clinical symptoms of, 81
- prevalence of, 78
- risk factors for, 80

Vitamin C fortificants, 130

Vitamin C fortification
- special foods, 130

Vitamin D
- bioavailability of, 83
- defined, 81

Vitamin D deficiency
- defined, 81

health consequences of, 84
osteomalacia, 81
prevalence of, 82
rickets, 81
risk factors for, 83
Vitamin D fortificants, 130
Vitamin D fortification
  efficacy trials, 20
  milk, 131
  rickets, 20
  special foods, 130
Voluntary fortification, 33, 250
  risks, 34

Water
  iodine fortification, 121
  methods of iodine fortification, 121
Western Pacific
  inadequate iodine nutrition, 54
  prevalence of vitamin A deficiency, 49
Wheat flour
  calcium fortification, 131
  iron fortification, 105
  vitamin A fortification, 19, 115
World Declaration on Nutrition, xviii
World Food Dietary Assessment System, 153
World Food Programme (WFP), fortification guidelines, 28
World Health Assembly, 11
World Health Organization (WHO), xvi

breast milk intakes, 169
CHOICE project, 208
iodine deficiency indicators, 54
salt iodization, 120
Vitamin and Mineral Nutrition Information System, 5
World Health Report, xiv
World Summit for Children, 11

Zambia
  vitamin A fortification, 14, 116
Zimbabwe
  prevalence of vitamin B_{12} deficiency, 66
Zinc
  bioavailability of, 59, 124
  defined, 57
  methods to increase absorption, 125
Zinc deficiency
  association with iron deficiency, 58
  defined, 57
  dermatitis, 61
  diarrhoea, 61
  health consequences of, 61
  mental disturbances, 61
  prevalence of, 57
  risk factors for, 59
Zinc fortificants
  defined, 124
Zinc fortification
  special foods, 125

www.ingramcontent.com/pod-product-compliance
Ingram Content Group UK Ltd.
Pitfield, Milton Keynes, MK11 3LW, UK
UKHW051249180426
11947UKWH00020B/1617

9 789241 594011